NEGOTIATING THE FRENCH POX IN EARLY MODERN GERMANY

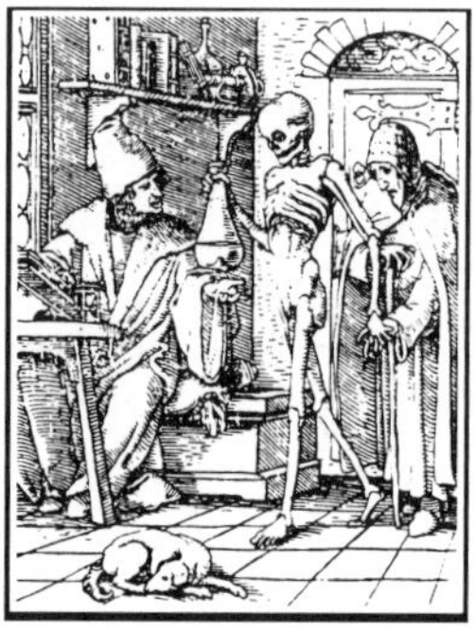

The History of Medicine in Context

Series Editors: Andrew Cunningham and Ole Peter Grell

Department of History and Philosophy of Science
University of Cambridge

Department of History
The Open University

Titles in this series include:

Contraception, Colonialism and Commerce
Birth Control in South India, 1920–1940
Sarah Hodges

Crafting Immunity
Working Histories of Clinical Immunology
Edited by Kenton Kroker, Jennifer Keelan and Pauline M.H. Mazumdar

Maritime Quarantine
The British Experience, c.1650–1900
John Booker

The Great Nation in Decline
Sex, Modernity and Health Crises in Revolutionary France c.*1750–1850*
Sean M. Quinlan

Negotiating the French Pox in Early Modern Germany

CLAUDIA STEIN
University of Warwick, UK

For Sander,
a real friend, a sound advisor
in all worldly matters and a
endless source of intellectual
inspiration.
Many thanks for all
of that
Claudia

ASHGATE

This revised English edition has been translated from the original German publication *Die Behandlung der Franzosenkrankheit in der Frühen Neuzeit am Beispiel Augsburg* © 2000 by Franz Steiner Verlag GmbH.

Published by
Ashgate Publishing Limited
Wey Court East
Union Road
Farnham
Surrey, GU9 7PT
England

Ashgate Publishing Company
Suite 420
101 Cherry Street
Burlington
VT 05401-4405
USA

www.ashgate.com

British Library Cataloguing in Publication Data
Stein, Claudia
Negotiating the French pox in early modern Germany. – (The history of medicine in context)
1. Syphilis – Germany – Augsburg – History – 16th century 2. Public health – Germany – Augsburg – History – 16th century 3. Health attitudes – Germany – Augsburg – History – 16th century 4. Health behavior – Germany – Augsburg – History – 16th century 5. Communicable diseases – Epidemiology – Case studies
I. Title
614.5'472'0943375'09031

Library of Congress Cataloging-in-Publication Data
Stein, Claudia.
Negotiating the French pox in early modern Germany / by Claudia Stein.
p. cm. — (The history of medicine in context)
Includes bibliographical references and index.
ISBN 978-0-7546-6008-8 (alk. paper)
1. Syphilis–Germany–Augsburg–History–16th century. 2. Syphilis–Germany–Augsburg–History–16th century. I. Title. II. Series.
[DNLM: 1. Syphilis–history–Germany. 2. Disease Outbreaks–history–Germany. 3. History, 16th Century–Germany. 4. History, 17th Century–Germany. 5. Syphilis–epidemiology–Germany. WC 160 S819n 2008]

RC201.6.G32A947 2008
614.5'4720943375–dc22

2008025984

ISBN 978 0 7546 6008 8

Mixed Sources
Product group from well-managed forests and other controlled sources
www.fsc.org Cert no. SA-COC-1565
© 1996 Forest Stewardship Council
FSC

Printed and bound in Great Britain by
MPG Books Ltd, Bodmin, Cornwall.

Contents

List of Illustrations and Table

Illustrations

Table

Acknowledgements

Like most academic studies, this one has been long in the making. I began by thinking that it would be a matter of merely converting my German text into English. I should have known that even with the help of a professional translator (Julian Forsyth, to whom I remain enormously grateful) it would never be so easy. And I should have realised that I wouldn't be able to leave alone as a 'faithful translation' ideas that I had begun to outgrow and that I was continuing to shed through the very process of transliteration. It would not be right, therefore, to say that in converting the original German version of my doctoral thesis into an English monograph I eliminated some material and added other, as prefaces to the like customarily announce. In the end, this was (is) a very different book from that which I handed to Julian. It inhabits a different mind and text, even if (cheating on myself somewhat) I have remained faithful to my original structure. I cannot honestly say that I have simply sought to refine much of the material with a view to rendering historical complexities clearer and the argument more precise. I have, but the business of doing so has resulted in a different book.

Opportunities to publish papers have helped in this, although the only publication in which the reader will find any direct borrowings from the material presented here (in the Introduction and Chapter 3) is that on 'The Meaning of Signs: Diagnosing the French Pox in Early Modern Augsburg', *Bulletin of the History of Medicine*, 80 (2006).

Unchanged is my heartfelt thanks to my benefactors. First, to the *Studienstiftung des Deutschen Volkes*, the *Europäische Kulturinstitut* in Augsburg, and the German Academic Exchange Service (DAAD), who provided me with the initial funding for my research. And, second, to the Wellcome Trust whose provision of a post-doctoral fellowship allowed me to rework my material and embark on other endeavours that greatly assisted me with reflecting on this one. The final draft of this book was written in the congenial atmosphere at the History Department at Warwick University, where, since 2003, I have been privileged to hold a Wellcome Trust lectureship in the History of Medicine.

Many librarians and archivists have had to put up with my endless requests and queries. For being so tolerant I am especially grateful to the staff of the Stadtarchiv and Staatsbibliothek Augsburg, particularly Hans-Jörg Künast, Helmut Zäh and Wolfgang Meyer; the Staatsbibliothek in Munich; the National Library of Medicine in Bethesda, Maryland; and the Wellcome and British Libraries in London. The time spent at the Fuggerarchiv in Dillingen with Franz Karg and Dana Koutnà will always remain a special memory. For their help in providing photographs and granting permission for reproduction, I am grateful to the Wellcome Library, London and the Städtische Kunstsammlungen Augsburg.

I have received tremendous help and encouragment from friends and colleagues. They have been generous in sharing their knowledge and in making me feel at home in the various places I lived during my research and writing. It was at the Stuttgart Institut für Geschichte der Medizin der Robert Bosch Stiftung with Robert Jütte and his staff that I first encountered the world of early modern medicine. Lorraine Daston and the staff and visiting scholars at the Max Planck Institute for the History of Science in Berlin opened up another world of thinking for me. The seminars, debates and conversations that I had there I cherish as among the most inspiring intellectual experiences of my life. Many of the people I met there became friends and I would like to thank them all for their support. My visit to the Fishbein Centre for the History of Science in Chicago and the History Department at the University of California, Berkeley was an indispensable first encounter with the Anglo-American world of scholarship, which I quickly came to realise was radically different from my German intellectual experience. Arnold Davidson's seminars in Chicago are largely responsible for my passion for Foucault. I am also especially grateful to Hal Cook and his staff at the Wellcome Trust Centre for the History of Medicine at UCL for providing me with a supportive and intellectually stimulating environment. To two of the many academic visitors at the Centre I owe special thanks: Mary Lindemann and Bruce Moran, both of whom became dear friends and gave me invaluable advice on the final manuscript. Finally, I owe enormous thanks to my colleagues in the History Department at Warwick University. They endured my ongoing conversations about 'the book' and helped me to feel comfortable in the land and language of Middlemarch. I also owe special thanks to Janet Dickinson, Rebecca Earle, Emma Lewis and Roger McGraw, who read final versions of the chapters. The same again goes to the team at the Warwick Centre of the History of Medicine: David Arnold, David Hardiman, Sarah Hodges, Colin Jones (now at Queen Mary College, London), Hilary Marland, Mathew Thomson, and Molly Rogers, together with all the undergraduate, graduate, and postdoctoral fellows whose happy company, generosity, and solid advice was so invaluable. Not least from them I have learned how to find my way around the bizarre world of British academia. For this too, not least, I am indebted to my friend Angela McShane who, never shy of pointing out my 'Germanness', was an endless source of information and excellent advice on all aspects of the customs and retentions of the English. Our friendship goes back to my first days at Warwick, suitcase in hand.

This book is dedicated to those I owe the most. I have had the good fortune of parents, Renate and Jürgen Stein, who are best friends and whose support and love has known no bounds. And – though it is more than 'and' – Roger Cooter: wordsmith, critic and companion whose insistence on the 'point of at it all' became the point of it all.

The shortcomings are all my own.

Claudia Stein
London 2008

List of Abbreviations/Note on the Text

fl.	Gulden = 60 Kreuzer (currency)
kr.	Kreuzer (currency)
StAA	Stadtarchiv Augsburg
StaBiA	Stadt- und Staatsbibliothek Augsburg

Note on the Text

While I preserved the orthographic particularities of the original sources (e.g. capitalisations, irregular spellings, diacriticals and punctuations) in the German version of the book, I have modernised the translation to make it easier for the English-speaking reader. However, ligatures and abbreviations are supplied in brackets.

Although Ulrich von Hutten's treatise is available in an English translation by Thomas Paynell, *De Morbo Gallico* (London, 1533), I translated from the German original from which Paynell's version departs considerably.

I have translated the titles of the German treatises and the original quotations. However, I quoted the original German titles in the footnotes and the bibliography to make it easier to identify them in library and archive catalogues. For the sixteenth-century German names and titles I tried to find English equivalents. Exceptions are the names of the three Augsburg pox hospitals, which I kept in German throughout the book because it makes it easier to tell them apart.

Claudia Stein

Introduction

In the chronicle of his hometown, the southern German imperial city of Augsburg, Hector Mülich gave prominence to three events in 1495. First, the generous donation of a silver bust of a saint to one of the city's churches; second (in great detail) the devastation caused by a fire in the nearby town of Gersthofen; and third, the dramatic highpoint of the year, the emergence of a mysterious disease:

> That year a great plague came into the land, which manifested itself in large pustules. It was termed the French pox on account of having first appeared in France; thereafter it spread throughout the world … causing much affliction and notable suffering, indescribable and as yet unknown to men, which neither doctors nor other healers could fathom. And [it is said] many people have the disease three or four years, and become very weak from it. In Augsburg they had built a house for times of plague in which the poor folks were put. And in the same building they now housed the poor suffering from the pox, so that all at once there were 125 persons housed there. And for the love of God they were given to eat and to drink. God preserve us from this great plague; no one has heard of it, knows where it comes from or how to guard against it.[1]

Mülich had no doubt who was to blame for this divine punishment: the French.[2] Many of his contemporaries shared his view, frequently tracing the national association to a specific historical event: the invasion of the Italian peninsula in 1494 by the armies of the French king, Charles VIII (1483–1498).[3] It was believed that the disease first erupted among Charles' mercenaries, who at the cessation of hostilities returned to their respective homelands, thus spreading the new plague throughout Europe. In the German lands the labels that were quickly ascribed to

1 For quote see Hector Mülich, *Chronik des Hector Mülich. Mit Zusätzen von Demel, Walter und Rem*, in *Die Chroniken der deutschen Städte vom 14. bis ins 16. Jahrhundert* (Leipzig, 1894), vol. 23, pp. 421–2; see also Paul von Stetten (the elder), *Geschichte der Heil. Röm. Reichs Freyen Stadt Augsburg Aus Bewährten JahrBüchern und Tüchtigen Urkunden gezogen und an das Licht gegeben* (2 vols, Frankfurt and Leipzig 1743/1758), vol. 1, p. 247.

2 For other explanatory strategies see William Eamon, 'Cannibalism and Contagion: Framing Syphilis in Counter-Reformation Italy', in *Early Science and Medicine* 3 (1998), pp. 1–31; Anna Foa, 'The New and the Old: The Spread of Syphilis (1494–1530)', in Edward Shorter and Guido Ruggiero (eds), *Sex and Gender in Historical Perspective* (Baltimore, 1990), pp. 26–45.

3 Jon Arrizabalaga, Roger French, and John Henderson, *The Great Pox: The French Disease in Renaissance Europe* (New Haven, 1997), pp. 20–25.

this hitherto unknown condition reflect this conviction, the most common being the French Disease (*Franzosenkrankheit*), French pox (*Franzosenpocken*), or the Latin equivalent, *morbus gallicus*.[4]

Scapegoating the French to expedite the search for the disease's geographical origin brought no one any closer to solving the question of how to confront and treat the pox. Learned medical treatises in both Latin and German soon proliferated, presenting cosmological and physiological interpretations, and offering various therapies.[5] Nor was the struggle to contend with the French pox confined to the world of letters. Impatient and despairing pox victims were soon hammering at the doors of charitable institutions, begging the authorities to act. The first municipality to do so was the imperial city of Augsburg. In 1495, the council opened a pox hospital, the *Blatterhaus*, which (as Mülich's chronicle notes) had originally been built for victims of the plague. Although other cities were quick to follow Augsburg's example, by the end of the sixteenth century no German community had as many specialised institutions for treating the pox as this merchant metropolis on the river Lech. Besides the *Blatterhaus*, two private hospitals (*Holzhäuser*) (opened in 1523–1524 and 1572) are known to have been founded by members of the merchant-banker family, the Fuggers.[6] All three hospitals offered free medical treatment to the city's poxed poor. This study examines these institutions in detail. It is concerned with their organisation and administration as well as admission processes. It also investigates whether the establishment of the pox hospitals differed from that of other health care institutions in the city. Moreover, the surviving hospital records also allow a reconstruction of the various medical cures

4 For the different names of the disease in the European languages see Iwan Bloch, *Der Ursprung der Syphilis: Eine medizinische und kulturgeschichtliche Untersuchung, part 1: Ursprung der Syphilis* (Jena, 1901), part 2: *Kritik der Lehre von der Altertumssyphilis* (Jena, 1911), here part 1, pp. 297–305.

5 For these works see Conrad Heinrich Fuchs, *Die ältesten deutschen Schriftsteller über die Lustseuche in Deutschland von 1495 bis 1510, nebst mehreren Anecdotis späterer Zeit, gesammelt und mit literaturhistorischen Notizen und einer kurzen Darstellung der epidemischen Syphilis in Deutschland* (Göttingen, 1843); Karl Sudhoff, *Graphische und typographische Erstlinge der Syphilisliteratur aus den Jahren 1495 und 1496* (Munich, 1912); ibid., *Aus der Frühgeschichte der Syphilis: Handschriften- und Inkunabelstudien epidemiologischer Untersuchung und kritische Gänge* (Leipzig, 1912); ibid., *Zehn Syphilisdrucke aus den Jahren 1495–1498* (Milan, 1924). Sudhoff's last work was translated into English by the American medical historian Charles Singer, *The Earliest Printed Literature on Syphilis: Being Ten Tractates from the Years 1495–1498: in Complete Facsimile with an Introduction and Other Accessory Material by Karl Sudhoff*, adapted by Charles Singer (Florence, 1925). Arrizabalaga/French/Henderson, *The Great Pox*, p. 8, have recently drawn attention to some of the problems of Singer's translation.

6 For a general overview on French pox hospitals in German cities see Robert Jütte, 'Syphilis and Confinement: Early Modern German Hospitals for Syphilitics', in Norbert Finzsch and Robert Jütte (eds), *Institutions of Confinement: Hospitals, Asylums, and Prisons in Western Europe and North America, 1500–1950* (Cambridge, 1996), pp. 97–116.

and offer rare and fascinating insights into the lives and sufferings of some of the patients before and after they fell ill with the pox.

But this work seeks to do more than reconstruct the socio-cultural reactions of early modern society to the pox, particularly the treatment of the disease in new hospitals. The first part investigates a question that few historians who have worked on the pox have dealt with seriously: What actually *was* the French Disease? Or, to frame this differently, how did people in the sixteenth century understand the physical reality of this new disease, and how did they explain its causes and symptoms? How did they perceive the relationship between their bodies and the pox, which also formed the rationale for the various treatments? This study aims at linking socio-cultural reactions to the pox in a particular location within the sixteenth-century conceptual understandings of this disease.

Venereal Syphilis or French Pox? An Overview

For the majority of historians the issue of the identity of the pox was never a question. With few exceptions, historical research identifies early modern accounts and visual representations of the pox with the modern disease entity of venereal syphilis.[7] Through retrospective diagnosis the sixteenth-century pox has become integral to the many 'Histories of Syphilis'.[8] These usually begin with the disease's alleged first appearance in Europe at the end of the fifteenth century and end with gloomy forebodings on the social impact of today's most threatening sexually-transmitted disease, AIDS.[9] The idea that venereal syphilis has its own history, the development of which can be traced back to its possible origins, is grounded in a specific view of disease shared by the authors of these 'histories', namely that diseases are stable, unchangeable 'scientific facts'.[10] By

7 For the modern entity of venereal syphilis see Jon Arrizabalaga, 'Syphilis', in Kenneth F. Kiple (ed.), *The Cambridge World History of Human Disease* (Cambridge, 1993), pp. 1025–1033. One of the few exceptions is the study by Arrizabalaga/French/Henderson, *The Great Pox*. For their methodological approach see pp. 1–3.

8 Older works in this tradition are W. M. A. Pusey, *The History and Epidemiology of Syphilis* (London, 1933); Wilhelm Frederik Robert Essed, *Over den Oorsprung der Syphilis: Een kritisch-historisch-epidemiologische Studie tevens ontwerp eener Theorie* (Amsterdam, 1933); Charles Clayton Dennie, *A History of Syphilis* (Springfield, 1962).

9 See for example J. David Oriel, *The Scars of Venus: A History of Venereology* (London and Berlin, 1994); Sheldon Watts, *Epidemics and History: Disease, Power and Imagination* (New Haven, 1997); Stefan Winkle, *Geißeln der Menschheit: Kulturgeschichte der Seuchen* (Düsseldorf and Zürich, 1997); Kevin Brown, *The Pox: The Life and Near Death of a Very Social Disease* (Phoenix Mill, 2006).

10 A recent example of this view is the article by Allan Brandt, 'Sexual Transmitted Diseases', in William F. Bynum and Roy Porter (eds), *Encyclopedia of History of Medicine* (2 vols, London, 1993), vol. 1, pp. 562–84. For an interesting discussion of the problems inherent to this view see Thomas Schlich, 'Die Herstellung wissenschaftlicher

affording a privileged epistemological status to present-day scientific knowledge, the modern concept of venereal syphilis is turned into a trans-historical object of universal validity. According to such accounts our modern notion of diseases is that of independent entities that can be clearly distinguished aetiologically, morphologically or symptomatically, and which remain more or less constant from patient to patient.[11]

This study takes a different approach. Informed by work in the history of science and medicine stemming from the groundbreaking study of the Polish bacteriologist Ludwik Fleck (1896–1961), it argues for an understanding of disease as a socio-cultural construct specific to a particular scientific and socio-cultural setting at a given time.[12] From this angle, the perception and understanding of disease is always subject to ongoing historical change; early modern views on the pox and today's on modern venereal syphilis are thus incommensurable. This does not mean, however, that the historian cannot detect resemblances between present knowledge and older opinions in their source material.[13] With respect to the early modern understandings of the French pox and modern views on venereal syphilis, the term 'syphilis' itself is illustrative. It was first deployed by the Veronese humanist and physician Girolamo Fracastoro (c. 1478–1553) in a poem *Syphilis sive morbus gallicus* (1530) (Syphilis or Morbus Gallicus) on the mythological origin of the new disease in the recently discovered New World.[14] In this Fracastoro had an indigenous shepherd named Syphilus shout blasphemous insults at the Sun-

Fakten als Thema der Geschichtsforschung', in Norbert Paul and Thomas Schlich (eds), *Medizingeschichte: Aufgaben, Probleme, Perspektiven* (Frankurt a. M. and New York, 1998), pp. 107–29.

11 Karl-Heinz Leven, 'Krankheiten – historische Deutung versus retrospektive Diagnose', in Norbert Paul and Thomas Schlich (eds), *Medizingeschichte: Aufgaben, Probleme, Perspektiven* (Frankfurt and New York, 1998), p. 161; Margret Pelling, 'Contagion/Germ Theory/Specificity', in William F. Bynum and Roy Porter (eds), *Encyclopedia of History of Medicine* (2 vols, London, 1993), vol. 1, p. 314; Schlich, 'Die Herstellung wissenschaftlicher Fakten', p. 114.

12 Ludwig Fleck, *The Genesis and Development of a Scientific Fact*, T. J. Trenn and R. K. Merton (eds), (Chicago, 1979). Fleck's book appeared first in German under the title *Entstehung und Entwicklung einer wissenschaftlichen Tatsache. Einführung in die Lehre vom Denkstil und Denkkollektiv* (Basel, 1935).

13 Here I follow Ian Hacking, *The Emergence of Probability: A Philosophical Study of the Early Ideas About Probability, Induction and Statistical Inference* (Cambridge, 1975), p. 21; see also ibid., *Presenting and Intervening: Introductory Topics in the Philosophy of Natural Science* (Cambridge, 1983), pp. 65–74.

14 However, the term syphilis was not widely used until the eighteenth century. Geoffrey Eatough, *Fracastoro's 'Syphilis': Introduction, Text, Translation and Notes* (Liverpool, 1984); G. L. Hendrikson, 'The "Syphilis" of Girolamo Fracastoro', *Bulletin of the History of Medicine* 2 (1934), pp. 515–46; Mary B. Campbell, 'Fracastoro's De Syphilis and the Discovery of the New World', in Daniel Segal (ed.), *Crossing Cultures: Essays in the Displacement of Western Civilization* (Tuscon, 1992), pp. 3–32.

god who, in return, punished the shepherd for this audacity with the new ailment. But despite the fact that the same term is still used today, Fracastoro's medical understanding of the terrible disease which afflicted his poem's hero cannot be measured against any of the central tenets of our modern conception of venereal syphilis.

The medical understanding which we today associate with the term syphilis is a recent invention and part and parcel of the genesis of a conceptualisation of the human body entirely different from that existing in the fifteenth and sixteenth centuries. As the French philosopher Michel Foucault argued, our perception of the human body and its diseases has undergone a dramatic change. 'For us the human body defines, by natural right, the space of origin and of distribution of disease.'[15] As he pointed out in *The Birth of the Clinic* (1963), this body is 'a space whose lines, volumes, surfaces, and routes are laid down, in accordance with a now familiar geometry, by the anatomical atlas. But this order of the solid, visible body is only one way – in all likelihood neither the first, nor the most fundamental – in which one spatialises disease. There have been, and will be, other distributions of illness'. And there were. As Foucault went on to show, our familiar 'self-evident' conception of the human body developed only gradually from the late eighteenth century. Crucial to this process was the discourse of anatomical pathology which emerged as a new scientific medical discipline during the eighteenth century and that gained supremacy in the nineteenth. The anatomically-trained eye of the physician probed the interior of the human form, acquiring knowledge of the functions of living organs through its intensive observation and investigation of the organs in the dead. This visual correlation between living and dead human matter had not previously existed in medicine, Foucault claimed. The clinical, dissecting gaze constituted as the 'body' only what it had learned to 'see'.

The genesis of the modern medical conception of venereal syphilis can be regarded as an example of the phenomenon Foucault referred to as the 'suzerainty of the gaze', which, he believed, became one of medicine's defining characteristics from the end of the eighteenth century.[16] Under the dominance of the 'new gaze' the understanding of the relationship between the body and its disease changed dramatically. It was only then, and, according to Foucault, for the first time in medical experience, that 'the space of configuration of the disease and the space of localisation of the illness in the body have been superimposed … the illness is articulated exactly on the body, and its logical distribution is carried out at once in terms of anatomical masses'.[17] Earlier centuries, as this study will show in detail, did not assume that disease and the human body shared the same space or that the causes and development of disease could (or should) be related to the body's anatomy.

---

15 For this quotation and the following, see Foucault, *Birth of the Clinic: An Archaeology of Medical Perception* (London and New York, 1993), p. 3.

16 Ibid., p. 4.

17 Ibid., pp. 3–4.

In the long term the new eighteenth-century conception of disease and its relationship to the body led to a normative understanding of the body. The great success of the science of bacteriology, established at the end of the nineteenth century, was based on this idea of corporeal standardisation, and through new laboratory practices bacteriologists strongly contributed to the further development of this conception.[18] The isolation of the syphilis agent was one of bacteriology's first successes. Following the 'discovery' of the pathogen for anthrax, cholera and tuberculosis, the specific cause of venereal syphilis (the bacterium 'treponema pallidum') was isolated in 1905 and examined under the microscope by the zoologist Fritz Schaudinn (1871–1906) and the physician Erich Hoffmann (1868–1959).[19] A year later the bacteriologist and serologist August Paul von Wassermann (1866–1925) described a serodiagnostic procedure to prove the existence of the agent, the test known as the Wassermann Reaction (WaR).[20]

'Seeing' the disease agent changed the diagnostic act for ever. Irrespective of the form the disease took within and on the surface of the body, its specific identity was from now on determined by the presence of the pathogen. From this point on, the complex and ancient doctrines of causality were abandoned in the construction of a wholly new pattern of causality.[21] Medical diagnostics underwent a dramatic shift from the classification of signs and symptoms observed at a patient's bedside to the laboratory-based diagnosis of causal organisms.[22] Thereafter a diagnosis could only be confirmed when the laboratory examination of the patient's bodily fluids and tissue proved the presence of the pallid, spiral-shaped bacterium.

The idea of monocausal disease agents opened up entirely new prospects for treating infectious diseases. For the first time in its history Western medicine

18 On German bacteriology see Christoph Gradmann, *Krankheit im Labor: Robert Koch und die medizinische Bakteriologie* (Göttingen, 2005).

19 Ernst Bäumler, *Amors vergifteter Pfeil. Kulturgeschichte einer verschwiegenen Krankheit* (Hamburg, 1976), pp. 135–6; Peter G. Hesse and Joachim S. Hohmann, *Friedrich Schaudinn, 1871–1906: Sein Leben und Wirken als Mikrobiologe Eine Biographie* (Frankfurt and New York, 1995), Jean Lindemann, 'Siegel, Schaudinn, Fleck and the Etiology of Syphilis', *Studies of History and Philosophy of Biological and Biomedical Sciences* 32 (2001), pp. 435–455.

20 Ilana Löwy, 'Testing for a Sexually Transmitted Disease, 1907–1970: The History of the Wassermann Reaction', in Virginia Berridge and Philipp Strong (eds), *AIDS and Contemporary History* (Cambridge, 1993), pp. 74–92.

21 Arrizabalaga/Henderson/French, *The Great Pox*, p. 2. For the emergence of this new conceptual approach to causality in medicine see K. Codell Carter, *The Rise of Causal Concepts of Disease* (Aldershot, 2003).

22 Paul Weindling, 'From Infections to Chronic Diseases: Changing Patterns of Sickness in the Nineteenth and Twentieth Centuries', in Andrew Wear (ed.), *Medicine in Society: Historical Essays* (Cambridge, 1992), p. 308; for this shift see also Andrew Cunningham, 'Transforming Plague: The Laboratory and the Identity of Infectious Disease', in Andrew Cunningham and Perry Williams (eds), *The Laboratory Revolution in Medicine* (Cambridge, 1992), pp. 209–43.

was able to chalk up notable successes in its battle against epidemics. After the successful transmission of the syphilis agent to animals, a frantic search for specimen cures began.[23] Syphilis treatment recorded what was perceived at the time to be its first significant success in 1909–1910, when the Georg-Speyer Institute of Pharmacology in Darmstadt, under the leadership of Nobel prize-winning chemist Paul Ehrlich, developed a chemotherapeutic cure for syphilis, the first 'specific', *Salvarsan*. Ehrlich's prediction for chemotherapeutic agents for each and every infectious disease – 'magic bullets' – was the promise of modern medicine.[24]

At the dawn of the twentieth century syphilis not only occupied the minds of German laboratory scientists. It was conspicuous by its presence in day-to-day political debate. The discussions about the *Lustsuche* (lust epidemic) and its perceived threat to the individual, the family, the state and the 'race' was one of the central themes of social and health policy in the German Empire.[25] Debate raged over its social causes, its dissemination, and the measures to combat it, the last concentrating primarily on the regulation of prostitutes, who were seen as one of the chief propagators of the 'sexual vice'. Not that this 'Syphilis hysteria' was a specifically German phenomenon. From 1899 doctors and lawyers, administrators, diplomats, church leaders, representatives of ethical and humanitarian movements, and women's organisations from all over the world met at a series of international conferences to collaborate on strategies to solve the acute problems posed by syphilis and prostitution.[26] Historians and medical practitioners with a passion for history contributed to these debates with wide-ranging studies on the 'History of Syphilis'.[27] The medical historian Karl Sudhoff (1876–1938),[28] the Berlin

23 Bäumler, *Amors vergifteter Pfeil*, chapters 4–6; Lutz Sauerteig, 'Die Eroberung des Gesundheitsmarktes: Pharmazeutische Industrie und Gesundheitswesen um die Jahrhundertwende', *Wirtschaft und Wissenschaft* 4 (1996), pp. 35–42.

24 For this see Allan Brandt, *No Magic Bullet: A Social History of Venereal Disease in the United States Since 1988* (New York and Oxford, 1985).

25 Lutz Sauerteig, 'Medizin und Moral in der Syphilisbekämpfung', *Jahrbuch des Instituts für Geschichte der Medizin der Robert Bosch Stiftung* 19 (2000), pp. 55–70; ibid., *Krankheit, Sexualität, Gesellschaft: Geschlechtskrankheiten und Gesundheitspolitik in Deutschland im 19. und 20. Jahrhundert* (Stuttgart, 1999), pp. 68–71.

26 For these conferences see *Sauerteig, Krankheit, Sexualität, Gesellschaft*, pp. 62–5; also Paul Weindling, 'The Politics of International Co-Ordination to Combat Sexually Transmitted Diseases, 1900–1980s', in Berridge/Strong, *AIDS and Contemporary History*, pp. 93–117.

27 Publications on the history of the pox before the late nineteenth century are not considered here because they rely on a different conception of disease causation and also differ in their conceptions of history writing. But for a discussion of some of the earlier works see Arrizabalaga/French/Henderson, *The Great Pox*, pp. 10–15; and Hans-Uwe Lammel, *Klio and Hippocrates. Eine Liason littéraire des 18. Jahrhunderts und die Folgen für die Wissenschaftskultur bis 1850 in Deutschland* (Stuttgart, 2006), pp. 149–77.

28 For the more than forty articles which Karl Sudhoff published on early modern syphilis see the bibliography by Grete Herbrand-Hochmuth, 'Systematisches Verzeichnis

specialist in skin and sexual diseases Iwan Bloch (1872–1922),[29] and the Viennese surgeon Karl Johann Proksch (1840–1923)[30] were among these pioneers. Their narratives were constructed around the conviction that modern scientific medicine would ultimately succeed in combating syphilis.[31] Deeply influenced by the ideals of German historicism, a school of thought that believed that all human activities (including the sciences) were defined by their history, all their efforts were devoted to the forensic task of collecting evidence on the presence of the disease in human history.[32] Such testimony, they were convinced, would help resolve once and forever the then current scientific and political debates over syphilis and other infectious diseases. No one was more certain about this than Sudhoff, who sought 'to achieve understanding of the epidemiological and clinical symptoms observed in earlier epidemics with the aid of all of today's historical, bacteriological, clinical, statistical and epidemiological methods, and to extract conclusions beneficial for today's understanding and treatment of infectious diseases'.[33]

These turn-of-the-century studies are still regarded as authoritative on the history of syphilis, not least because of the wealth of primary sources that they drew on.

---

der Arbeiten Karl Sudhoffs', *Sudhoffs Archiv* 27 (1934), pp. 134–86; and Rudolf Zaundik, 'Bibliographie Karl Sudhoffs: Nachtrag für die Jahre 1933–1938', *Sudhoffs Archiv* 31 (1938), pp. 343–4; on Sudhoff's views on history writing see Gundolf Keil, 'Sudhoffs Sicht vom deutschen Mittelalter', *Nachrichtenblatt der Deutschen Gesellschaft der Medizin, Naturwissenschaften und Technik e.V.* 31 (1981), pp. 94–129; Thomas Rütten, 'Karl Sudhoff and the "Fall" of German Medical History', in Frank Huisman and John Harley Warner (eds), *Locating Medical History: The Stories and Their Meaning* (Baltimore and London, 2004), pp. 95–114; on biographical details see also Dirk Rodekirchen and Heike Fleddermann, *Karl Sudhoff 1853–1938: Zwei Arbeiten zur Geschichte der Medizin und der Zahnheilkunde. Mit einem Essay 'Paracelsus und der gläserne Mensch'* (dissertations, Cologne, 1991).

29 Bernhard Egger, *Iwan Bloch und die Konstituierung der Sexualwissenschaften als eigene Disziplin* (dissertation, Düsseldorf, 1988).

30 Not a great deal is known about the life of this Viennese surgeon (Wundarzt). For some information see Erna Lesky, *Die Wiener medizinische Schule im 19. Jahrhundert* (Graz, 1965). Proksch's most important works are *Die Geschichte der venerischen Krankheiten* (2 vols, Bonn, 1895), and *Die Litteratur über die venerischen Krankheiten von den ersten Schriften über Syphilis aus dem Ende des fünfzehnten Jahrhunderts bis zum Jahre 1889* (5 vols, Bonn, 1889–1900).

31 Iwan Bloch, *Das erste Auftreten der Syphilis (Lustseuche) in der europäischen Kulturwelt: gewürdigt in seiner weltgeschichtlichen Bedeutung, dargestellt nach Anfang, Verlauf und voraussichtlichem Ende* (Jena, 1904), p. 33. Already in 1876 Proksch believed in the existence of a distinct 'syphilitic virus' waiting to be 'discovered'. See Johann Karl Proksch, 'Ein Beitrag zu den Sammelwerken der ältesten Schriften über Syphilis', *Medicinisch-chirurgisches Central-Blatt* 11/47 (1876), p. 7.

32 Georg G. Iggers, 'Historicism: The History and Meaning of the Term', *Journal for the History of Ideas* 56 (1995), pp. 129–52.

33 Karl Sudhoff and Georg Sticker (eds), *Zur historischen Biologie der Krankheitserreger: Materialien, Studien und Abhandlungen* (Gießen, 1910), p. 6.

Two themes in particular captured these men's attention and have continued to do so ever since: the geographical origins of 'syphilis'[34] and its impact on the moral and scientific landscape of early modern Europe. The first concern triggered an extensive and ongoing scholarly debate between those who considered the disease to be imported from the Americas after 1492, and those who did not.[35] Among the latter were Sudhoff and Proksch who argued that venereal syphilis had always existed on the European continent, although under different names.[36]

The second concern, the alleged influence of 'syphilis' on the moral and scientific development of sixteenth-century Europe, is more central to this study: it was already a matter of intense analysis at the turn of the twentieth century. Iwan Bloch scrutinised a vast amount of historical material for evidence of the impact of 'syphilis' on sexual behaviour and moral attitudes in the early modern period.[37] Inspired by Jacob Burckhardt's (1818–1897) interpretation of the Renaissance as the historical moment in which the modern individual was 'born', Bloch claimed that the sudden outbreak of 'syphilis' contributed significantly to that development.[38] His argument was based on his conviction that the sexual transmission of the pox had already been identified and was widely acknowledged

34 I put the term in quotations marks to draw attention to the anachronistic nature of such labelling. I shall use in my own work the sixteenth-century term 'pox'.

35 Bloch considered the idea that the French pox was native to Europe since antiquity as 'the greatest error ever spread in the history of medicine'. See Bloch, *Der Ursprung der Syphilis*, part 1, p. VI. This long-smouldering debate over the origin of the pox is given new impetus, every now and again, by modern microbiological examinations of paleopathological finds. However, it is unlikely that a definite answer will be provided in the near future. An interesting article on the virtues and pitfalls of paleopathology for a history of disease see Bruno Latour, 'On the Partical Existence of Existing and Non-Existing Objects', in Lorraine Daston (ed.), *Biographies of Scientific Objects* (Chicago, 2000), pp. 247–69.

36 For an overview see Francisco Guerra, 'The Dispute over Syphilis Europe Versus America', *Clio Medica* 13 (1978), pp. 39–61; Ann Carmichael, 'Syphilis and the Columbian Exchange: Was the New Disease Really New?' in Mario G. Marques and John Cule (eds), *The Great Maritime Discoveries and the World Health* (Lissabon, 1991), pp. 189–90.

37 Bloch coined the term Sexualwissenschaft (science of sexuality), which he defines as the 'science of the sexual, meaning the appearance and influences of sexuality in regard to the physical and spiritual, as well as to individual and social relations'. See Iwan Bloch, 'Aufgaben und Ziele der Sexualwissenschaft', *Zeitschrift für Sexualwissenschaft* 1 (1914–15), pp. 2–11; see also Egger, *Iwan Bloch*, pp. 94–7.

38 Jacob Burckhardt, *Die Kultur der Renaissance in Italien/Die Kunst der Renaissance in Italien* (Munich, 1997); Bloch, *Ursprung der Syphilis*, vol. 1, p. 6; also ibid., *Das Auftreten der Syphilis*, p. 6; Iwan Bloch and Georg Loewenstein, *Prostitution* (2 vols, Berlin, 1912/25), vol. 1, pp. 31–3. Bloch's academic adversaries Sudhoff and Proksch strongly disagreed with him on this point. As they believed syphilis to be indigenous to the European continent long before the fifteenth century, they refuted the idea that it caused any immediate or lasting cultural impact.

in the sixteenth century.[39] This awareness of the sexual origin of the disease, he argued, considerably altered the behaviour between the sexes, which had been far less inhibited in pre-medieval and medieval times. Fear of infection through sexual intercourse, he contended, led to a distancing of men and women. Their sexual behaviour became more responsible, and thus helped to ensure that they developed into more independent, rational, and more culturally advanced individuals.[40] The closure of the municipal brothels, the stigmatisation of prostitutes, and the abolition of the public baths which are reported in sixteenth-century European sources were all interpreted by Bloch as a direct response to the sudden appearance of French pox and the influence it exerted on human behaviour and social mores.

Bloch's arguments were echoed by many German cultural historians at the turn of the twentieth century, and are still in vogue.[41] As one recent monograph put it,

> [t]hen came the shock, at the moment when the Renaissance was beginning to unfold its petals into full bloom. The epidemic proportions of the new plague and the virulence of its effects turned the promiscuous habits of the time into a mortal danger. The bath houses were the first to suffer, and their closure was followed by restrictive measures directed against prostitutes and brothels in all cities in Europe.[42]

The continuous repetition of these old interpretations is all the more astonishing in view of the many other studies that have refuted such claims. It has been shown, for instance, that the closure of public baths and brothels in sixteenth-century German towns had little to do with the appearance of the French pox. Instead, the closures were intrinsically related to increasing economic difficulties besetting

---

39 Bloch/Loewenstein, *Prostitution*, vol. 1, p. 6.

40 Ibid., pp. 5–6.

41 On the emergence of German Kulturgeschichte see Roger Chickering, *Karl Lamprecht: A German Academic Life* (1856–1915) (Atlantic Highlands, 1993). For turn-of-the-century examples see Josef Schrank, *Die Geschichte der Prostitution in Wien, in historischer, administrativer und hygienischer Beziehung* (Wien, 1886); Wilhelm Rudeck, *Geschichte der öffentlichen Sittlichkeit in Deutschland* (Jena, 1897); Alfred Martin, *Deutsches Badewesen in vergangenen Tagen* (Jena, 1906); W. Sorge, *Geschichte der Prostitution* (Berlin, 1920); Alfons Fischer, *Geschichte des deutschen Gesundheitswesens* [1933] (reprint Hildesheim, 1965); Max Bauer, *Das Geschlechtsleben in deutscher Vergangenheit* (Dresden, 1930).

42 Johannes Fabricius, *Syphilis in Shakespeare's England* (London, 1994), p. 17. The alleged 'shock of syphilis' is also used to explain other early modern historical phenomena such as the witch trials. See S. Andreski, 'The Syphilitic Shock: A New Explanation of the "Great Witch Craze" of the 16th- and 17th-Centuries in the Light of Medicine and Psychiatry', *Encounter* 58/5 (1982), pp. 7–26.

brothel-owners and, more importantly, the propagation and implementation of new and stricter moral standards introduced with the Reformation.[43]

But old habits die hard, and studies investigating the alleged socio-cultural impact of the pox continue to be produced. In fact, since the appearance of AIDS in the early 1980s, such studies have enjoyed something of a renaissance. And AIDS has also revived another strain in these 'pox impact'-studies: the identification of historical sources that support an interpretation of its catalytic effect on sixteenth-century medical theory and practice. It is not surprising that the origins of this interest are traceable to the moment when bacteriology celebrated its first great victories. At the end of the nineteenth century, Karl Johann Proksch was one of the first to claim that the unexpected appearance of the new disease seriously challenged early modern medical practice. According to him the event stirred practitioners into action and compelled them to arrive at ideas different from those to be found in the ancient medical literature. Their 'scientific research' into the nature of the new disease supposedly triggered revolutionary results. For the first time in the entire history of medicine, Proksch rejoiced, its practitioners were able to successfully distinguish one specific disease from another. And this crucial step in the understanding of disease aetiology not only contributed to weakening ancient traditions in medical practice and learning, but also prepared the ground for the emergence of modern scientific practice.[44] Some recent authors are even more celebratory: one proclaimed that '[t]he epidemic shocked the dormant medical mind of Western Europe into action and brought about a transition from magic to rational medicine'.[45] With great enthusiasm, similarly positivistically-minded scholars have devoted attention to the supposed 'pioneers of rational science' among the early modern medical profession.[46] According to these narratives the Italian academic physician Girolamo Fracastoro 'foresaw' the discovery of microbes, while the Swiss-born medical practitioner Paracelsus (1493/4–1541) is celebrated as the forerunner of modern biochemical research.[47]

43 Lyndal Roper, *The Holy Household: Women and Morals in Early Modern Augsburg* (Oxford, 1991); Peter Schuster, *Das Frauenhaus. Städtische Bordelle in Deutschland 1350–1600* (Paderborn, 1992), pp. 129–31; Beate Schuster, *Die freien Frauen. Dirnen und Frauenhäuser im 15. und 16. Jahrhundert* (Frankfurt and New York, 1995), pp. 342–50. For an analysis of sixteenth-century literature in relation to the pox see Walter Tilmann, *Unkeuschheit und Werk der Liebe. Diskurse über Sexualität am Beginn der Neuzeit in Deutschland* (Berlin 1998), pp. 396–415.

44 Proksch, *Geschichte der venerischen Krankheiten*, vol. 1, p. 4.

45 Fabricius, *Syphilis in Shakespeare's England*, p. 59.

46 Leven, 'Krankheiten', p. 157; Arrizabalaga/French/Henderson, *The Great Pox*, p. 7

47 See, for instance, Oriel, *Venus*, p. 15, and Fabricius, *Syphilis in Shakespeare's England*, p. 32; for a much more sophisticated and balanced interpretation of Fracastoro's ideas see Vivian Nutton, 'Perception of Fracastoro's Theory of Contagion: The Seeds that Fell Among Thorns?', *Osiris* 6 (1990), pp. 196–234.

Thanks to the efforts of social historians of medicine and medical anthropologists these 'progress stories' of modern medicine have been seriously questioned.[48] We now know more fully the many ways in which past societies and cultures dealt with sickness and what it meant to be ill, or to recover from illness in different cultural settings.[49] Some of these social historical perspectives have been applied to the study of the French pox where particular emphasis has been placed on the interaction between medicine and society by examining the perspective of the patients and hospital histories.[50] Such studies successfully challenge the widespread assumption that before the eighteenth century hospitals were not infirmaries for the seriously ill but merely repositories for the community's poor, foreigners and the chronically sick. The archival records of these institutions tell otherwise: most early modern hospitals drew their patients predominantly from the community's poor, and hence functioned as an integral part of every city's poor relief economy. Moreover (and more important for this study) they show that the *cure* of the poor sick had been the overriding concern at hospitals from as far

48 For the aims of a social history of medicine see Arthur Imhoff and Oivid Larsen (eds), *Sozialgeschichte und Medizin. Probleme einer quantifizierenden Quellenbearbeitung in der Sozial- und Medizingeschichte* (Oslo and Stuttgart, 1976); Alfons Labisch, 'Zur Sozialgeschichte der Medizin: Methodologische Überlegungen und Forschungsbericht', *Archiv für Sozialgeschichte* 20 (1980), pp. 431–69; Alfons Labisch and Reinhard Spree, 'Neuere Entwicklungen und aktuelle Trends in der Sozialgeschichte der Medizin in Deutschland – Rückschau und Ausblick', *Vierteljahrschrift für Sozial- und Wirtschaftsgeschichte* 84 (1997), pp. 171–210; 305–21; Walter G. Rödel, 'Mensch und Gesundheit in der Geschichte der Neuzeit: Notizen zu einem Forschungsprojekt', *Medizinhistorisches Journal* 19 (1984), pp. 138–47; Robert Jütte, 'Sozialgeschichte der Medizin: Inhalte – Methoden – Ziele', *Medizin, Gesellschaft und Geschichte* 9 (1990), pp. 149–63; Martin Dinges, 'Social History of Medicine in Germany and France in the Late Twentieth Century: From the History of Medicine Towards a History of Health', Huisman/Warner (eds), *Locating Medical History*, pp. 209–36.

49 For a detailed discussion of these studies see Annemarie Kinzelbach, *Gesundbleiben, Krankwerden, Armsein in der frühneuzeitlichen Gesellschaft. Gesunde und Kranke in den Reichsstädten Überlingen und Ulm, 1500–1700* (Stuttgart, 1995), pp. 11–20.

50 Maries J. Van Lieburg, 'De syfilitische patiënt in de geschiedenis van het Nederlandse ziekenhuiswezen vóór 1900', *Tjdschrift voor Soziale Geschiedenis* 8 (1982), pp. 156–79. Van Lieburg's study was inspired by two earlier publications written by the medical historian Owsei Temkin, 'On the History of "Morality and Syphilis"', in ibid., *The Double Face of Janus* (London, 1977), pp. 472–84, and ibid., 'Therapeutic Trends and the Treatment of Syphilis before 1900', in ibid., *The Double Face of Janus* (London, 1977), pp. 518–24. For the history of hospitals see the still useful essay collection by Lindsay Granshaw and Roy Porter (eds), *The Hospital in History* (London and New York, 1989); also Guenter Risse, *Mending Bodies, Saving Souls: A History of Hospitals* (Oxford, 1999); and now John Henderson, *Renaissance Hospitals: Healing the Body and Healing the Souls* (Oxford, 2006).

back as the Middle Ages.[51] Studies drawing on these sources predominantly focus on the social, economic and legal considerations that governed the admission of the patients, their treatment and length of their stay. That the nature of an inmate's illness might have played a vital part in these administrative processes is not generally considered. Colin Jones has drawn attention to this shortcoming and showed in a study on early modern French hospitals that these institutions specialised in the treatment of specific disease phenomena, and thus 'practised as much medical *ex*clusion as *in*clusion, as much filtering out as filtering in' on the basis of a patient's physical condition.[52] In line with this argument, Robert Jütte and other medical historians have singled out the sixteenth-century pox hospitals as one of the most significant examples of this trend. Weren't these brand new institutions set up for the treatment of a new specific disease?[53] In fact, some scholars have claimed that pox hospitals were 'pre-modern clinics', presenting the most decisive step forward towards the modern specialised hospital.[54] The utility

51 Early modern poor relief and health care is a favourite topic among social historians of medicine. See, for example, Robert Jütte, *Patient und Heiler in der vorindustriellen Gesellschaft. Krankheit – und Gesundheitsverhalten im frühneuzeitlichen Köln* (habilitation thesis, Bielefeld, 1989); Jonathan Barry and Colin Jones (eds), *Medicine and Charity Before the Welfare State* (London and New York, 1991), pp. 26–37. See for the importance of treatment in hospitals, for example, Ulrich Knefelkamp, *Das Heilig-Geist-Spital in Nürnberg vom 14.–17. Jahrhundert. Geschichte, Struktur, Alltag* (Nuremberg, 1989); Luise Windemuth, *Das Hospital als Träger der Armenfürsorge im Mittelalter* (Stuttgart, 1995).

52 Colin Jones, 'The Construction of the Hospital Patient in Early Modern France', in Norbert Finzsch and Robert Jütte (eds), *Institutions of Confinement: Hospitals, Asylums, and Prisons in Western Europe and North America, 1500–1950* (Cambridge, 1996), p. 60.

53 Karl Sudhoff first drew attention to the importance of these institutions for the general history of hospitals. See Karl Sudhoff, 'Wendepunkt im Krankenhauswesen des Abendlandes', *Archiv für Geschichte der Medizin* 21 (1929), pp. 246–7; see also René Burgun, 'Mésure contre la Syphilis à Strasbourg (1495–1789): Das Blatterhaus', in Georges Livet and Georges Schaff (eds) *Médicine et assiance en Alsace XVIe–XXe siècle* (Strasbourg, 1976), pp. 62–7; Anneliese Seiz, 'Das Ulmer Blatter-Haus im Seelhaus im Gries: Ein Beitrag zur Geschichte des öffentlichen Gesundheitswesens in Ulm', *Ulm und Oberschwaben: Zeitschrift für Geschichte und Kunst* 44 (1982), pp. 366–71; Helmut Puff, 'Das Hamburger Hiobshospital in der frühen Neuzeit', *Hamburger Zustände: Jahrbuch zur Geschichte der Region Hamburg* 1 (1988), pp. 183–207; María Luz López Terrada, 'El mal de siment en la Valencia del siglo XVI: Imágenes del morbo gallico en un a ciudad mediterránea europea', *Dynamis* 11 (1991), pp. 119–46; ibid., 'El Tratamiento de la sifilis en un hospital renacentista: La sala del mal de siment del hospital general de Valencia', *Asclepio* XLI (1989), pp. 19–50; Anita Malamani, 'Notizie sul mal franscese e gli ospedale degli incurabilie in età moderna', *Critica Storica* 15 (1978), pp. 193–216; Arrrizabalaga/French/Henderson, *The Great Pox*, pp. 145–233; Kevin Siena, *Venereal Disease, Hospitals, and the Urban Poor: London's 'Foul Wards', 1600–1800* (Rochester, 2004); ibid., *Sin of the Flesh: Responding to Sexual Disease in Early Modern Europe* (Toronto, 2005).

54 Jütte, 'Syphilis and Confinement', pp. 114–15; Kinzelbach, 'Böse Blattern', p. 57.

of these bold claims will be tested against the evidence stemming from the rich and original archival remains of the three Augsburg pox hospitals.

Methodological Approach

Leaving aside whether or not the pox can be identified with modern venereal syphilis, the first chapter of this study concentrates on investigating its sixteenth-century physical identity. Methodologically, it follows Andrew Cunningham, who has proposed a new approach for historians in understanding the identity of past diseases.[55] He claims that neither the outdated strategy of retrospective diagnosis nor the more recent fashion for studying changing 'disease concepts' actually brings us closer to the identity of diseases in the past. Unlike retrospective diagnosis, the notion of 'disease concepts' takes into account that diseases are not stable, historical entities, but changing socio-cultural constructions.[56] But, Cunningham warns, a danger lurks in this acknowledgement. Too often the 'concept of disease' is understood as more-or-less exclusively the result of mental activity.[57] Instead, he suggests, we should turn our attention towards 'disease concepts in action' – that is to the diagnostic act itself. It is through the questions that are asked and answered during the act of diagnosis, he continues, and through the practices applied by those involved in this operation, that the identity of disease (past and present) may be established.[58]

Also methodologically important for this study are the works of Ian Maclean and Nancy Siraisi, who have independently explored philosophical discussions on disease identification in early modern Latin treatises on medical semiology.[59] Their erudite analyses are helpful in comprehending early modern conceptions of disease definition and distinction. Maclean shows how these definitions were ultimately based on a completely different understanding from today of the meaning of sensible bodily signs and their relation to disease and its causes; and Siraisi draws attention to the multiplicity and complexity of the phenomena that early modern medical diagnosis had to reckon with, and which accounted for 'the flexibility of definition and classification possible even in the case of well known

55 Andrew Cunningham, 'Identifying Diseases in the Past: Cutting through the Gordian Knot', *Asclepio* 54 (2002), pp. 13–34.

56 As an example Cunningham quotes Adrian Wilson, 'On the History of Disease-Concepts: the Case of Pleurisy', *History of Science* 38 (2000), pp. 271–319.

57 Cunningham, 'Identifying Disease', pp. 15–16.

58 Therefore, Cunningham claims, all diseases possess an 'operational identity'. See ibid, p. 16. For this operational identity of diseases see also ibid., 'Transforming Plague', p. 213.

59 Ian Maclean, *Logic, Signs and Nature in the Renaissance: The Case of Learned Medicine* (Cambridge, 2002), pp. 282–4; Nancy Siraisi, 'Disease and Symptom as Problematic Concepts in Renaissance Medicine', in Eckhard Kessler and Ian Maclean (eds), *Res et Verba in the Renaissance* (Wiesbaden, 2002), pp. 217–40. I am grateful to Nancy Siraisi for allowing me to read an earlier draft of this paper.

and relatively well understood ailments'.[60] However, Siraisi as well as Maclean base their claims on investigations of highly theoretical philosophical treatises mainly written by university-trained physicians. How these theoretical reflections were applied to and were, at the same time, shaped by daily medical practice is not their concern.

This study brings these two areas closer together: the world of medical reasoning on the meaning of physical signs and the daily practice of diagnosing and treating them. In order to revive the relationship between the pox and the sixteenth-century 'medical gaze', a strict separation between 'theory' and 'experience' of the pox will be avoided. The deeper structures of visibility – 'the codes of knowledge' as Foucault called them (and which this study targets) – informed both fields and bound them together.[61] Only when styles of reasoning in medical semiotics are investigated in tandem with the various practices in deciphering and treating physical symptoms in a specific locality, this study suggests, may we glimpse at what people in the late fifteenth and sixteenth century took to be the physical identity of the pox.[62] In looking through the lens of the three Augsburg pox hospitals, this study endeavours to capture the 'pox concept in action'.

The participants in the examinations of the Augsburg pox hospitals differed widely in their social status and vocational background. Nevertheless, they shared similar views and practices about the functioning of the human body and its diseases, if not necessarily its treatment. This study demonstrates that the sick, their medical practitioners and the witnesses present at the clinical encounter in Augsburg's pox hospitals all spoke essentially the same language; they were equal partners in a 'unitarian medical world'.[63] The rich and detailed archival records from which the medical world of early modern Augsburg can be reconstructed demonstrate that the sick, regardless of their social and/or intellectual backgrounds, not only diagnosed their own individual bodily signs and symptoms, but also considered themselves competent judges of medical success.[64] The mindset of the ailing individuals presenting themselves at the three hospitals in Augsburg was not a *tabula rasa* on which the institution's appointed medical practitioners stamped their conceptual ideas about disease. On the contrary, the mind of the sick was a dynamic space for interior visualisation and story-telling which every healer,

60 Siraisi, 'Disease and Symptom', p. 239.

61 Foucault, *Birth of Clinic*, pp. 90–91.

62 In my understanding of 'styles of reasoning' I follow Ian Hacking, *Historical Ontology* (Cambridge, 2001), pp. 178–99; also Arnold I. Davidson, *The Emergence of Sexuality: Historical Epistemology and the Formation of Concept* (Cambridge, MA, 2002), especially chapter 5.

63 Colin Jones and Laurence Brockliss, *The Medical World of Early Modern France* (Cambridge, 1997), p. 237, have coined this expression to describe the distribution of medical knowledge and practice in early modern France.

64 My findings match those of Gianna Pomata for early modern Bologna. See her brilliant study, *Contracting a Cure: Patients, Healers and the Law in Early Modern Bologna* (Baltimore, 1998), p. 123.

university-trained or otherwise, took into account. Integral, and often intertwined parts of the clinical encounter in the hospitals, included taking the sick person's history thorough a physical examination. The diagnostic results of these 'medical portraits,' as they have come to be called,[65] constituted a merger between the medical practitioners' 'sketches' of the patient's condition and the practitioner's own knowledge and experience in treating the pox. The final diagnosis was a picture of disease that seemed a meaningful and explanatory reflection of the patient's condition to all the parties involved in the diagnostic act.

To grasp the unitarian medical world in Augsburg in the late fifteenth and sixteenth century this study draws both on surviving hospital records revealing the daily diagnostic and therapeutic practices at the pox hospitals (between 1495–1632), and on vernacular German pox treatises and pamphlets published between 1496 and 1620. I am aware that, with regard to vernacular sources, this approach is methodologically problematic, not least because we can never know if any of the inmates or even the practitioners, staff or administrators knew of the contents of these publications or were aware of their existence, even though some of them were authored by Augsburg citizens. Still, as Michael Gieseke has suggested, vernacular texts can teach us much about shared medical worlds.[66] Like the 'medical portraits' painted from the clinical encounter, vernacular texts were the products of collective consent. Penned predominantly by those in the medical trade, but with differing intellectual and social backgrounds, vernacular German medical texts aimed at instructing the 'common man' (*gemeinen Mann*),[67] the stratum of early modern society that did not read Latin easily or at all. To reach this audience a vernacular author had to take into account and build upon the reader's own knowledge and practical skills. As Adrian Johns has pointed out, early modern audiences for printed materials on the natural world and the human body were not receptacles, but agents of appropriation who had their own means to determine the credibility and trustworthiness of a text – a relationship not unlike that between patients and medical practitioners.[68] In order to become a

65 Brian Nance, *Turquet de Mayerne as Baroque Physician: The Art of Medical Portraiture* (Amsterdam and New York, 2001), p. 78.

66 Michael Giesecke, *Der Buchdruck in der Frühen Neuzeit. Eine historische Fallstudie über die Durchsetzung neuer Informations– und Kommunikationstechniken* (Frankfurt, 1998), pp. 527–41. For early modern England, see Andrew Wear, *Knowledge and Practice in English Medicine, 1550–1680* (Cambridge, 2000), and Mary E. Fissell, *Patients, Power, and the Poor in Eighteenth-Century Bristol* (Cambridge, 1991); ibid., *Vernacular Bodies: The Politics of Reproduction in Early Modern England* (Oxford, 2004).

67 For a discussion of the term see Peter Blickle, *Deutsche Untertanen. Ein Widerspruch* (Göttingen, 1981), pp. 15–18.

68 Adrian Johns, *The Nature of the Book: Print and Knowledge in the Making* (Chicago, 1998), pp. 31–43. Intersubjective trust as a key element in the making of early modern knowledge about the natural world has been investigated by Steven Shapin in his monograph *Social History of Truth: Civility and Science in Seventeenth-Century England* (Chicago, 1994).

'bestseller' – a consideration that played in the minds of both author and publisher – a vernacular medical book had to have the right balance between 'instruction' and 'recognition'. As Giesecke has argued, vernacular German authors achieved this by downplaying complicated scholastic methodology while emphasising the practical application of the advice they offered. German-writing authors shared with those publishing in Latin the same stock of knowledge about the natural world and the human body, and accepted the same underlying logic,[69] but they demoted the highly theoretical scholastic principle of argumentation and proof ('why') to second place behind the description of its possible practical uses ('how'). Vernacular medical treatises are therefore a crucial source for this study's concern with the practical dimension of the diagnosis of the pox and its treatment, as well as the styles of reasoning that informed them.

My methodological approach to these texts is 'archaeological' in the Foucaultian sense. I am interested in laying bare similarities, that is, in unearthing underlying medical ideas and practices shared by German writers on the pox. This focus on the *shared* features of texts makes the individual agenda of each author (and their possible differences) less important for the purpose of this study.

Ten treatises and pamphlets form the core of the study. They all aimed, or so they claimed, at informing the 'common man' in order to save him from the clumsy and inexperienced hands of dangerous pox doctors (*Franzosenartzten*) who 'treated poor patients very badly – indeed threatened to rip them off both their money and health'.[70] The earliest of these treatises, *A Pretty Treatise on the Origin of the Evil French Pox, Called the Wild Warts. Also a Regimen on How to Conduct Oneself During this Time*, was printed in Augsburg in 1496.[71] It was written by Joseph Grünpeck (1472–1533) who later became court historian to the emperor Maximilian I (1459–1519). In 1496 he was teaching rhetoric at the University of Ingolstadt in Bavaria. It was over a decade before another pox treatise appeared, this time, in Pforzheim: *A Useful Regime Against the French*

69 Giesecke, *Buchdruck*, pp. 555–6.

70 Knobloch, *De Lue Venerea*, Vorrede.

71 *Ein hübscher Tractat von dem vrsprung der Bösen Franzos, das man nennet die Wylden wärtzen. Auch ein Regiment wie man sich regiren soll in diser zeyt* (Augsburg, 1496). This was a translation of Grünpeck's Latin treatise published earlier. Russell is wrong about the publishing dates; see Paul A. Russell, 'Syphilis, God's Scourge or Nature's Vengeance? The German Printed Response to a Public Problem in the Early Sixteenth Century', *Archiv für Reformationsgeschichte* 80 (1989), p. 293. For the correct dates see Sudhoff, *Zehn Syphilisdrucke*, p. XXV; and for a reprint of the tract see ibid., pp. 71–115. It was during his time at the imperial court that Grünpeck caught the pox himself and published another Latin tract dealing with his personal suffering from the disease. It is not included here because it was never published in German. For Grünpeck's biography see Albin Czerny, 'Der Humanist und Historiograph Kaiser Maximilians I. Joseph Grünpeck', *Archiv für österreichische Geschichte* 73 (1888), pp. 315–64.

Evil Pox, Which Asks a Number of Pertinent Questions (1509).[72] Its author was Alexander Seitz (1470–1540), a physician in the Swabian town of Marbach.[73] This was a response to an earlier enquiry by Elisabeth Schott, Abbess of the nearby Cistercian convent at Lichtenstern, who had sent Seitz six questions concerning the 'lamentable and poisonous disease of the wicked French pox, which now afflicts and corrupts the human race so wretchedly'.[74] It was nearly a decade after that, in 1518, that an Augsburg print shop (owned jointly by the merchant and apothecary Max Wirsung [also Wirsing] and the academic physician Sigmund Grimm [c. 1480–1532]) produced an anonymous pamphlet, *A Tried and Tested Prescription of a Wood Called Guaiacanum.*[75] Here was the first detailed description in the German vernacular instructing on how to prepare and administer this new 'wonder drug' imported from the New World. Guaiacum was soon to become the most frequently used remedy for the French pox next to mercury. Hot on the heels of this publication followed another laudation on guaiacum's miraculous healing properties, also published in Augsburg, *On the Miraculous Medicine Called Guaiacum Wood, and How to Cure the French Disease or Pox* (1519).[76] Its author was the imperial knight and humanist Ulrich von Hutten (1488–1523), who in 1519 was notorious throughout the German territories for his harsh criticism of the Roman Catholic Church.[77] Von Hutten had first-hand experience with the pox: since 1510 his body had been ravaged by it, and he was miraculously cured by the new 'wonder drug' during a stay in Augsburg in 1518. In twenty-six

72 *Ein nutzlich regiment wider die bösen frantzosen mit etliche[n] clugen fragstucken* (Pforzheim, 1509). I shall quote from the reprinted version in Peter Ukena (ed.), *Alexander Seitz sämtliche Schriften* (Göttingen, 1970), vol. 1, pp. 7–29.

73 For Seitz see Albert Moll, 'Doktor Alexander Seitz aus Marbach und seine Schrift über die Lustseuche vom Jahre 1509' (Stuttgart, 1825); Karl Schottenloher, *Doktor Alexander Seitz und seine Schriften: Ein Kleinbild aus dem Münchner Ärzteleben des XVI. Jahrhunderts* (München, 1925).

74 Ukena, *Alexander Seitz*, p. 7.

75 *Ein bevert rezept von ainem holtz genannt Guaiacanum* (Augsburg, 1518). I shall use a reprint of this tract from 1519 published by the Augsburg printer Hans of Erfurt with a slightly altered title, *Hienach volgt ain bevert recept von ainem holtz genannt Guaiacanum wechst in Antilles in ainer Insel gehaisen la isola spagnola: fast hailsam für all alt schäden vnd die kranckhait der Frantzosen* (Augsburg, 1519). For the various editions of this print see Vöttinger–Pletz, *Lignum Sanctum*, pp. 33–5. For the sixteenth-century world of printing in Augsburg see Hans-Jörg Künast, *'Gedruckt in Augsburg'. Buchdruck und Buchhandel in Augsburg zwischen 1468 und 1555* (Tübingen, 1997).

76 *Von der wunderbarliche[n] artzney des holtz Guaiacum genant, und wie man die frantzosen oder blatteren heilen sol* (Augsburg, 1519). Von Hutten first published his tract in Latin and Thomas Murner translated it a year later into German. For both texts see Eduard Böcking (ed.), *Ulrich von Hutten: Schriften* (Leipzig, 1861), vol. 5, pp. 399–497.

77 For the changing historical judgement on Ulrich von Hutten's political activism see Wilhelm Kreutz, *Die Deutschen und Ulrich von Hutten: Rezeption von Autor und Werk seit dem 16. Jahrhundert* (Munich, 1984).

chapters von Hutten describes his lengthy suffering and what he believed to be his guaiacum cure. Six years after von Hutten's celebratory treatise, in 1525, another anonymous tract was published in Strasbourg praising the medicinal properties of the wood: this brief work, *A Clear Account On How to Heal Old Wounds, Holes and Ulcers with the Wood Guaiaco. So Easy that Everybody Can Do It Requiring Very Little Money*, was a bestseller reprinted many times with slightly altered titles and illustrations.[78] Four years later appeared a treatise which did not share these strong beliefs in the healing properties of the wood from the New World: *A Useful Regimen for Countering the Widespread and Unclean French Disease* (1529), penned by Magnus Hundt (1449–after 1529), who at the time of the publication was a minister in Leipzig. His book was based on his experiences in treating the pox as a physician in the Saxon mining town of Joachimstal.[79] Broader in outlook was a, *Newly Invented and Tried and Tested Medicine, Help and Advice ... for Expelling, Healing and Curing the French Pox* (Strasbourg, 1541),[80] by Walter Hermann Ryff (c. 1500–1548). Ryff was not only one of the most prolific, but also the most contentious, authors in the German vernacular on medical and natural philosophical topics in the sixteenth century, and was often accused of plagiarism. His tract on the pox (as many of his others) was a translation of *De ligni sancti multiplici medicina et vini exhibitione*, published in Rome in 1537 by the Neapolitan physician and papal surgeon Alfonso Ferri (1500–1595). It became an extremely popular treatise on the pox and served as a model for Franz Renner,

78 *Ein clarer bericht wie man alte schaden, löcher vnd bülen heylen soll mit dem holtz Guaiaco also leycht das es ein yeder thun mag vmb ein kleynen costen* (Strasbourg, 1525). For the different editions see Vöttinger–Pletz, *Lignum Sanctum*, pp. 36–8.

79 *Eyn kurtzes vnd sehr nutzlichs Regiment [...] wider die weltleuftige vn[d] vnsauber kranckheit der Frantzosen* (Magedburg, 1529) As Hundt published treatises on various topics, including theology, his identity was a matter of discussion among historians of medicine. Proksch, for example, believed in the existence of two academics named Magnus Hundt. Having checked most of available publications under that name I came to the conclusion that there was only one doctor Hundt. He had spent several years as a physician in the Saxon mining town of Joachimsthal before he moved to Magdeburg. For Hundt see *Bibliographie hervorragender Ärzte*, vol. 21, p. 34; *Allgemeines Gelehrten Lexikon*, vol. II, cols 1773–1774, and *Allgemeine Deutsche Bibliographie*, vol. 13, p. 392.

80 *New erfundne heylsam und bewärte artzney gewusse hilff unnd radt ... die Frantzosen oder bösen blatern, ... gründtlichen vnd gentzlichen zu vertreiben heylen vnd Curieren* (Strasbourg, 1541). For the different editions of this tract see Josef Benzing, 'Walter H. Ryff und sein Werk: Eine Bibliographie', *Philobiblion* 2 (1958), pp. 126–55; 203–25. Here I am using the edition published by Samuel Emmel in Strasbourg in 1559. Ryff's works (often translations of other authors) were enormously popular and enjoyed many editions. His proliferation raised suspicion among some of his contemporaries such as the medical professor Leonhart Fuchs who reproached him for plagiarism. For a recent re-evaluation of Ryff see William Eamon, *Science and the Secrets of Nature: Books on Secrets in Medieval and Early Modern Culture* (Princeton, 1994), pp. 96–8. For the early modern understanding of authorship and plagiarism see Johns, *Nature of the Book*.

who condensed his experience as a barber-surgeon in Nuremberg into an even more popular treatise: *A New Well-Reasoned, Helpful and Useful Little Handbook of General Practice of All Internal and External Medication Against the Frightening Repulsive French Disease* (first published in 1548 and continuously reprinted to 1609).[81] Possibly because of the enormous success of Renner's book, no further such treatises appeared for nearly fifty years. Published in 1594 by the Arnstadt physician Johannes Wittich (1537–?),[82] *On Ligno Guayaco, Miracle Tree Called Res Nova; on China Ex Occidentali India; on Sarsaparilla; on the Fennel Wood Sassafras, and the Kidney Wood Called Lignum Nephriticum* dealt not only with guaiacum, but also with other imports from the New World considered to be therapeutically effective against the pox.[83] The final treatise I consider in this study is *De Lue Venerea, a Short History of the French Disease*, published in 1620 by Tobias Knobloch, a physician from Ansbach and personal physician to a widowed Princess of Brandenburg.[84]

An obvious omission from this list of pox authors is Paracelsus (1493/4–1541), who wrote several pox treatises in the German vernacular. As in his other writings, these seized the opportunity to trumpet disdain for the Hippocratic–Galenic ideals and practices held dear by most of his colleagues.[85] It is precisely for this reason that his pox writings are excluded here. To introduce them would necessitate comparing them with those of other pox authors, and hence emphasise difference in sixteenth-century medical theory in relation to the pox. But my aim is, rather, to trace the constitutive elements of a unitarian medical world shared by the authors of the available sixteenth-century vernacular literature on the pox and the practitioners, staff and inmates in Augsburg's three pox hospitals. The hospital

---

81 *Ein new wol gegründet nützlichs vnnd halysams handtbüchlein gemeiner Pratick aller innerlicher und eusserlicher Erztney so wider die erschröckliche, abscheuliche Krankheit der Frantzosen* (Nuremberg, 1559). For the history of the various editions see Proksch, *Die Literatur über die venerischen Krankheiten*, p. 84. I shall use the editions from 1559 and 1609 which are the same in content but have slightly different titles.

82 For Wittich's biography see *Allgemeine Deutsche Biographie*, vol. 43, p. 63.

83 Here I use the reprint from 1603. *Von dem Ligno Guayaco, Wunderbaum, res nova genandt; von der china ex occidentali india; von der Sarsaparilla; von dem Fenchelholtz Sassafras, und von dem Grießholtz, so man Lignum Nephriticum nenne* (Arnstadt, 1603).

84 *De Lue Venerea. Von Frantzoson kurtzen Bericht* (Giessen, 1620). On Knobloch see *Lexikon der gelehrten Ärzte*, vol. 4, p. 559.

85 See Gundolf Keil and Willelm F. Daems, 'Paracelsus und die "Franzosen": Betrachtungen zur Venerologie Hohenheims, I: Pathologie und nosologisches Konzept', *Nova Acta Paracelsica* IX (1977), pp. 99–151. See also Karl Sudhoff, 'Über Hohenheims Syphilisschriften', *Münchner medizinsche Wochenschrift* 59 (1902), p. 1899; Johann Daniel Achelis, 'Über die Syphilisschriften des Theophrastus von Hohenheim: Die Pathologie der Syphilis', *Sitzungsberichte der Heidelberger Akademie der Wissenschaften, Mathematisch-Naturwissenschaftliche Klasse* 9 (1938), pp. 3–42. See also Arrizabalaga/French/Henderson, *The Great Pox*, pp. 103–4; Allen G. Debus, *The Chemical Philosophy: Paracelsian Science and Medicine in the Sixteenth and Seventeenth Centuries* (2 vols, New York, 1977), p. 52.

sources available reveal in fact no Paracelsian influence, nor does the analysis of the medical practice at the three Augsburg hospitals reflect any significant enthusiasm for the medical ideas of the self-styled *Luther medicorum*.[86] I have no need, therefore (nor inclination), to add to the vast literature that celebrates Paracelsus as one of the heroes and revolutionary figures of early modern medicine and science.[87]

By reviving the unitarian medical world which instructed the 'diagnostic act' at the Augsburg pox hospitals, this study seeks to fill a gap in the existing literature on the French pox. While social and cultural historians have illuminated the quotidian experience of the new illness in the late fifteenth and sixteenth century, they have largely ignored its epistemological status and meaning. Most studies continue to identify the French pox with venereal syphilis, even though some historians mention in passing that early modern contemporaries perceived the pox within the context of Galenic humoral pathology. Other historians, more interested in the world of medical ideas, have analysed the thinking of learned practitioners on the pox, but they rarely engage with the daily practice of its treatment.[88] By contrast, this study aims at formulating the ways in which the epistemological understanding of the pox – its nosological picture, so to speak – shaped and was shaped by medical and socio-cultural practices in a specific local setting.

86 In a characteristically bombastic passage Paracelsus drew attention to the parallels between himself and Martin Luther. See Debus, *Chemical Philosophy*, p. 52.

87 See, for instance, Walter Pagel, *Das medizinische Weltbild des Paracelsus. Seine Zusammenhänge mit Neuplatonismus und Gnosis* (Wiesbaden, 1962), ibid., *Paracelsus: An Introduction to Philosophical Medicine in the Era of the Renaissance*, 2nd edn (Basel and New York, 1982); Charles Webster, 'Alchemical and Paracelsian Medicine', in ibid., *Health, Medicine and Morality in the Sixteenth-Century* (Cambridge, 1979), pp. 300–333; ibid., 'Paracelsus: Medicine as Popular Protest', in Ole Peter Grell and Andrew Cunningham (eds), *Medicine and the Reformation* (London, 1993), pp. 57–77; Udo Benzenhöfer (ed.), *Paracelsus* (Darmstadt, 1993). For interesting thoughts on the 'Paracelsian myth' see Bruce T. Moran, 'Paracelsus und seine internationale Rezeption in der frühenNeuzeit: Beitrage zur Geschichte des Paracelsismus', *Bulletin of the History of Medicine* 75 (2001), pp. 125–7.

88 For a recent example of this fine scholarship see Jon Arrizabalaga, 'Medical Responses to the "French Disease" in Europe at the Turn of the Sixteenth Century', in Siena, *Sins of the Flesh*, pp. 33–55.

Chapter 1
What was the French Pox?

Prima Causa: God

For sixteenth-century contemporaries, coping with illness involved coming to terms with one's Maker, the Lord and Creator of the universe. In only six days, Genesis told them, the Almighty created the world and gave to all things within it a specific meaning and purpose. Until man's Fall from Grace, all living beings in this carefree, heavenly paradise lived in harmonious togetherness. Humankind, made in God's image and thus the crown of His creation, enjoyed universal knowledge and was free from all physical suffering. But Eve's bite of the apple destroyed all this; not only was the right to stay in the Garden of Eden lost, but so too, through her disobedience, did the human body become an object of shame and subject to pain and disease, decay and mortality.[1]

Thus for early modern Christians disease was a constant reminder of this *Ur*-sin that had tainted mankind forever and from which no one could ever hope to be redeemed. But disease was also understood as an immediate reaction of God, His divine punishment, *flagitium Dei*, with which He chastised the daily performed sins of mankind. No one regarded illness as something random or coincidental. In the context of divine will, disease always had a higher purpose. It was a sign from God, and it was man's duty to decipher and interpret its message.[2]

There was little need for debate among the authors under investigation here about the *prima causa*, the most fundamental reason for the outbreak of the new disease. That 'the primary and most common cause of these plagues derives from the will of God' was the unshakeable conviction not only of Joseph Grünpeck, but of all the other authors of the pox treatises.[3] However, as to which particular sin had put the Almighty in the mood for this dreadful punishment, opinions varied considerably. One cannot help wondering whether in fact each author advanced

1 Klaus Schreiner, 'Si homo non pecasset ... Der Sündenfall Adams und Evas in seiner Bedeutung für die soziale, seelische und körperliche Verfaßtheit des Menschen', in ibid. and Norbert Schnitzler (eds), *Gepeinigt, begehrt, vergessen. Symbolik und Sozialbezug des Körpers im späten Mittelalter und in der frühen Neuzeit* (Munich, 1992), pp. 41–2.

2 For sin and disease see Darrel W. Amundsen, *Medicine, Society, and Faith in the Ancient and Medieval Worlds* (Baltimore, 1996); Mary Lindemann, *Medicine and Society in Early Modern Europe* (Cambridge, 1999), pp. 206–12; Ole Peter Grell and Andrew Cunningham, *The Four Horsemen of the Apocalypse: Religion, War, Famine and Death in Reformation Europe* (Cambridge, 2000), chapter 5.

3 Sudhoff, *Grünpeck*, p. 84.

his own 'favourite sin', the one he considered most reprehensible, to the forefront of his debate. Thus, according to the Nuremberg barber-surgeon Franz Renner, God had brought the new plague down on humanity 'without doubt to punish the sins of fornication and excessive drunkenness'.[4] Yet the Ansbach doctor, Tobias Knobloch, deemed drunkenness a lesser evil. For him it was the 'shameful lust of mankind' which had compelled the Lord to resort to such drastic measures.[5] The pox was merely the 'justa Dei vindicta, the just and rightful punishment of eternal Almighty God' for the most shameful of all imaginable sins. Since the creation of the world, Knobloch ranted, the carnal evil grew steadily and had reached such proportions among his own contemporaries that 'many wrongly consider it a virtue'. Joseph Grünpeck, by contrast, expressed the view that fornication, though significant, was only one of three cardinal sins to be avoided at all cost, reminding his readers that arrogance and greed were at least as reprehensible and therefore to be shunned just as vigorously.[6]

But as all my authors hastened to add, there was hope for mankind because the Almighty was as much a merciful God as a vengeful one. Just as He had inflicted the pox upon humans, it lay exclusively within His power to relieve them of it and allow their wretched bodies to heal. For this to happen, wrote Magnus Hundt, each sufferer must understand and accept that his or her illness was first and foremost 'God's punishment for disobedience' and a testing of individual faith.[7] Not to accept one's own responsibility, or, even worse, to lose faith in God during the course of one's illness, could have potentially fatal consequences. After all, only the Almighty had the power to alleviate human affliction through His infinite Grace and Mercy. So as not to endanger recovery, Magnus Hundt thus advised that every pox sufferer was to make peace with God before beginning treatment. The Nuremberg barber-surgeon Franz Renner also warned his readers against abandoning their faith, however much God might appear to be testing it. So as not to be plagued with such a disease for the duration of his or her entire life,

4 Renner, *Artzneybüchlein*, Foreword IIv.

5 For this and the following quotation, Knobloch, *De Lue Venerea*, p. 30.

6 Sudhoff, *Grünpeck*, p. 84; for sexual intercourse as sinful act in relation to the pox see Walter, *Sexualität*, pp. 396–415; more general Vern L. Bullough, 'Sex in History', in Jacqueline Murray and Konrad Eisenbichler (eds), *Desire and Discipline: Sex and Sexuality in the Premodern West* (Toronto, 1996); Richard Davenport-Himes, *Sex, Death and Punishment: Attitudes to Sex and Sexuality in Britain Since the Renaissance* (London, 1990).

7 For the following see Hundt, *Nutzbarlichs Regiment*, p. 3a–b. For the relationship between Christian faith and medicine see Ronald L. Numbers and Darrel W. Amundsen (eds), *Caring and Curing: Health and Medicine in the Western Religious Traditions* (New York and London, 1986); Andrew Wear, 'Religious Beliefs and Medicine in Early Modern England', in Hilary Marland and Margaret Pelling (eds), *The Task of Healing: Medicine, Religion and Gender in England and the Netherlands, 1450–1800* (Rotterdam, 1996), pp. 145–69; Ole Peter Grell and Andrew Cunningham, *Religio Medici: Medicine and Religion in Seventeenth-Century England* (Aldershot, 1996).

each sufferer must 'acknowledge his sins, renounce evil, do penance and call upon the Lord as the supreme physician to grant him forgiveness and mercy'.[8] Renner promised his readers that their faith would be rewarded because the Lord was 'so good, so gracious, so merciful that He shall not inflict greater suffering than he [the sufferer], with God's help and mercy, is able to bear'.[9]

A sure sign of this divine grace and mercy, these authors all agreed, was the arrival of a new miraculous drug from the New World, the wood guaiacum. Why else, they wondered, would it reach Europe at precisely the moment when it was most urgently needed? The anonymous author of *A Clear Account* expressed in writing what the others most probably believed as well, namely that

> God, our Redeemer, comforted the lonely afflicted with a noteworthy medicine, previously hidden from the doctors, called Guaiacum wood, which the loving Father has sent from foreign lands. The effect of this wood, in the disease already cited and other diseases, is so miraculous that it can only be a special gift of God, who shall never abandon His children in their fears when they call on Him.[10]

The authors attached great importance to prayers and repentance as an indispensable precondition for the effectiveness of any treatment. However, they by no means intended to instil in their readers a stoic fatalism. The acceptance of illness as God's punishment, as a warning or as a test of faith was not to result in the sufferers rejecting all medical treatment as meaningless. From the earliest times Christianity had taught that God in His infinite mercy mitigated the punishment of the Fall and gave to mankind the means to alleviate illness through medication.[11]

The duty of every Christian was thus to look after and maintain his or her body (as the home of the immortal soul) and to seek medical advice in the event of illness. Deliberately neglecting health and rejecting medical help was tantamount to wilfully shortening the life span allotted by God, an almost unsurpassable act of negligence that was equated with the sin of suicide.[12] That at least was how the Marbach physician Alexander Seitz expressed it in his reply to Abbess Elisabeth's request. She had asked him whether there was in fact any point in attempting to cure the pox, since it was generally recognised as God's rightful punishment for

8 Renner, *Handbüchlein*, fol. IVv; fol. XIv–XIIr.

9 Ibid., fol. XIv.

10 Anonymous, *Ein clarer bericht*, fol. Av.

11 Andrew Wear, *Knowledge and Practice*, pp. 30–31. For Islamic views on this question, which are very different see Michael Dols, *The Black Death in the Middle East* (Princeton, 1977).

12 For suicide in the early modern period see Kathy Stuart, *Defiled Trades and Social Outcasts: Honor and Ritual Pollution in Early Modern Germany* (Cambridge, 1999), pp. 197–200; David Lederer, 'The Dishonorable Dead: Perception of Suicide in Early Modern Germany', in Sibylle Backmann et al. (eds), *Ehrkonzepte in der frühen Neuzeit. Identitäten und Ausgrenzungen* (Berlin, 1998), pp. 349–65.

the sins of mankind. Seitz could not at all agree with this line of reasoning, not least because it called his entire profession into question. On no account, he assured the doubting abbess, should a patient 'suffering from this or any other serious illness rely entirely on healing powers of nature or God alone to cure him'.[13] Drawing on both the Holy Scriptures and the opinions of a number of ancient medical authorities, Seitz explained that in the struggle with dangerous and venomous ailments the human body's natural inclination to survive should be accompanied and supported by 'permissible remedies'.[14] It was deeply regrettable, he continued, that due to the Fall mankind had lost the knowledge of most of nature's secrets. However, God in His wisdom and goodness had granted physicians understanding of how to extract the secret healing powers hidden in stones and herbs once again to comfort and help their fellow men. Seitz even quoted the Bible to prove the extent to which the medical profession deserved particular honour and respect. 'We read in Ecclesiastes XXXVIII: Honour the physician, for God has created him from necessity'.[15] Indeed, the Creator expected mankind to make full use of the cures He had provided for, as Seitz urgently reminded the abbess, everything that the 'planter of all virtue' had brought into being in the act of creation was there with a purpose. So those who, on falling ill, laid their hands in their laps and trusted blindly in divine grace were, in Seitz's view, acting against the will of God in rejecting His merciful gifts; indeed, they were wilfully harming themselves. In the event of their death they would be solely responsible and, as the abbess knew full well, Seitz reminded her, suicide was 'not a minor sin'.[16]

As for the physician, Seitz continued, it was both his duty and in his professional interest to offer his patients not just treatments but comforting words, and to sustain them in their faith, for it was generally acknowledged that 'medicine could cure if supported by faith'.[17] Without spiritual encouragement, a patient's spirits could be all too 'frightened and depressed' and therefore not particularly receptive to the medicine's healing properties. Indeed, obviously drawing on his own experiences, Seitz warned that 'the patient often dies an unnatural death, as soon as he finds himself without encouragement'. The cures applied by the medical practitioner could only be properly effective if his patients were strengthened in their faith and their fears were calmed, for 'if a man has true faith his inner strength is unleashed, and turned eager to absorb the medicine'.

When Seitz published his treatise in 1509, the 'true faith' to which he referred was the one propagated by the Roman Catholic Church.[18] However, only a few years later, due to the first challenges of the Reformation, the question of faith

---

13 Ukena, *Alexander Seitz*, pp. 19–20.

14 Ibid., p. 20.

15 Ibid., pp. 19–20.

16 Ibid.

17 For this and the following quotations see ibid., p. 20.

18 For Seitz's changing religious attitudes see Moll, *Alexander Seitz*; Schottenloher, 'Alexander Seitz'.

became the subject of intense and fierce public controversies all over the German-speaking lands.[19] Some interesting aspects of the early debate can be gleaned from the treatise penned by the reform-minded knight and publicist Ulrich von Hutten.[20] In his account, *On the Miraculous Medicine Called Guaiacum Wood*, predominantly a gripping personal report of his own suffering from the pox, von Hutten also discusses the role and value of relics in the cure of disease, a widespread belief and practice strongly endorsed by the Catholic Church but increasingly criticised by the supporters of Protestant reform.[21]

Rome had never explicitly taught that saints could cure diseases but, despite that, their relics were ascribed healing powers in the event of illness and played a significant intermediary role between the sick and God in Catholic religion.[22] The specific benefits of relics were largely determined by the illnesses that this or that saint had allegedly endured in his or her lifetime. All sorts of 'special saints' existed for eye infections, sore throats, toothache, childlessness, paralysis and so on. Patron saints of the new French pox were those who were already believed to have successfully interceded for various kinds of illnesses manifesting themselves on the skin. Thus the Biblical Job, who suffered from skin rashes, was inundated with prayers and supplications, which is why one occasionally finds the pox referred to as the 'Disease of St Job'.[23] Another 'French pox-specialist' was St Rochus who, together with St Sebastian, was also frequently invoked in the event of plague. Specific geographic locations also soon acquired special importance for pox sufferers through the reports and rumours of alleged healing miracles that had happened there. Sometimes such miracles even inspired the establishment of an entirely new place of pilgrimage, such as at the city of Mörchingen in Lorraine

19 For an overview of the various religious reform movements see Steven Ozment, *The Age of Reform, 1250–1550: An Intellectual and Religious History of Late Medieval and Reformation Europe* (New Haven, 1980); also the articles in Thomas A. Brady, Heiko Oberman, and James D. Tracy (eds), *Handbook of European History 1400–1600: Late Middle Ages, Renaissance and Reformation*, vol. 2: *Programs and Outcomes* (Leiden, 1995), pp. 61–93.

20 It would be interesting to trace Hutten's social and political ideas in this treatise. Until now it has only been used as an example of the early modern experience of illness. See Michael Peschke, *Ulrich von Hutten (1488–1523) als Kranker und als medizinischer Schriftsteller* (Cologne, 1985); see also Lewis Jillings, 'The Aggression of a Cured Syphilitic: Ulrich von Hutten Projection of His Disease as a Metaphor', *The German Quarterly* 68 (1995), pp. 1–18.

21 For the role of wonders and miracles in early modern culture see Lorraine Daston and Katharine Park, *Wonders and the Order of Nature, 1150–1750* (New York, 1999).

22 For the role of miracles in early modern medicine see Nancy Siraisi, *The Clock and the Mirror: Girolamo Cardano and Renaissance Medicine* (Princeton, 1997), pp. 149–94.

23 Leprosy was also occasionally called St Job's disease. See Arrizabalaga/French/Henderson, *The Great Pox*, p. 52; for the figure of Job in Jewish and Christian tradition see S. Terrien, 'Job', in M. Eliade (ed.), *The Encyclopedia of Religion*, vol. 8, pp. 97–100.

(France), which attracted large numbers of pilgrims worshipping the relatively unknown Irish saint St Fiacrius.[24]

It is interesting to note that von Hutten, although he ridiculed some of the excesses of the 'miracle business', did not call into question the belief in relics *per se*. He was firmly convinced that prayers to the 'right' saint such as St Rochus could be most effective in curing the pox.[25] What worried and excited him were the profits he believed the Catholic Church was making out of the gullibility of its flock. Within the reform-minded circles to which von Hutten belonged, strong criticism of the mother Church's greed for profits was particularly strident. The chief object of reproach was the selling of indulgences, the widespread practice that exempted sinners from heavy acts of penance in return for alms or other services to the Church.[26]

Von Hutten was convinced that the Church was squeezing money out of pox sufferers by exploiting their belief in miracles and that its representatives were not averse to telling lies in their relentless pursuit of profit. To that end church dignitaries, von Hutten claimed, disseminated amongst the populace the miraculous story of a certain monk, Evagrius[27] (very probably von Hutten meant the Irish saint Fiacrius), who allegedly suffered from a skin condition after having lived in solitude for several years, feeding himself upon raw and unhealthy foodstuff.[28] The tale of Evagrius, von Hutten continued, had caused many God-fearing and pious pox victims to undertake long journeys to the church of the supposed saint in France, at great cost to their pockets and to their already fragile health. Von Hutten noted maliciously that he was hardly surprised that their hopes for a miracle cure were so rarely fulfilled, since it was not even certain that the monk in question had ever existed.[29] Von Hutten's suspicion that the Catholic Church had simply invented St Evagrius in order to get its hands on the money and property of its believers stemmed from his deep general mistrust of the official representatives of Rome, and particularly of their claim to possess the sole authority in interpreting the Holy

24 Luzian Pfleger, 'Das Auftreten der Syphilis in Straßburg, Geiler von Kaysersberg und der Kult des hl. Fiakrius', *Zeitschrift für Geschichte des Oberrheins* 72 (1918), pp. 153–73.

25 Böcking, *Hutten*, p. 401. For the continuation of the belief in miracles in post-Reformation England see Alexandra Walsham, 'Miracles in Post-Reformation England', in Kate Cooper and Jeremy Gregory (eds), *Signs, Wonders, Miracles: Representations of Divine Power in the Life of the Church* (London, 2005); ibid., 'Miracles and the Counter Reformation Mission to England, *Historical Journal* 46, 4 (2003), pp. 779–815.

26 Heinz Schilling, *Aufbruch und Krise: Deutschland 1517–1648*, 4th edn (Berlin, 1998), pp. 96–8.

27 Here I follow Bloch's view. See Bloch *Ursprung*, p. 80; also Pfleger, *Geiler*, p. 172.

28 Böcking, *Hutten*, p. 400.

29 Ibid., p. 401. The French church that is mentioned by von Hutten is probably the one in Mörchingen.

Scriptures.[30] With their repugnant speeches, von Hutten ranted, the Catholic clergy was trying to persuade people that the world 'had never been more wicked than now'.[31] In response to such unsurpassed iniquity, they made their flock believe that God was compelled to punish mankind and send them the pox, one of the greatest plagues since the creation of the world. Although von Hutten (like all the other pox authors) had no doubt that divine will was the primary cause for the scourge of the pox, he rejected this official interpretation by Rome's officials. If one took the trouble to read the Scriptures and the ancient historians, as he had done at great depth, von Hutten reassured his readership, one soon arrived at the conclusion that the present times were by no means the most iniquitous in human history. With its concocted tales of mankind's unparalleled wickedness, the Church was basically pursuing the same goal as it was with its invention of the tale of the saintly monk Evagrius, von Hutten argued: It fanned people's anxieties about their health in the pursuit of its own selfish ends.

Von Hutten's tract exposes the emerging rift that would separate the Catholic and Protestant valuations of miracle cures from the end of the seventeenth century onwards. While many Protestant theologians became convinced that the age of miracles began and ended with Biblical times, Catholic theologians believed that miracles could still happen here and now.[32] These differing interpretations owed something to the fact that, in contrast to Catholic doctrine, Protestant teachings regarded neither the individual's outward or visible 'good works', nor the prominent role of the church as an intermediary between God and man, as fruitful foundations on which sinners inflicted with disease might expect to be cured. Faith in miracles, the reformers believed, would only sustain sufferers in false hopes about their recovery. The believer's inner redemption through faith and grace was increasingly seen in Protestant theology as a matter to be resolved exclusively between the individual and his God. In the eyes of the reformers, only faith and inner redemption could absolve an individual of his or her sins. Holy relics and reports of miracle cures thus seemed to Protestant contemporaries increasingly suspect.[33]

30 For von Hutten's attitudes towards the Catholic Church see David Friedrich Strauß, *Ulrich von Hutten* (Bonn, 1895); and the more recent work by Kreutz, *Ulrich von Hutten*.

31 For this quotation and the following see Böcking, *Hutten*, p. 402.

32 Lorraine Daston, 'Wunder, Naturgesetze und die wissenschaftliche Revolution des 17. Jahrhunderts', *Jahrbuch der Akademie der Wissenschaften zu Göttingen* (1991), pp. 99–122.

33 Carter Lindberg, 'The Lutheran Tradition', in Numbers/Amundsen, *Western Religious Traditions*, pp. 173–203.

Secunda Causa: Astrology

The conviction that French pox ultimately derived from the will of God was closely connected with the prevailing belief in the influence of the heavens on all matters of importance in human existence. As Joseph Grünpeck explained to his readers, God had given the stars and planets power to 'influence human creatures and order and regulate all things'.[34] In fact, all the authors under discussion took the judgements of astrologers very seriously, even if, in their writings, they tackled the subject with varying degrees of thoroughness.[35] The 'astra have no small influence on the course and causation of diseases', Tobias Knobloch explained to his readers.[36] And the barber-surgeon Franz Renner, who referred his readers to the academically-trained and 'more experienced astronomis and medicis' for more detailed information on the subject, made it clear that in his daily practice certainty about the constellation of the stars at the moment of the patient's birth was an essential precondition to beginning treatment.[37] How would one otherwise be able to judge confidently, Renner asked, what the patient 'had been born with and given by nature'? Without astrological information, he personally would never risk either diagnosis or cure.

But what 'world view' lay at the root of this belief in the influence of the heavens on human health and disease? The works assessed in this study yield a number of ancient natural-philosophical principles as underpinning this

34 Sudhoff, *Grünpeck*, p. 93. Recent scholarship claims that there was little difference between Catholics and Protestants with regard to their belief in medical astrology. See, for example, Sachiko Kusukawa, 'Aspectio divinorum operum: Melanchthon and Astrology for Lutheran Medics', in Ole Peter Grell and Andrew Cunningham (eds), *Medicine and the Reformation* (London and New York, 1993), pp. 33–56; for a more general look at early modern astronomy/astrology see Notker R. Hammerstein, 'The Battle of the Booklets: Prognostic Tradition and Proclamation of the World in Early Sixteenth-Century Germany', in Paola Zambelli (ed.), *'Astrologi Hallucinati': Stars and the End of the World in Luther's Time* (Berlin and New York, 1986), pp. 129–51; Eugenio Garin, *Astrology in the Renaissance: The Zodiac of Life* (London, 1983); Krystof Pomian, 'Astrology as a Naturalistic Theology of History' in Paola Zambelli, *'Astrologi Hallucinati'*, pp. 29–43.

35 For an overview of the discussions related to the appearance of the pox see Wolf-Dieter Müller-Jahncke, *Astrologische-magische Theorie und Praxis in der Heilkunde der Frühen Neuzeit* (Stuttgart, 1985), pp. 117–22; Catrien Santing, 'Medizin und Humanismus: Die Einsichten des Nürnbergischen Stadtarztes Theodoricus Ulsenius über Morbus Gallicus', *Sudhoffs Archiv* 79 (1995), pp. 139–49.

36 Knobloch, *De Lues Venerea*, p. 11.

37 Renner, *Handbüchlein*, fol. 6r.

understanding. Most prominent is the notion of a two-sphere cosmos (one above and one below the moon) with the earth at its centre.This idea originated with Plato and was further developed by Aristotle and other ancient natural philosophers and astronomers, most notably Claudius Ptolemy (83–161 AD) in his astronomical work *Almagest*. The latter remained influential over the entire sixteenth century, despite the new heliocentric theories of Copernicus.[38] According to that particular understanding of the cosmos, all natural phenomena in the sphere above the moon (the superlunary sphere) were believed to be perfect, timeless and unchangeable. This superlunary world consisted of a single element, the quintessence or ether. Around the outermost stars and planets, which orbited within this sphere and created the unchanging music of eternity, there arched the uppermost heaven, the so-called Empireum. According to Christian astrologers the Empireum not only held the universe together, but was the residence of God and the elect. From ancient times, astrologers/astronomers (a distinction between the two is hard to make for the early modern period) grouped particular clusters of stars in the superlunary sphere as star signs, which were mathematically calculated and delineated. Together they formed the Zodiac, which itself was divided into twelve planetary 'heavenly houses' which, with the aid of astronomical tables, could predict both the movements of the stars and planets, specific constellations and prognosticate their influence on human destiny. This close relationship between the stars and human activity was grounded in the conviction that the superlunary sphere continuously influenced, or as Joseph Grünpeck, following Aristotle, put it, 'ruled over', the world inhabited by mankind (the sublunary sphere).[39]

This world beneath the moon was the realm of the four elements (earth, water, fire, air) and according to Aristotelian natural philosophy was a place of imperfection, continuous change and decay. It was thought that, in common with the other living things on earth, the human body consisted of these four basic elements and their corresponding qualities (dry, moist, hot and cold). Each individual was made up of a distinct composition of these elements and qualities, to which were also associated the four bodily humours: blood (moist/hot), yellow bile (hot/dry), black bile (dry/cold), phlegm (moist/cold).[40] This idiosyncratic mixture was the

38 Copernicus' (1473–1543) famous work *De Revolutionibus Orbium Coelestium Libri Six*, propagating the heliocentric worldview, was published in 1543. However, it took a long time for his ideas to be widely adopted. For the slow acceptance of Copernican ideas see Robert S. Westman, 'The Copernicans and the Churches', in David C. Lindberg and Ronald L. Numbers (eds), *God and Nature: Historical Essays on the Encounter between Christianity and Science* (Berkeley, 1986), pp. 76–113. For the influence of Aristotle's ideas on medicine see Charles B. Schmidt, 'Aristotle among the Physicians', in Andrew Wear, Roger K. French, I. M. Lonie (eds), *The Medical Renaissance of the Sixteenth Century* (Cambridge, 1985), pp. 2–15.

39 Sudhoff, *Grünpeck*, p. 93.

40 For the development of the theory of the four humours see Raymond Klibansky, Erwin Panofsky and Fritz Saxl, *Saturn and Melancholy: Studies in the History of Natural Philosophy, Religion, and Art* (London, 1964), pp. 3–123. See also G. Harig, *Bestimmung*

individual's natural 'temperament' or 'complexion', the main four being choleric, melancholic, sanguine and phlegmatic.[41] Any alteration in the innate balance of one's innate complexion carried with it the risk of illness.

Such an alteration could be brought about by the stars and planets in the superlunary sphere, which, as God's servants and at his command, were able to alter the elements and qualities of the sublunary sphere. This necessarily affected also the composition of the human complexion. All authors agreed that the element of air was particularly susceptible to such planetary influences, since it was, Magnus Hundt explained, 'more inclined to such change than the other elements. Since air is qualitatively warm and moist, poisonous foul changes may easily occur'.[42] Ulrich von Hutten also considered corrupt or pestilential vapours (miasma) to be one of the chief causes of French pox, explaining that all the 'stargazers' he had asked attributed these pox-provoking changes in the composition of air to an midnight conjunction of Saturn and Mars and to two previous eclipses of the Sun.[43]

The widespread concept of the micro-macrocosm supported this notion of cosmic influences on human health. According to this understanding, the human body (inhabiting the sublunar sphere) comprised the 'little world' or microcosm. At the same time, the human body (the microcosm) was a fixed component of the 'great world' that surrounded him, the so-called macrocosm, which included the eternal superlunary spheres.[44] It was taken for granted that between these two worlds there existed a close relationship and a similarity in the forces, matter, and elements that constituted them. It was further understood that every detail of the 'microscopic' world of the human body had a corresponding 'macroscopic' counterpart. The human body was considered to be a reflection of the macrocosm, mirroring the proportions of the heavenly sphere. The macrocosm was mirrored in the human body and man was in concord with the cosmos or, as Mary Lindemann has put it: 'In astrological medicine man is said to be a Microcosm (or little

---

und Intensität im medizinischen System Galens (Berlin, 1974), pp. 45–51; Erich Schöner, *Das Viererschema in der antiken Humoralpathologie* (Wiesbaden, 1964).

41 Since the twelfth century the Latin term 'complexio' increasingly supplanted the Greek term 'temperament' or 'krasis'. See Per-Gunnar Ottosson, *Scholastic Medicine and Philosophy: A Study of Commentaries on Galen's Tegni (ca. 1300–1450)* (Naples, 1984), pp. 129–31; 134–6.

42 Hundt, *Nutzbarlichs Regiment*, p. 4b.

43 Böcking, *Hutten*, p. 404. For miasma theory in general see Caroline Hannaway, 'Environment and Miasmata', in William F. Bynum and Roy Porter (eds), *Companion,* vol. 1, pp. 292–308; for miasma theories in the eighteenth century see the inspiring study by Alain Corbin, *The Foul and the Fragrant: Odor and the French Social Imagination* (Leamington Spa, 1986).

44 David C. Lindberg, *The Beginnings of Western Science: The European Scientific Tradition in Philosophy, Religious, and Institutional Context, 600 B. C. to A. D. 1450* (Chicago, 1992), pp. 47–50.

world) and in him the Almighty has imprinted his own image.'[45] The parallels, correspondences and analogies between the micro- and macrocosm that astrology had to take into account were innumerable. In the sixteenth century, astrology-versed medical practitioners were busy drawing connections between their patients' sensible physical signs, age and daily habits, and the vast amount of phenomena in the surrounding macrocosm, such as their star signs, the planetary positions at the time they fell ill, the four seasons and directions, and so on, producing great numbers of diagrams and horoscopes to calculate the most propitious times for treatment (or avoidance of it).[46] It was, for example, vitally important to rule out those days of the year for cure when medical intervention might be particularly dangerous on account of a patient's individual planetary constellation.[47] Such calculations would also offer insights into which planet – or sinister planetary conjunction – was directly responsible for the affliction. On the basis of similar astrological calculations certain diseases were perceived as closely related, as 'friends or neighbouring each other'.[48] Ulrich von Hutten, for example, believed that a great number of ailments that were similar in their physical appearance to that of the pox were also astrologically related to it. Among these he counted 'tumours, leprosy, scabia, and all kinds of evil scabs and boils with whatever could afflict man's body as well as podagra and many infirmities of the hands and other limbs'.[49]

It is tempting for a modern reader to dismiss this overwhelming and widespread belief in the influence of stars and planets on the outbreak and spread of French pox as fatalism. The authors of the tracts under discussion, however, saw it quite differently. Despite their belief that a person's character and innate 'inclination' towards certain diseases were determined at birth by the heavens, they were equally convinced that the individual could strive – with God's help – to resist such dispositions. They even saw it as every man's duty to pre-empt, resist and successfully avert illness through a proper regimen of life. The stars and planets were only the servants of God, mere instruments of His divine power. Without His will they were powerless.[50] Joseph Grünpeck exemplifies this way of thinking.

45 Lindemann, *Medicine and Society*, p. 20.

46 Allan Chapman, 'Astrological Medicine', in Charles Webster (ed.), *Medicine and Mortality*, pp. 175–300. For the 'Renaissance episteme' see Michel Foucault, *The Order of Things: An Archaeology of the Human Sciences* (London, 2003), pp. 3–50.

47 Many German medical practitioners did not practice between 23 July and 24 August. This period, reigned by the star Sirius, was called the 'dog days' (*Hundstage*). It was believed to bring climatic change followed by natural catastrophes and diseases and was considered dangerous for all kinds of medical treatment.

48 Böcking, *Hutten*, p. 406.

49 Ibid., p. 404.

50 Medical horoscopes were considered preventive, not an expression of fatalism. See Chapman, 'Medical Astrology', p. 275: 'The preventive medical horoscope aimed at instructing man how to act, so that free will could alley with nature in the preservation of health.'

Great conjunctions, Grünpeck explains, such as those between the cold-moist planet Saturn and the moist-warm planet Jupiter, could produce death, infertility and political upheaval. 'From movements in the heavens, such as changes from one sign to another, as from wet to dry and cold to warm, he continued, may come great events.'[51] Anyone born under the signs of Saturn and Jupiter, as well as those born in the year of an eclipse of the sun, were fundamentally more inclined towards 'the evil French Disease' than others.[52] But Grünpeck qualified this assertion by assuring his readers that anyone dispositioned in such a way by birth would of course not inevitably succumb to pox, but with God's help could successfully prevent it: 'Of this I must warn the reader, that I do not ascribe anything to necessity, but only to natural causes and inclination, which his free will with God's help may freely withstand. The power of Almighty God, with the will of the individual, may counter such inclination.'[53] Thus, Grünpeck concluded, it often transpired that people with an astrological disposition to a particular disease could go through life without ever catching it.

While for Joseph Grünpeck and the other authors astrology was vital for making the sudden outbreak of the pox comprehensible as well as for determining its future course, their belief in the power of the Almighty and cosmic influences did not automatically lead them to pay less attention to the possible natural causes of disease.[54] Diseases like the French Pox had of course to be deciphered at the physical, not just the cosmological level.

Medical Semiotics and the Concept of a Physical Sign

No one described the many physical symptoms accompanying the French pox more vividly than Ulrich von Hutten who had suffered himself from it for over nine years:

> First of all I had no use of my left foot, for there had this disease lurked more than eight years. And upon my kneecap there were stinking oozing ulcers and great pains … It would not bear much covering with clothes and if I went to bear

51 Sudhoff, *Grünpeck*, p. 94. For the great importance of the conjunction of Saturn and Jupiter see Grafton, *Cosmos*, p. 9. Grafton points out that the fact that Saturn and Jupiter reach conjunction every twenty years was used by Persian, Jewish, Arabic and European astrologers in turn to fix and account for great turning points in world history, like the rise of new religions, or to predict history's end.

52 Sudhoff, *Grünpeck*, p. 104.

53 Ibid., p. 100.

54 For the magical-astrological practices of early modern healers see Michael MacDonald, *Mystical Bedlam: Madness, Anxiety, and Healing in Seventeenth-Century England* (Cambridge, 1981); also David Lederer, *Madness, Religion and the State in Early Modern Europe* (Cambridge, 2006).

> upon my foot the pain was insufferable ... I was so weak in both calves of my legs that I could not walk for long. And my left side was hurting so much that I did not dare to raise the arm. And my right shoulder had become so weak, and showed a swelling of the size of an egg. On the left side of my body I also had a sore though not painful but producing a foul and stinking matter as if it was cancer … On the back of my head I had a running sore, and I could not bear any touching of that.[55]

Tumours, boils, open, oozing and festering or hardened eruptions of the skin, accompanied by unbearable pain that came mostly at night, were only some of the legion of physical signs that wracked and enfeebled the knight's body year upon year.[56] From the pens of the learned physicians and barber-surgeons analysed in this study we have other quite graphic and affecting descriptions of similar physical changes. Historians, as the introduction to this study has shown, tend to equate these sixteenth-century descriptions of the pox with our modern clinical picture of venereal syphilis. However, what these attempts at restrospective diagnosis do not take into account at all is the fact that all these descriptions were based on a radically different understanding of a physical sign and how it relates to disease.

Today in Western medicine physical signs generally serve to indicate a specific nosological entity. When we talk about disease we have in mind some particular conditions.[57] The term 'disease' commonly refers to a pattern of signs that somehow hang together and recur, in more or less the same way, in successive individuals. It is only the recurrence of a pattern of events, a number of elements combined in a definite relationship, chronological and geographical, which we label a disease. A disease consists of a congeries of signs – no single sign, by itself, makes a disease entity. On the basis of this understanding, modern medicine tends to differentiate between subjective 'symptoms' that are only felt by the sick individual, and objective 'signs', which can be also sensed by another person.[58] The latter is usually the physician who is expected to organise the 'chaos' of subjective symptoms and to arrange them into a logical, coherent order, associated with a specific disease entity, described in a medical textbook or visually represented in the anatomical atlas. It appears as if there is no hidden meaning beyond the visible

55 Böcking, *Hutten*, pp. 483–4.

56 Von Hutten's illness raised concerns and pity among his friends. One even suggested to him to commit suicide and thus end his unbearable suffering. See Böcking, *Hutten*, p. 482.

57 For the following see Lester King, 'What is a Disease?' in Arthur Caplan et al. (eds), *Concepts of Health and Disease: Interdisciplinary Perspective* (Reading, MA, 1981), p. 112.

58 Andrew Wear, *Knowledge and Practice*, p. 127. Not all European languages, however, distinguish between 'objective signs' and 'subjective symptoms'. In the German language, for instance, the terms 'sign' and 'symptom' are used synonymously.

sign or symptom; it seems entirely transparent to the calculating and authoritative gaze and the language of the doctor.[59]

Our conception of a sign and its more or less fixed and predefined relationship to a specific disease would have struck all the sixteenth-century pox authors as bizarre. For them, disease and physical signs were bound together by a different code; crucially, they followed a different structure of sensibility. The way they perceived and interpreted the body's physical reality provided no space for our radical distinction between superior (in regard to its 'truth' value), objective bodily knowledge 'owned' by the medical practitioner and (the subordinated subjective bodily knowledge felt by the patient. Every diagnosis was inextricably bound up with the disease experience of the ailing individual or, as Andrew Wear has put it, '[t]he description of the patient's subjective symptoms or feelings, the patient's story as it were, were also made part of the description of the disease … .'[60]

The most striking difference to our modern sign conception is that early modern contemporaries perceived any physical sign as relatively open to interpretation and its possible meanings as pointing in very different directions.[61] As the medical historian Roger French has pointed out, the meaning of a physical sign was not restricted as a signifier of a specific disease entity; in fact, it could even be that it was not related to disease at all but 'to cause … or to accidental results of a cause'.[62] In sixteenth-century medicine cause and disease were not necessarily related, as Ian Maclean has exemplified through the writings of the famous sixteenth-century Italian physician Girolamo Cardano (1501–1576). Cardano, Maclean explains, differentiated between 'pure signs' (such as bad colour), signs that were simultaneously causes (he cites pain and wakefulness as examples), signs that were identical to illness (such as epilepsy and jaundice), and signs which were both causes and illnesses.[63] Moreover, a bodily sign could point to one of the three possible states of the human body (natural, non-natural, unnatural), in which the patient happened to be at the time of the examination.[64] But physical signs not only provided information about a patient's present physical condition. They also

59 Foucault has argued that this reorganisation of the medical gaze slowly emerges during the eighteenth century. See *Birth of the Clinic*, p. 91.

60 Wear, *Knowledge and Practice*, p. 128; see also for a discussion on ontological and holistic views of disease Pelling, 'Contagion', p. 315.

61 I can only offer a rather superficial account of this very complicated matter. I shall not distinguish between the terms 'symptom' and 'sign' as the German authors seem to have used them interchangeably. For a detailed analysis of this important question in Latin medical treatises see Maclean, *Logic, Signs, and Nature*.

62 Roger French, 'Sign Conceptions in Medicine from the Renaissance to the Early 19th Century', in Roland Posner, Klaus Robering and Thomas A. Sebeok (eds), *Semiotik: Ein Handbuch zu den zeichentheoretischen Grundlagen von Natur und Kultur* (Berlin and New York, 1997), vol. 2, col. 1357.

63 Ian Maclean, *Logic, Signs, and Nature*, p. 282.

64 Ingo Wilhelm Müller, *Humoralmedizin: Physiologische, pathologische und therapeutische Grundlagen der galenistischen Heilkunst* (Heidelberg, 1993), pp. 87–93.

possessed a historical dimension and provided clues about past or future physical experiences and possible developments of disease. Michel Foucault summarised these different temporal connotations of a sign as follows: 'The sign announces: the prognostic sign, what will happen; the anamnestic sign, what has happened; the diagnostic sign, what is now taking place.'[65]

This understanding of a physical sign as an ambiguous signifier was by no means confined to the academic medical elite but was shared by many in early modern German society.[66] A clue as to how widespread this view actually may be found in detailed discussions on the interpretation of bodily signs in the many vernacular medical books written for the 'common man', such as the *Mirror of Medicine* (Spiegel der Artzney), a sixteenth-century bestseller. The author, Strasbourg physician Lorenz Fries (c. 1482–1530), used the example of uroscopy to explain to his readers some of the meanings of signs.[67]

> These signs are of three kinds: some are called Demonstrativa, these show the current state of health or illness such as urine which is of average colour, thickness or thinness, with a regular cloud on the bottom. This [urine] indicates present health, while [urine] contrary to these [signs] indicates present sickness. Other signs are called Rememorativa, these indicate past sickness or health and are most useful to the doctor. So for example when a sick person's urine indicates loss of health the doctor may understand what his natural complexion is. The third kind [of signs] are called Prognostica and signify future health or sickness as when urine containing a green circle and blue bubbles foretells a stroke.[68]

But why could a physical sign take on so many meanings? And what underlying conceptual understanding accounted for this interpretative openness? Again Fries's *Mirror of Medicine* offers a first clue. He submits that 'a sign is a thing that insinuates something through the senses'.[69] In other words, the meaning of a physical sign was not exhausted by its sensual perception. Fries seemed to say that the sensual experience of a bodily sign alone holds no definite meaning in itself. His definition points to some kind of meaning-giving domain beyond the actual physically sensible sign.

Recent work on the sense of sight and embodiment in the Middle-Ages and the early modern period helps us to get closer to the different understanding of

---

65 Foucault, *Birth of the Clinic*, p. 90.

66 I agree here with Maclean who has claimed this recently in his *Logic, Sign, and Nature*, p. 227.

67 For uroscopy see Johanna Bleker, 'Die Kunst des Harnsehens – ein vornehm und nötig Gliedmaß der schönen Artzney', *Hippokrates* 41 (1970), pp. 385–95.

68 Fries, *Spiegel der Artzney* (Strasbourg, 1532), p. XXXIXr. Most pox authors follow his distinction. See for instance, Knobloch, *De Lue Venerea*, p. 44.

69 Fries, *Spiegel der Artzney*, p. XXXIX: 'Das ist ein ding das etwas durch die sinnlichkeit [zu] verstehen gibt'.

sensibility and, hence, to what Fries might have had in mind.[70] Medieval visual culture, it has been argued, can only be grasped if we allow ourselves to embrace the idea that in the past the visual was not solely visible. We have to account for an 'invisibility of vision'.[71] For medieval and early modern contemporaries, vision extended in fact beyond mere sense perception and included extra-sensory realms (terrestrial and spiritual conceptions and ideologies) of the world. What is missing from this particular understanding of the visible from a modern perspective is the perceptual correlate of an objective world, that is, the distinction between an objective and subjective gaze (the objectifying gaze). Of course the 'medical gaze' accessing the sick body during the clinical encounter comprises more than just the visual perception of a bodily sign and includes the sense of touch, taste, smell and hearing. But I would argue that, very much like the sense of sight, these sense perceptions too derived their ultimate meaning from realms beyond the immediately sensible. Lorenz Fries would probably have agreed.

His definition of a physical sign, at least, was ultimately couched in Aristotelian natural philosophy whose main tenets, as Mary Fissell has demonstrated for early modern England, circulated widely in early modern society (along with other conceptual ideas deriving from classical and medieval scholarship).[72] Aristotle was explicitly acknowledged by Fries at the beginning of his chapter on 'Signs of Disease' as the great Greek philosopher who maintained that 'all art should begin from the things which are the most sensible to us'.[73] Fries drew here on the Aristotelian idea that the process of acquiring knowledge of any natural object began with all the senses.[74] From repeated sense experience followed memory; and from memory, by process of intuition, the experienced investigator of nature was supposed to be able to grasp the universal feature of things, their nature or essence (the universalia). Once he possessed this universal definition he could put it to use as the premise for deductive demonstrations. Thus, certain knowledge about the French pox for example, was (for the academic physician at least) to be gained by a process that began with sense experience. However, what was learned by this inductive process did not acquire the status of certain and universal knowledge until it was put into deductive form. The end product of this process,

70 See Suzannah Biernoff, *Sight and Embodiment in the Middle Ages* (Houndmills, 2002); also Carolly Erickson, *The Medieval Vision: Essays in History and Perception* (New York, 1976).

71 Biernoff, *Sight and Embodiment*, p. 3.

72 Mary Fissell, *Vernacular Bodies: The Politics of Early Modern England* (Oxford, 2004); G. E. R. Lloyd, *Aristotle: The Growth and Structure of His Thought* (Cambridge, 1968). On Aristotelian natural philosophy and its early modern critics see Keith Hutchison, 'Dormative Virtues, Scholastic Qualities, and the New Philosophies', *History of Science* 29 (1991), pp. 245–278; for the many different versions of Aristotelianism see Charles B. Schmitt, *Aristotle in the Renaissance* (Cambridge, MA, 1983).

73 Fries, *Spiegel der Artzney*, p. XXXIX: 'Dz man in jede kunst anfangen soll von den dingen die uns im kuendlichsten sind'.

74 For the following see Lindberg, *Western Science*, pp. 39–51, p. 50.

then, was a deductive demonstration based on the universal definition of a natural object, such as the French Disease.

The Aristotelian notion of a physical sign as indicative of something else, something hidden and not directly accessible to the senses, was supported and reinforced by the early modern idea of a dualistic body, a major symbolic opposition in Western medicine from its first formulation in the ancient Greek Hippocratic treatises.[75] As Barbara Duden has shown in her seminal study of the patients of the German physician Storck, the inner body was considered a place of hidden and secret activities until far into the eighteenth century.[76] Only through the physical signs on the surface of the skin could a sick individual and his or her medical practitioner speculate about the secrets happening inside. However, to get an idea of what was going on inside was vital for the diagnosis of the pox and the following treatment.

The Causes of the Pox and Its Matter

The aim of every clinical encounter was to decipher via the sensible physical signs the invisible secret properties of the French Disease: its natural causes, the composition of its matter and its idiosyncratic nature. Only on the basis of this knowledge, all authors firmly believed, could an effective treatment be proposed for each individual sufferer.[77]

In the first few years of the spread of the disease, however, there seems to have been a lack of consensus about these important questions; a state of affairs that, with the benefit of hindsight, was bemoaned by von Hutten in 1519: 'But as to its nature and its location, there was much fruitless questioning, much argument and contradiction, and many diverse opinions were anxiously disputed.'[78] These ongoing debates, which seemed to have plagued learned medical practitioners more than others, were fuelled by the increasing realisation that the pox was a new

75 Gianna Pomata, *Contracting a Cure: Patients, Healers, and the Law in Early Modern Bologna* (Baltimore, 1998), p. 132; also Marie-Christine Pouchelle, *The Body and Surgery in the Middle Ages* (New Brunswick, 1990).

76 Barbara Duden, *The Woman Beneath the Skin: A Doctor's Patients in Eighteenth-Century Germany* (Cambridge, MA, 1992).

77 For the dangers of treatment without knowledge of these matters see Ukena, *Alexander Seitz*, p. 58.

78 Böcking, *Hutten*, p. 405. For the early discussions on the nature of the French Disease in Italy and German see Arrizabalaga/French/Henderson, *The Great Pox*, pp. 56–112; John Arrizabalaga and Roger French, 'Coping with the French Disease: University Practitioners' Strategies and Tactics in the Transition from the Fifteenth to the Sixteenth Century', in Roger French et al., *Medicine from the Black Death to the French Disease* (Aldershot, 1998), pp. 248–87; Russell, 'Syphilis', pp. 286–307; Claudia Stein, 'Der Leipziger Streit (1497–1501) über die Ursachen der Franzosenkrankheit und ihre Behandlung im Augsburger Blatterhaus' in Stefan Oehmig (ed.), *Medizin und Sozialwesen in Mitteldeutschland in der Reformationzeit* (Leipzig, 2007), pp. 156–78.

and hitherto unknown disease phenomenon. University-trained physicians could not therefore, as was their tradition, turn to authoritative disease descriptions by ancient medical authors for advice on how to interpret the physical reality of the pox.[79] Our authors' writings show, however, that this initial diagnostic uncertainty, still prominent in Grünpeck's treatise of 1496, was quickly remedied.[80] By 1509 Alexander Seitz felt confident enough to define the material composition of the pox as follows: '[t]he matter of this disease is none other than salted, corroded, coagulated blood which is harmful to the good natural blood', he wrote to Abbess Elisabeth, citing the 'well-founded opinion of highly learned physicians'.[81] And von Hutten himself could report that, after lengthy discussions, the doctors agreed that the matter of the disease lay concealed in 'contaminated, burned or otherwise evil blood'.[82]

But what exactly is to be understood by 'evil and contaminated blood'? How did it differ from 'natural blood', and how could 'good blood' suddenly turn 'evil'? To untangle these rather complicated issues it is useful to begin with the observation that within the early modern understanding of bodily functioning the term 'blood' designated two different and distinct things. 'Blood' (or sanguinis) together with red or yellow bile (also choler), black bile (or melancholy) and phlegm, was one of the four bodily fluids or humours thought to be essential to the functioning of the body. These four humours, in turn, were believed to be fused in 'blood', the actual fluid found in the veins. This blood, incorporating with it the other humours, fulfilled an important function in the body's economy: it was the body's nutrition.[83]

Alexander Seitz considered it important for his readers to understand how the body's 'good or natural' nutritional blood was produced before he would lead them through the various physiological scenarios that could possibly be responsible for turning this 'good' and nutritious blood into the poisonous matter of the French pox. Thus, he explained, all ingested food was first transformed to some kind of nutritious fluid (chyle) in the stomach. Subsequently, it was transported to the liver and there concocted (literally 'cooked') into the four humours, blood, the two biles and phlegm. Various further stages of concoction followed, purifying the nutritional blood of superfluities, which were then excreted. Finally this purified end product was sent through the body with the help of the liver to nourish its various parts and organs. This purification of nutritional blood (Seitz compared this process with the fermentation of young wine) was absolutely vital because it

79 For the authority of ancient text over the practice of learned medicine see Maclean, *Logic, Signs, and Nature*, pp. 191–3.

80 Sudhoff, *Grünpeck*, pp. 73–4. In the following I shall restrict myself to those causes most frequently mentioned in the treatises.

81 Ukena, *Seitz*, pp. 9–10.

82 Böcking, *Hutten*, p. 404; see also Renner, *Handbüchlein*, fol. VIIr.

83 Nancy Siraisi, *Medieval and Early Renaissance Medicine: An Introduction to Knowledge and Practice* (Chicago, 1990), p. 106.

was during this process that the composition of the four humours in the nutritional blood was adjusted to the innate individual complexion (or temperament) of each individual.[84] Responsible for the purification of the nutritional blood, Seitz told the Abbess Elizabeth, were specific organs, which the Almighty God, as the 'planter of all virtue and careful architect of His creation', had chosen and ordered to filter harmful, excess substances from the nutritional blood.[85] Thus, the spleen for example, would attract any superfluous yellow bile or 'raging yellow foam', he explained. And while the gall bladder would purge the nutritional blood of excess black bile, the lungs would draw off excrescent phlegm, and the liver was responsible for, extracting superfluous excess of the humour blood.

If, however, be it through the obstruction of veins leading to or from one of the purifying organs or, indeed, through a general 'weakening' of such an organ's God-given powers, these rectifying processes were disrupted, a person's complexion could become imbalanced, Seitz warned. Illness was then likely to follow. Invoking his long-standing experiences as a medical practitioner, Seitz reported that an excess of phlegm in the nutritional blood resulting from the malfunctioning of the purifying properties of the lungs or kidneys, for example, could lead to dropsy or a one-day fever. Excess of choler in the complexion might grow into a three-day fever or even jaundice, and a weakening of the spleen's rectifying powers could possibly develop into cancer or even leprosy. However, it was the obstruction and deficiency of the liver and/or gall bladder, Seitz maintained, that was the root cause for the accumulation of the poisonous matter of the dreaded French pox in the nutritional blood.

Not all the authors shared Seitz's view, instead associating the formation of the pox matter with irregularities in the functioning of the spleen and/or lung or brain. If they disagreed on the specific organ(s) responsible, they all agreed that the formation of the 'salted, burned, and coagulated' matter of the French pox was related to an unnatural excess of black bile and/or phlegm in the human complexion. Hidden in the nutritional blood and distributed via the liver throughout the body, the morbid pox matter had ample possibility to 'take root' in the body, the Magdeburg physician Magnus Hundt explained.[86] But luckily its efforts were not always rewarded, he continued, because the corrupted fluid frequently encountered vigorous resistance from those body parts and organs that refused to accept the unbalanced nutritional blood as nourishment and went to any length to fight and get rid of it. Often, Hundt explained, 'they [the body parts] drive it [the morbid matter] into the skin which is then damaged by its sharpness and turns into poisoned scabies which is called the French pox'.[87]

84 Ibid., p. 10; Renner, *Handbüchlein*, fol. VIIv; for the widespread use of the vine-metaphor see Pouchelle, *Body & Surgery*, pp. 154–8.

85 For the following see Ukena, *Alexander Seitz*, p. 10.

86 Hundt, *Nutzbarlichs Regiment*, p. 19r–v. For a similar explanation see Knobloch, *De Lue Venerea*, p. 1; Renner, *Handbüchlein*, fol. VII; Böcking, *Hutten*, p. 404.

87 Hundt, *Nutzbarlichs Regiment*, p. 19r–v.

Physiological causes could also account for the sudden and precarious imbalance in the nutritional blood. All authors deemed a wrong or imbalanced diet to be just as dangerous as the malfunction of one of the purifying organs. Seitz warned his reader never to touch any foodstuff whose complexional composition came close to that of the pox matter (i.e. moist, cold and acid). To help his readers to choose simultaneously balanced *and* pox-preventing daily meals, he provided long lists of foods at the end of his treatise which were to be avoided at all costs. Among the foodstuff listed one finds the meat of animals 'which like to dwell by water' and all kinds of water birds or fish whose preferred habitats were standing or stagnant ponds.[88] Moreover, Seitz cautioned against the consumption of older game such as hare, deer, geese and cranes, or legumes such as beans, peas, and in particular lentils. Particularly detrimental to the humoral balance in Seitz's view were hot dishes, in particular spicy vegetables like radish, onions or garlic. Mustard and especially salt was to be avoided under all circumstances because it obstructed the pores of the skin.[89]

But not only the consumption of wrong foods could yield dramatic results. Too much of it was also dangerous, Seitz pointed out, particularly if the pox matter had already rooted in the body, 'for the more the unclean body consumes, the more the sickness will increase and as Galienus spoke, even if one pours good wine into a stinking barrel, it will not turn into anything good'.[90] And von Hutten was convinced that his fellow-German's well-known excessive eating habits were responsible for the widespreadness of the pox in his beloved fatherland.[91] However, as the Arnstadt physician Johannes Wittich was quick to point out to his readership, restricting one's food intake was not the solution to the problem. Drawing on his own experiences of war-related food shortages, he stressed that periods of hunger were equally detrimental to one's natural humoral balance and threatened to bring about a rapid increase in melancholic fluids.[92] Seitz offers his readers the Galenic explanation of how this came about. If the body, he explained, is denied food 'the stomach (which wants to be fed) attracts much humid, slimy matter from all over the body for its nutrition and becomes polluted …; the whole body is poisoned because the stomach fed itself with feculence'.[93]

Our authors wasted much ink discussing how the pox originated 'from one's own blood', but, at the same time, they were well aware that 'a person may contract such a disease externally and be infected by another'.[94] Significantly, how

88 For the following see Ukena, *Alexander Seitz*, pp. 22–3.

89 Ukena, *Alexander Seitz,* p. 22. All authors warned against salt. Von Hutten devoted a whole chapter to its dangers during the pox cure. See Böcking, *Hutten*, chapter 16; pp. 448–51.

90 Ukena, *Alexander Seitz*, p. 25. Böcking, *Hutten*, p. 403.

91 Böcking, *Hutten*, p. 403.

92 Wittich, *Ligno Guayaco*, fol. B2r.

93 Ukena, *Alexander Seitz*, p. 25.

94 Ibid., p. 11.

they imagined the exact mechanism of such an infection (whether they thought of transferable atom- or germ-like organisms like their contemporary Italian colleague Girolamo Fracastoro did) does not become clear from their writings.[95] Within the framework of Hippocratic-Galenic medicine, which stressed the quantities and qualities of fluids, this question was not obvious enough for them to investigate. But all warned their readers of possible sources of infection. The greatest danger, in their view, lay in the direct contact with the various bodily fluids and excretions of those who were already suffering from the pox. And there is a concrete physiological explanation for this observed 'fluid phobia' among all pox authors. Sweat, saliva, semen or urine were all considered to be by-products of the various concoctions of nutritional blood.[96] If the latter was contaminated (as in the case of French pox) these fluids and excretions were necessarily affected, and the immediate contact with them presented a danger to others. But the contaminated matter, Seitz explained, could also 'conceal itself' for long periods outside the body in the clothes or bed linen.[97] The barber-surgeon Renner thus advised his readers under no circumstances ever to exchange clothes or share a bed with a pox sufferer or to even use their bed linen. Contact with the residues of sweat and other contaminated bodily fluids that might still be hidden there could easily lead to a healthy person being infected with the 'French poison', he warned.[98] This is also why sexual intercourse or 'daily copulation' also harboured grave dangers, according to the Nuremberg barber-surgeon. As the body heated up during 'the act of lying with such an unclean person', the pores of the skin would open up and contaminated sweat could thus easily be transferred to a healthy body.[99] For the same reasons extra caution had to be exercised in using eating and drinking utensils previously used by pox victims. Knobloch therefore advised his readers to make absolutely sure that their daily meals were not prepared by 'infected' cooks who had contaminated the foodstuff by touching it and serving it in unclean vessels.[100] Even in bakeries Knobloch sniffed the dangers of infection, for example, when pox-suffering bakers kneaded the fresh dough with their contaminated fists or, even worse, when some drops of their contaminated sweat or saliva might fall into it. One must also be careful in one's daily dealings with money, wrote Knobloch, as coins may carry the poison. Money passed through so many hands, he explained, 'one may be pure, the other impure'. He therefore advised that coins should never be given to small children, as they were in the habit of putting them in their mouths. By far the greatest source of danger, in the opinion of all the authors, was the public bath. One could never be certain, wrote Franz Renner, whether a pox victim was not mingling with the other healthy

95 For Fracastoro's ideas see Nutton, 'Fracastoro's Theory of Contagion', pp. 196–234.

96 For more details see Siraisi, *Renaissance Medicine*, p. 105.

97 Ukena, *Alexander Seitz*, p. 11.

98 Renner, *Handbüchlein*, fol. IIIIr.

99 Ibid.

100 For the following see Knobloch, *De Lue Venerea*, pp. 18–19.

bathers and endangered them through his or her contaminated sweat.[101] Moreover, drawing on his personal experience, he claimed, that given many bath owners were often using their cupping and bleeding instruments on several different clients without cleaning them in-between, the contamination could very easily be transferred to another customer. Daily medical practice had taught Knobloch and Renner that the pox could also be passed on from parents to their offspring through contaminated male and female semen.[102] Renner lamented that he had seen all too often how newborn babies came into the world with symptoms of the disease all over their precious small bodies.[103] Some of them, Tobias Knobloch reported, were so 'covered' that – in spite of the most loving attention from their parents and every effort by the medical practitioners – they often died soon after birth.[104] Infants faced another great danger: infection through the contaminated breast milk of a pox-infected wet-nurse, a phenomenon Knobloch had observed frequently.[105] Again, these particular modes of infection were explained through the close relationship between breast milk/semen and nutritional blood. Very much like saliva or sweat, both were considered by-products of the various concoctions of nutritional blood.[106] Once this was corrupted by the poisonous pox matter, semen and breast milk were as well and would potentially contaminate the foetus in the mother's womb or the infant suckling at the wet-nurse's breast. But what were the physical signs that indicated to Knobloch and Renner that an infant was actually infected with the pox? What were the pox signs?

The Signs of the Pox

Convinced that every human being possessed an innate, unique blend of the four humours fused in the nutritional blood, the authors also considered the contamination of these vital fluids a highly individual issue. From case to case the pox would manifest itself differently, they all agreed, in a vast variety of symptoms and signs. In fact, the sheer number of physical signs that could be associated with the pox provoked von Hutten to the despairing comment that 'you might almost imagine that all diseases are contained in the pox'.[107] And Knobloch boasted that in the course of his long medical practice he had encountered more than three

101 Renner, *Handbüchlein*, fol. IIIIr.

102 According to Aristotelian and Galenic theory both parents produced semen. For medieval and early modern ideas on reproduction and heredity see Joan Cadden, *Meanings of Sex Differences in the Middle Ages: Medicine, Science and Culture* (Cambridge, 1993), chapter IV.

103 Ibid., fol. IIr–v. The idea that the pox would be passed on from parents to children is mentioned by several authors.

104 Knobloch, *De Lue Venerea*, pp. 17–18.

105 Ibid., p. 17.

106 Siraisi, *Renaissance Medicine*, pp. 78–80; Thomas Laqueur, *Making Sex: Body and Gender from the Greeks to Freud* (Cambridge, MA, 1992), pp. 35–45.

107 Böcking, *Hutten*, p. 405; also Renner, *Handbüchlein*, fol. VIr–VIIr.

hundred different 'species' of French Disease.[108] Solely because it would take too long, he explained, and, moreover, a too detailed description of all the possible signs would sow unnecessary confusions in the minds of his readers, 'we will leave many unreported and only remark on a few'.

In line with the tenets of humoral pathology, Knobloch then went on to distinguish four kinds of French Disease: the melancholic, phlegmatic, choleric and sanguine pox. With sufficient experience, Knobloch stated, it was possible to decipher by the form, colour, size, smell and consistency of the individual physical sign from which of these four kinds an individual might be suffering. From his personal experience the choleric species of the French Disease, for example, could be easily identified by their hard and reddish boils, covered by a yellow lid.[109] An additional hint was that this pox type tended not to suppurate but manifested itself all over the body in 'guzzling lichen'. The melancholic type of the pox, on the contrary, only rarely spread all over the body. It developed more slowly than the sanguine type, Knobloch professed, and manifested itself in 'big blue or greyish cones'. Both types, however, were 'extremely stubborn' and difficult to treat for the practitioner because they shared the vexing tendency to temporarily disappear from the surface of the skin only to reappear after some time somewhere else on the body. Like Knobloch, the other authors confined themselves to describing four general types of pox, however, without necessarily assigning the same symptoms and signs to each type.[110] Moreover, they were well aware 'that such poison does not confine itself to one body fluid but may also from time to time attack two, three or all four'.[111] But nobody wished to deal with these complicated cases in detail, again, to avoid bewilderment in their readers. The Magdeburg physician Magnus Hundt just recommended that in case it was suspected that more than one humour was contaminated, the sufferer must, under all circumstances, call upon the trained eye and experienced judgement of a medical practitioner because the diagnosis would be extremely difficult and long-winded.[112]

Apart from visible changes on the surface of the skin, all authors associated great pain with the pox. According to humoral theory, pain resulted either from a rapid change to the body's material structure, such as injuries through stabbing or hitting, for example.[113] Or, and this was the reason for extreme pains in the course of the pox, it could emerge from a transformation of the body's qualitative

108 For this quotation and the following see Knobloch, *De Lue Venerea*, p. 32.

109 For the following see ibid., p. 33.

110 See for example Renner, *Handbüchlein*, fol. VIr–VIIr; and Alexander Seitz in Ukena, *Alexander Seitz*, pp. 11–12.

111 Knobloch, *De Lue Venerea*, p. 34.

112 Hundt, *Nutzbarlichs Regiment*, p. 20r. Alexander Seitz is the only one who tried to describe the signs deriving from such 'mixed' pox matter to the Abbess Elisabeth but not without pointing out the great difficulties of doing so. See Ukena, *Alexander Seitz*, p. 12.

113 For this see Fries, *Spiegel der Artzney*, fol. XXXIXa.

composition, a 'rapid change in the complexion', as Fries explained.[114] That pox victims complained about particularly agonising pain, he continued, was due to the disease's unusually aggressive and poisonous matter, an exceptionally 'acid moisture, which penetrates all limbs'. Pain associated with the French pox was distinguished by two characteristics. First, the victims were under the impression that pain incessantly moved all over the body. Alexander Seitz related this phenomenon to the idea to be found in Galen's writings according to which pain was some kind of material substance. '[P]ain that travels back and forth', he explained to the Abbess Elisabeth Schott, 'is nothing more than a vapour or wind, according to Galen'.[115] This pain vapour was rooted in the poisonous disease-matter itself. Sometimes the matter would expel the vapour and would then 'chase' it throughout the body's veins. At the onset of the pox, this mobile pain vapour or wind could still be effectively treated and perhaps even driven out of the body by 'rubbing with warm cloths or cupping glasses', Seitz suggested to the abbess. But if such measures failed, it had to be feared that, sooner or later, the poisonous pain vapour would get stuck somewhere in the very small veins and, under the pressure of being trapped, would transform itself into a 'substance very much like the one from which it originated'. This 'vapour-turned-disease matter' could cause great destruction to the materiality of the inner organs of the body and was, according to Seitz, the true cause of the 'inner pox' that he had witnessed many times during his anatomy lessons at the university of Padua.[116] Knobloch was equally adamant that all pain must be countered at the very onset of the disease, otherwise the affected limbs and body parts would become accustomed to it, cease to fight it effectively and finally succumb to its malign influence, becoming 'crippled … and ruined completely'.[117]

How was the crippling of limbs through pain explained? Franz Renner was particularly interested in this question because he had observed this phenomenon many times in his medical practice. Indeed, he claimed that it was the impossibility of finding anything written on this subject in vernacular German that motivated

114 For the Galenic pain concept see Rosa Maria Moreno Rodriguez and Luis García-Ballester, 'El dolor en la teoria y la practica medicas de Galeno', *Dynamis* 2 (1982), pp. 3–24; Rudolph S. Siegel, *Galen on Sense of Perception: His Doctrines, Observations and Experiments on Vision, Hearing, Smell, Taste, Touch and Pain, and their Historical Sources* (Basel, 1970), pp. 174–93. For the cultural specificity of pain and its perception see Ester Cohen, 'Towards a History of European Physical Sensibility: Pain in the Later Middle Ages', *Science in Context* 8 (1995), pp. 47–74; also Roselyne Rey, *The History of Pain*, 2nd edn (Cambridge, MA, 1998); Elaine Scarry, *The Body in Pain: The Making and the Unmaking of the World* (New York, 1985); and Jakob Tanner, 'Körpererfahrung, Schmerz und die Konstruktion des Kulturellen', *Historische Anthropologie* 2 (1994), pp. 489–502.

115 For this quotation and the following see Ukena, *Alexander Seitz*, p. 13.

116 Ibid., p. 12. For his studies in Italy see ibid., p. 8.

117 Knobloch, *De Lue Venerea*, p. 136.

his treatise.[118] According to Renner, pain-vapour, stemming from the acid and poisonous pox matter, extracted all the natural moisture from the ligaments, tendons, veins or nerves, resulting in the loss of their innate natural suppleness and elasticity. These would then simply 'shrivel and become too short', resulting in restricted mobility and sometimes even complete paralysis of the pox sufferer.

The Nuremberg barber-surgeon also offered a detailed, but standard explication for the second characteristic peculiar to the pains of the pox – the increase of intensity during the night.[119] While the pores of the skin were wide open during the day, so that 'impure humours' could easily exit, at night the pores 'close and are blocked so that such humours cannot escape or find a way out'. Consequently, the pain-vapours produced by the evil acid pox matter became trapped in the body and started to run wild, trying to find an escape. This resulted in almost unbearable feelings of pain for the sufferer, Renner concluded. Tobias Knobloch could not agree more with this explanation: 'In the night's cooler temperatures the pores close, so that nature cannot expel these poisonous vapours, which are then stronger.'[120] Furthermore, argued Knobloch, the intensity of the pain was also affected by the weather. If it was cold and damp the pains increased, he warned his readers, 'for the pains are then caused not only by the closing of the pores, but the corrupt internal moisture is increased by the outside damp, giving rise to even greater agonies'.[121]

The list of symptoms related to the pox provided by the authors reveal a particular understanding of physical signs. Sensible signs always indicated a change in the body, but the authors seem not to have linked any sign automatically to a particular disease. Signs such as pain were granted some kind of independent status, as the French historian of medicine Rosalyne Rey explained. Pain in early modern medicine, she argued, was viewed neither as an alarm signal nor as a sentinel; for an early modern medical practitioner, it was neither a state that announced an illness to come nor even a prodrome: it could also be a disorder itself.[122]

The disappearance of pain was therefore not inevitably a sign of recovery from the pox. Lorenz Fries even warned his readers explicitly against such a treacherous association. He had often observed doctors treating the 'ulcers of the French pox' with salves to alleviate the pain and deluding themselves thinking that, once they had stopped the pains 'the bell was cast'.[123] Such a conclusion was not only gravely inaccurate; it was potentially fatal, Fries warned. Only when a disease's natural causes hidden in the invisible inner body had been identified and successfully

118 See Renner, *Handbüchlein*, fol. CLXXXIIIv. For the following quotations see ibid., fol. CLVIIv.

119 For the following see ibid., fol. Vr–v.

120 Knobloch, *De Lue Venerea*, p. 136.

121 Ibid., p. 137.

122 Rey, *Pain*, p. 27. See also Duden, *Beneath the Skin*, p. 177.

123 For the following see Fries, *Spiegel der Artzney*, fol. XXXIIIv.

eradicated through the application of appropriate medication, could one hope for an improvement in the sufferer's condition. After all, Fries told his readers, the alleviation of pain could just as easily be a sign that the body had become accustomed to the pox-matter, and had given up fighting against it. Though the patient might no longer feel pain, the pox, the great trickster, was still present and could spread even more freely and secretly. In such cases, warned Fries, the consequences could be grave and the worst had to be expected. From his own experience Ulrich von Hutten was only too ready to concur with Fries' gloomy prognosis. Until he had been treated with guaiacum wood, the knight reported, he had been given many different medicines to relieve and stop the pains. However, none of them succeeded to 'root out the cause of the pain', which had returned every single time.[124]

Many of the authors devoted considerable attention to detailed descriptions of the various symptoms and signs of the pox. However, it is worth remembering that within the realm of early modern medical semiotics the materiality of a physical sign had no meaning in itself. It solely possessed an indicating character; it was a mere pointer to something else, hidden from view, buried within the depth of the body. To make a sign 'speak', to identify its meaning and define its relationship to the pox, it was necessary to introduce another important element into the diagnostic act: the sufferer's disease narrative.

The Art of Interpreting Signs

The decipherment of physical signs was a task undertaken by the pox sufferer in conjunction with a medical practitioner of his or her choice. The practitioner would inquire – if not already well acquainted with the person – about the latter's daily habits and past and present disease histories.[125] Close family members or friends could be consulted in order to reconstruct as complete a picture as possible. What the practitioners were looking for was any suggestion of irregularity in the sufferer's lifestyle, or possible deviations from his/her daily routines, as this could provide an explanation for ill-health.

The pox authors were well aware that their writings could not substitute for actual clinical encounters. This is why they constantly emphasised that the reader should always (with the help of a medical practitioner) adapt their advice to his or her own individual temperament, disease history, and lifestyle. Important factors for consideration were, in the words of the anonymous author of the treatise *A Tried and Tested Prescription*, 'the physical shape, youth or age, weakness or strength of the person, and whether the ravages and crippling effects of the disease were old

124 Böcking, *Hutten*, p. 413.

125 For the equality of medical practitioners and patients during the act of diagnosis and the possibility that several 'disease narratives' could be constructed simultaneously see Wear, *Knowledge and Practice*, pp. 133–6.

or new, great or small'.[126] Alas, the kind of information that was exchanged in the healer–patient encounter cannot be gleaned from the authors' writings. Fries, in his *Mirror of Medicine*, does, however, point to areas where the conversation might have gone. Indeed, he provides his readers with a long list of daily habits that he recommends them to mention during the consultation with medical practitioners in order to provide the basis for the best possible diagnosis. His list was loosely based on the so-called ancient six non-naturals, those influences the human body was incessantly exposed to, such as air, evacuation and retention, food and drink, motion and rest, sleeping and waking, and the passions.[127] Any alteration of the daily habits in relation to these six non-naturals could trigger substantial change in a person's natural complexion, and might thus be responsible for causing the pox. Therefore the patient, should mention,

> whether the diseases had appeared first on the fields or in the house, whether you felt cold or too hot, whether you were dressed or naked, how you dealt with drink and food – whether you have eaten at favourable times or not, or whether you had fasten too long or eaten too much, whether you have prepared the food wrongly or eaten an inappropriate foodstuff, or whether it was prepared inappropriately – whether you have been waking a lot or slept. Also whether you were lazy or worked, or whether you are used to be lazy and whether you worked the moment you fell ill. Whether you have been angry, melancholic, frightened.[128]

Remarkable in Fries's list is the attention it accords to the tiniest details in the patient's habits and disease history. It is interesting that phenomena like emotions, which to our modern medical understanding belong in the sphere of the psyche, are clearly, for Fries, concrete physical manifestations that directly affected and changed the composition of the elemental fluids. Indeed, in all the writings analysed here emotions like anger, shock or fear are considered as immediate and actual physical causes of disease. Anger was deemed dangerous because it could lead to a sudden overheating of all four humours, potentially resulting in inflammations and violent fever. Shock, fear and sadness threatened to provoke the opposite bodily reaction: the sick lost colour, pulse slowed and became weaker; the body cooled and the fluids dried up. Barbara Duden has shown that until well into the eighteenth century women and men perceived the functioning of their bodies not as separate and distinguishable from their social environment as we are used to understanding them today, but rather at the very centre of, and intrinsically interconnected with, all forms of social interaction.[129] A heated argument with

126 Anonymous, *Ain bevert recept*, fol. AVv.

127 L. J. Rather, 'The Six Things "Non-natural": A Note on the Origins and Fate of a Doctrine and Phrase', in *Clio Medica* 3 (1968), pp. 337–47.

128 Fries, *Spiegel der Artzney*, fol. IVr.

129 Duden, *Beneath the Skin*, p. 16; see also Pomata, *Contracting a Cure*, pp. 132–5.

a neighbour, a violent shock or feelings of sadness or melancholy were just as likely to be thought conducive to the pox as visiting the municipal baths or eating contaminated food.

To avoid catching the French pox in the first place, or to prevent an already existing condition from deteriorating, all the authors thus advised their readers to avoid abrupt emotional swings. During treatment, the anonymous author of *A Tried and Tested Prescription* advised, to lift the sufferer's spirits 'if possible by singing, playing the lute, and other things that give him pleasure'.[130] 'Fantasy or gloom' should be avoided under all circumstances. Any anxieties that arose could be dispelled by cheerful conversation, though it was vital to ensure that the sick person 'does not become irritated' by the chosen topic. Walter Ryff had similar advice: 'Furthermore, he [the sick] should drive out all worry, sorrow, suffering or bad temper, and ward off all afflictions of the spirit through which the body may fall sick.'[131] The sick person was to stay sunny and cheerful and be pleasantly entertained by his friends and relations. Magnus Hundt warned that particular care should be taken with pox sufferers of a melancholy complexion, 'as nothing is more harmful than a sad and suffering disposition, for it dries a man out to his bones and saps all his strength'.[132] For such individuals, the pleasures of light conversation, singing, lute-playing and being read to should be supplemented by visual delights such as framed pictures on the walls, 'so that their spirits be enlivened and their senses strengthened by the sight of green fields and woodland, and by pretty, cheerful paintings and portraits'.

While the authors attached great importance to the emotions, the difference between the sexes is scarcely touched upon. Alexander Seitz discussed it only in passing, despite the fact that his treatise was supposedly intended for a female readership, the Abbess Elizabeth Schott and 'all the sisters in her convent'.[133] It would be too simple to explain this neglect of the female body by observing that these works were all written by male authors, and were mainly directed at a male readership who were unlikely to pay much attention to the diagnosis and treatment of women. Misogynistic tendencies of individual authors cannot be excluded, of course, even if there is no definite textual evidence for them in their pox treatises. But as grounds for ignoring the female body in these writings, they are of only secondary importance, if indeed important at all. Rather, the main reason for this seeming exclusion is that, in sixteenth-century medicine, the physiological differences between the sexes had only minimal impact on the diagnosis and treatment of diseases like the pox. The most significant difference between women

130 For the following quotations see *Ain bevert recept*, fol. AIIIIr. For the important role of music in early modern therapeutics see Werner Friedrich Kümmel, *Medizin und Musik* (Munich, 1977); Peregrine Horden (ed.), *Music as Medicine: The History of Music Therapy Since Antiquity* (Aldershot, 2000).

131 Ryff, *New erfundne Artzney*, fol. CIIIr.

132 For the following see Hundt, *Nutzbarlichs Regiment*, p. 12r.

133 Ukena, *Alexander Seitz*, p. 11.

and men, the one that was of primary importance in interpreting physical signs, was the fundamental difference in their humoral complexions: in women, the elements of water and phlegm with their cold and moist qualities were held to be far more dominant than in men.[134] What is more, a woman's body, through monthly bleeding and its production of breast milk (which, as we have seen, was thought to be a by-product of the concoction of nutritional blood) was believed to be able to purge itself regularly of tainted bodily fluids, a process that was not available to men.

Such reasoning was not an 'invention' of the sixteenth century, but a central premise of ancient Aristotelian natural philosophy, which was common ground for all the authors in this study. No doubt they would have concurred with Fries's brief definition in his chapter 'On the Difference Between Men and Women', where the physiological differences between the sexes are briefly summarised thus:

> First, the man is hotter and drier than the woman; the woman is colder and moister than the man. You should therefore understand, if a man is of cold and wet complexion, he is nonetheless hotter and drier than a woman of hot and dry complexion. The man does not have as much surplus fluid as a woman, neither does the man by nature drive out excess fluid as does the woman. The man is purged through the eyes, through the nose, through the mouth, through vomiting, through his stools, through urine, through sweat, through the act of love, through the hair. But the woman has more, that is the time of her flowering [menstruation] and the milk. There are also differences in the constitution of the body and in number and location of certain parts what is more, women are quicker to anger than men are, they are not as brave as men although some can be mightily cross.[135]

The authors believed that the warmth and dryness of the male body made it more susceptible to pox. In this dry environment the disease's cold, moist, morbid matter found more 'nourishment' than in a woman's body, which was qualitatively similar to the disease matter itself. What is more, the poison could spread more freely in the male body. Through menstruation, the monthly 'woman's ailment … in which the woman's fluids find their natural outlet', the tainted nutritional blood was expelled from the female body, as Seitz explained to Abbess Elisabeth

---

134 For a balanced discussion of the differences between the sexes in medieval and early modern thought see Cadden, *Sexual Differences*; also Joan Cadden, 'Und er schuf Mann und Weib: Geschlecht und Wissenschaft im Werk der Hildegard von Bingen', in Barbara Orland and Elvira Scheich (eds), *Geschlecht der Natur. Feministische Beiträge zur Geschichte und Theorie der Naturwissenschaften* (Frankfurt, 1995), pp. 224–39; Laqueur, *Making Sex*. For a critic of Laqueur's one-sex model see the introduction of Katharine Park, *The Secrets of Women: Gender, Generation and the Origins of Human Dissection* (Cambridge, MA, 2006).

135 Fries, *Spiegel der Artzney*, fol. XIIr.

Schott.[136] That was the reason why a woman 'could contract or be infected with the disease from or by an outside party', he continued, but a 'woman only rarely generates the disease within herself'. The Ansbach physician Knobloch could not agree more with this view and added that it could therefore be extremely dangerous for women to miss their monthly period, whether it 'keeps itself hidden through unregulated eating, drinking, anger or old age'.[137] Then, very much like in men, evil and poisoned blood would accumulate, Knobloch and Seitz predicted, promoting in turn the rapid distribution and entrenchment of morbid pox matter within the female body.[138]

The Pox-Body Relationship

The peculiarity of signs, their general interpretive openness, accounted for a particular understanding of the relationship between the pox and the body which differs completely from today's view. For us, the human body ultimately defines the space of origin and distribution of disease, which is generally defined as a recurrent pattern of symptoms and events assembled in a specific chronological and geographical order and thus etiologically, morphologically and symptomatically distinguishable from other diseases. Disease, as we tend to understand it, is an entity that evolves and introduces new events in itself and at its own insistence.

However, for all the authors under consideration, the pox and the body *did not* possess a common, previously defined space; they communicated solely through the non-spatial elements of the sick individual's humours and qualities.[139] The set of physical signs that linked both was believed to be neither constant nor necessary. Neither the medical practitioner nor the sick necessarily viewed bodily signs and the pox as mutually dependent components in a specific disease entity called 'the pox'.[140] From the treatises emerges a picture similar to what Foucault described for the preclinical period: 'the nosological picture involves a figure of the disease that is neither the chain of causes and effects nor the chronological series of events nor its visible trajectory in the human body'.[141]

This is also why the localisation of the pox in a particular organ or body part during, for example, a post-mortem examination was of relatively little importance compared to its diagnosis in a living body.[142] Although some authors identified

---

136 For the following see Ukena, *Alexander Seitz*, p. 11.

137 Knobloch, *De Lue Venerea*, p. 28.

138 Ibid.; Ukena, *Alexander Seitz*, p. 11.

139 Foucault, *Birth of the Clinic*, p. 13.

140 Wolfgang Eich, *Medizinische Semiotik (1750–1850): Ein Beitrag zur Geschichte des Zeichenbegriffs in der Medizin* (Freiburg, 1986).

141 Foucault, *Birth of the Clinic*, p. 4.

142 For early modern anatomy see, for example, Roger French, *The Anatomical Tradition* (London, 1993); Andrea Carlino, *Books of the Body: The Anatomical Ritual and*

certain body parts as one of the possible topographic locations of the pox, they never conceived them as its material cause. The dissecting knife of a sixteenth-century anatomist could expose changes in a corpse's internal organs and interpret them as one of the causes (or a result) of the pox but such exposure did not provide definitive answers to the effect of the pox in a living body. It was impossible for a body from which the spirits and natural heat had departed after death to provide reliable information on the physiological processes going on inside a living human being.[143] There was no way for a medical practitioner to tell for certain what went on in the unfathomable depths of the body. Whatever a dissection might reveal was thus considered inconclusive or even misleading 'because it represents a post-mortem change in the body, not a true reflection of the normal situation'.[144] This is why Seitz, who recalled seeing pox signs inside a dissected corpse during his anatomy lectures at the medical faculty in Padua, drew no further conclusions as to understanding and treating the disease in his daily medical practice.[145] Visually perceived changes in an organ or other part of a dead body was for Seitz only one sign among many that, through further careful investigation, could potentially be interpreted as a symptom of the pox. But on no account was it necessarily relevant to understand the workings of the disease in his living patients, something Seitz had to come to grips with under all circumstances in order to be able to choose the appropriate treatment.

As the body and the French pox did not possess a common space the morbid matter of the pox circulated freely and travelled from one affected body part to another. It could even remain hidden for a time in a chosen location, without revealing itself through visible symptoms. Von Hutten knew this only too well from his many years of painful personal experience. Time and again it had ravaged previously unaffected areas of his skin, and the poison had manifested itself in the greatest variety of symptoms. It had sought out hiding places 'where it can take a long rest'.[146] There it resided, almost unnoticed, as if entrenched in its fortress, until it was ready to 'leave its castle' and reconquer the body.

But the pox was not just a 'homeless' disease in the understanding of von Hutten and his fellow pox authors. It also escaped time. In sixteenth-century

---

Renaissance Learning (Chicago, 1999); Jonathan Sawday, *The Body Emblazoned: Dissection and the Human Body in Renaissance Culture* (London, 1995); Karin Stuckenbrock, *'Der zerstückte Körper': Zur Sozialgeschichte der anatomischen Sektionen in der frühen Neuzeit (1650–1800)* (Stuttgart, 2001); Park, *Secrets of Women.*

143 For the function of spirits and 'calor innatus' see Siraisi, *Renaissance Medicine*, pp. 107–9.

144 Jerome J. Bylebyl, 'The Medical Side of Harvey's Discovery: The Normal and the Abnormal', in ibid., *William Harvey and His Age: The Professional the Social Context of the Discovery of the Circulation* (Baltimore, 1979), p. 32; 89; see also ibid., 'The Manifest and the Hidden in the Renaissance Clinic', in W. F. Bynum and Roy Porter (eds), *Medicine and the Five Senses* (Cambridge, 1993), pp. 40–60.

145 For this quotation and the following see Ukena, *Alexander Seitz*, p. 12.

146 For this quotation and the following see Böcking, *Hutten*, p. 406.

medicine the temporal did not play the role that it plays today.[147] It was admitted that a disease may last, and that its various episodes or phases may appear in turn. Medical practitioners have calculated the critical days of a disease since antiquity, and have known the significant values of arterial pulsation.[148] According to this reasoning, the authors thus separated different phases or states of the pox. Each disease episode was defined by a different degree of quantity of assumed pox matter. In the first phase, only small amounts of morbid matter were present in the body and still lacked, according to the authors, the power to subdue it entirely. In this phase it was believed that it was still relatively easy to expel the corrupt matter through bleeding, evacuation or sweating. If such measures failed to check the spread of the disease during its first phase, the tussle between body and pox could be expected to intensify in the second. This confrontation, often described as a 'struggle' by the authors, culminated in the pox's climax, observable when the growth in physical symptoms suddenly came to a hold. At this stage the so-called 'crisis' was suspected, the turning point either towards improvement or deterioration in a sufferer's condition.[149] The imminence of the crisis announced itself through the appearance of a variety of specific physical changes, such as severe headaches, mental confusion, an irregular pulse, and increased urination. The pox authors agreed on one thing: the deeper and longer the pox 'took root' in the sufferer's body and the more nutritional blood it succeeded in contaminating, the more difficult it became for the body to sustain the struggle. In the upcoming 'crisis', it had to be feared that 'the disease might then defeat nature', with potentially tragic consequences. As Renner predicted, if the disease was victorious and brought the nature of the body to its knees, the patient 'would naturally have little hope of recovery'.[150] In the worst case scenario this meant the death of the patient. If this was averted, however, the fourth and last phase of the disease could bring about his or her gradual recovery.

Since the time span of each phase was dependent on the individual's complexion and lifestyle, none of the authors made any judgement on the pox's likely duration. Their writings make clear, however, that they considered individuals of a wet and cold temperament not only less susceptible to the French pox, but also expected their sufferings to be both less dramatic and of shorter duration. As their humoral mixture resembled the cold-wet composition of the disease itself,

147 Foucault, *Birth of the Clinic*, p. 12: 'Time is integrated as a nosological constant, not as an organic variable. The time of the body does not affect, and still less determines, the time of the disease.'

148 For the problem of measuring time in medicine see Werner Friedrich Kümmel, 'Der Puls und das Problem der Zeitmessung in der Geschichte der Medizin', *Medizinhistorisches Journal* 9 (1974), pp. 1–22. For an interesting sociological account on the concept of time in history see Norbert Elias, *Über die Zeit*, 5th edn (Frankfurt, 1994).

149 For an analysis of the concept of medical crisis in the work of the French physician Jean Fernel (1497–1558) see Müller, *Humoralpathologie*, pp. 108–9.

150 Renner, *Handbüchlein*, fol. Xr.

Seitz explained, the latter could find insufficient nourishment to spread and 'take root'.[151] Conversely, their bodies were less likely to experience it as a 'threat' and felt thus less inclined to fight against it. A dramatic 'struggle' between pox and body was much more likely to occur in individuals of a hot-dry disposition. The cold-wet morbid matter of the pox was especially 'repugnant' and 'hateful' to their natural complexion, he explained, which was also why their bodies struggled so hard to rid themselves of the disease matter. Von Hutten attributed his own wretched nine-year sufferings to the fact that he was of a particularly 'dry and warm complexion'.[152] A further cause, he believed, lay in his intellectual activity for, as a doctor friend reputedly told him, 'those who were raised delicately and were devoted to books are healed of illness more slowly than others'. He was quick to clarify, however, that his treatise was only concerned with his personal experience of the disease, and that more general conclusions about the disease's duration could not therefore be extracted from it.[153]

Von Hutten's caution with regard to the disease's staying power was not exceptional. Tobias Knobloch goes so far as to refuse any debate upon the subject matter, convinced that 'the time cannot be set'.[154] Since every pox victim had a unique individual complexion, no one could foresee on what day the crisis, the climax of the struggle between morbid disease matter and the nature of the body, might occur, nor how intensely it would develop and with what outcome. Magnus Hundt was similarly vague in his prognosis: 'According to the complexion of the body, and the quality and quantity of the poisonous matter, some get rid of the disease soon, some slowly, and many drag themselves to the grave.'[155]

From our modern perspective, perhaps the strangest characteristic of the sixteenth-century pox was its ability to morph into other diseases. As von Hutten explained to his readers, the pox preference was for mutating into diseases with which it was believed to be astrologically related, thus 'at times this disease can develop into heavy podagra or apoplexy. Many sufferers become leprous, for it is believed that the pox and leprosy are friends or neighbours, because the two illnesses have common causes and the pox often ends in leprosy'.[156] In Hundt's view, the French pox, if not promptly treated, could develop into incurable 'flesh-devouring fistulas, cancer and boils'.[157] And Knobloch claimed to have witnessed on several occasions that the pox had mutated, almost from

151 For this and the following quotations see Ukena, *Alexander Seitz*, p. 10.

152 For this and the following quotation see Böcking, *Hutten*, p. 476.

153 Ibid., pp. 475–6.

154 Knobloch, *De Lue Venerea*, p. 123.

155 Hundt, *Nutzbarlichs Regiment*, p. 19v.

156 Böcking, *Hutten*, p. 406.

157 Hundt, *Nutzbarlichs Regiment*, p. 19v. In Hundt's description it becomes obvious that changes which we today identify as symptoms belonging to a disease entity could be considered independent illnesses.

one day to the next, into apoplexy or the dreaded dropsy.[158] Like the humanist von Hutten, the barber-surgeon Renner observed a very close 'kinship' between podagra and the pox. Moreover, he observed that through incorrect treatment more 'harmful illnesses such as asthma, phtisis, paralysis, palsy and trembling of the limbs' could result.[159]

The idea of the metamorphosis of diseases is rooted in the early modern conception of a physical sign and how its relationship to disease was understood. As mentioned earlier, no physical sign was automatically and exclusively assigned to the pox. The diagnostic gaze went beyond the immediately sensible and was directed upon what was going on in the invisible depth of the sick person's body. Via the sensible sign, the medical practitioner aimed at grasping the extent to which the quality and quantity of an ailing individual's bodily fluids differed from his or her natural complexion. Moreover, he had to define the hidden nature and essence of the disease. It was this underlying metaphysical concept of disease that accounted for a certain constancy and permanence of it, even if the physical signs associated with it differed from case to case. The absence of any standardised measurement and the fact that invisible realms had to be included into the interpretation of sensible signs, meant that the transition from one disease to another was fluid, the border line between them flexible.[160] The metamorphosis of disease, the flexibility and fluidity of its definition in early modern medicine was inevitable, due to a completely different organisation of medical knowledge, in which the relationship between the visible and invisible was perceived fundamentally different from today. We shall see in subsequent chapters, that the metamorphosis of diseases was not just a theoretical concept. In the Augsburg pox hospitals physical signs could be perceived on one day as indicative of the French pox, and on the next, of leprosy. Moreover, in some cases, the patient was believed to suffer from the pox *and* leprosy simultaneously.

The meaning of a physical sign was always temporary. The decisive moment, which turned a physical sign into a sign of the French pox, was the clinical encounter between the medical practitioner and the sick person. During the act of diagnosis both parties constructed the individual's disease narrative, which ultimately linked his or her physical signs to the French pox (or any other disease). This disease narrative, however, was never fixed, but could be altered at any moment in time.

Treating the Pox

The concept of 'essence' or 'nature' (in Greek, 'physis'), which has already surfaced several times in this study, was one of the cornerstones of the disease narrative. But what was the body's or the disease's nature, the understanding of which was

158 Knobloch, *De Lue Venerea*, p. 82.

159 Renner, *Handbüchlein*, fol. X.

160 Nance, *Medical Portraiture*, p. 98.

considered vital before any treatment could begin? 'Nature', Fries explained, 'is nothing less than an implanted force in all the things, which dwell under the moon. This force drives a thing to do the things in the way it does them or inspires it to strive for it'.[161] Again Fries' source for his short definition was the 'prince' of all philosophers, Aristotle. Each natural object in the terrestrial sphere of the Aristotelian earth-centred and two-folded cosmos was endowed with an individual inner force. This nature or essence was unique to that object and strove incessantly to provide or to reinforce its specific character, the particular behaviour of the thing. In sixteenth-century Christian Western society this force was believed to have been implanted by God in the act of divine creation.[162]

The task of the human body's nature was to preserve the individual balance of the humours and qualities and to avert potential disruptions. If the humours were already in a state of imbalance, nature's duty was to re-establish the complexion's 'natural condition'. In such cases, the nature of the body 'struggled' – as all the pox authors maintained – with the nature of the disease. The latter strove to subdue the patient's nature so that its poisonous substance could 'take root' all over the body. But the nature of the body was by no means defenceless against these incursions. It possessed natural defence mechanisms: the expulsion and excretion of corrupt and diseased matter through the body's various orifices: the mouth, nose, eyes, ears, nipples, armpits, anus, genitals and pores.[163]

However, in order not to lose this battle against the disease, the nature of the body had to be aided. And that is where the medical practitioner stepped in, guided by 'ratio and experientia', as Seitz explained.[164]As nature's servant and support, his barber-surgeon colleague Renner maintained, it was incumbent on the practitioner to sustain the sufferer's nature and direct it to the appropriate course.[165] To do so, it was especially advantageous (the pox authors explained) if the practitioner had treated the sufferer for some years, since he was then better acquainted with the characteristics of the sufferer's individual nature. On no account should a medical practitioner disregard, or worse, try to subdue the individual characteristics of the

161 Fries, *Spiegel der Artzney*, p. IIIr.

162 In a collective sense the term 'physis' or 'nature' denotes the ensemble of all natural objects, which possessed such a nature. See David C. Lindberg, *The Beginnings of Western Science: The European Scientific Tradition in Philosophical, Religious, and Institutional Context, 600 B.C. to A.D. 1450* (Chicago, 1992), p. 281. For the notion of 'nature' in medicine see the still useful article by Max Neuburger, 'An Historical Study of the Concept of Nature from a Medical Standpoint', *Isis* 35 (1944), pp. 16–28; for a more general account see Leonard Barkan, *Nature's Work of Art: The Human Body as Image of the World* (New Haven, 1975); and Lorraine Daston, 'The Nature of Nature in Early Modern Europe', *Configurations* 6 (1998), pp. 149–72.

163 For the various places of expulsion see Ukena, *Alexander Seitz*, p. 19.

164 Ibid.; for an explanation of these two terms see Maclean, *Logic, Signs, and Nature*, pp. 191–200.

165 Renner, *Handbüchlein*, fol. Xr.

patient's nature, or bend them to his will, warned Seitz.[166] Instead, mindful of his own strengths and weaknesses, the practitioner was to incorporate them in his deliberations before drawing up an appropriate course of treatment.

For their part, pox sufferers were to seek the services of a medical practitioner as soon as possible. As Knobloch warned, 'the deeper this plague takes roots, the more violently it roars and rages in the human body, for this plague is like a wolf who comes upon a stall full of sheep and does not depart unless driven from thence or until all the sheep have been strangled'.[167] Renner similarly exhorted his readers not to prevaricate so long that 'the illness has the upper hand and no further help can be expected'.[168] He warned that they would then 'be themselves guilty of the harm to their own bodies and rush headlong into their own degradation since they did not in good time undertake what was appropriate'.

Renner believed he had discovered why so many pox victims were wary of visiting medical practitioners. His daily encounters with pox victims taught him that some were 'ashamed of their affliction and cannot suffer that others should point it out to them'.[169] To prevent their neighbours and friends becoming aware of their condition, they often 'despised and made light of all decent remedies' that a practitioner might otherwise have prescribed for them in time. Seitz had another explanation for this 'doctor phobia': it was less the social consequences that the individual feared, he explained, than the financial expense that a visit to the doctor entailed. Most people, he complained to Abbess Elizabeth, were more worried about their livestock than their own health, 'for often one of them has a sick cow in a stable, and would rather spend money on curing it than on his own illness so much he blindly hates his own life and health'.[170]

There were various options open to the medical practitioner for supporting the sufferer's nature and assisting the body to discharge the disease's morbid matter. Firstly, he could reduce the proportion of contaminated nutritional blood through cupping, bloodletting or purging.[171] The great disadvantage of the first two methods was that they removed not only contaminated but also healthy blood, thus weakening the patient's nature and possibly hampering it in its struggle against the pox. The pox authors disagreed deeply as to whether, when and how often a pox sufferer should be bled.[172] Though most of them did not regard bloodletting as harmful, an exception was Seitz, who rejected it out of hand. Since it temporarily

166 For the following see Ukena, *Alexander Seitz*, p. 20.

167 Knobloch, *De Lue Venerea*, p. 40.

168 For this and the following quotation see Renner, *Handbüchlein*, p. Xr.

169 Ibid., fol. XIv.

170 Ukena, *Alexander Seitz*, p. 21.

171 For a description of the various bloodletting techniques see Robert Jütte, *Ärzte, Heiler and Patienten. Medizinischer Alltag in der frühen Neuzeit* (Munich and Zurich, 1991), pp. 71–3.

172 Similar discussion about the pros and cons of bloodletting can be found in plague tracts.

emptied the veins, Seitz argued, the vacuum thus created would provoke the liver into redoubled efforts to refill the empty veins with freshly produced nutritional blood. If the latter was contaminated by the poisonous pox matter, bloodletting ensured its faster distribution. For this reason, Seitz warned, bloodletting should be authorised only in exceptional cases.

While cupping and bleeding indiscriminately removed whatever was in the veins, purging – the selective excretion of harmful substances, usually through vomiting and evacuation of the bowels – was directly targeted against the specific diseased matter. Evacuation through purgatives, in the form of syrups, drinks, pills or enemas, could occur spontaneously or be artificially induced.[173] It was the authors' unanimous opinion that purgation should only be carried out under the supervision of a qualified medical practitioner, since the complexion and lifestyle of the pox victims must be taken into consideration when choosing the appropriate remedy and dosage. Admittedly, even the most conscientious execution of a purge could not prevent substances essential for the patient's health being evacuated at the same time – an unfortunate circumstance of which Renner gave fair warning in rhyme: 'When a healer purges to just the bad expel, he loses the healthy bits as well.'[174]

Bleeding, cupping and purging were not considered sufficient in themselves to expel the morbid matter once and for all, but they were an essential preparatory stage in advance of actual treatment. Reducing morbid matter in this way could effect temporary relief or even disappearance of symptoms. That did not mean, however, that the pox had been 'defeated'. Tobias Knobloch warned against such possible misconceptions: '[t]his plague is so constituted that it can remain in a person's body for 10, 15, even 20 or 30 years and only then cause all kinds of unpleasantness. Such poison is like a freshly cut-down tree for when such a tree has been cut-down and still fresh in the trunk and roots it commonly several years after if not from the trunk then from the roots sprouts anew little branches or shoots'.[175] To 'expel' the diseased matter from the body once and for all, its natural causes had to be removed. In other words, the qualitative imbalance in the nutritional blood had to be corrected and its unique harmonious balance restored through carefully targeted remedies. The first priority in choosing any vegetable, animal or mineral remedy was that its qualities should be directly opposed to that of the disease (the Galenic contraria principle).[176] The effect of the medication could be immediate or potential, slumbering as it were until the warmth of the body awakened its healing properties or 'occult qualities'.[177] As the majority of

173 For a long list of cheap and expensive purgatives see Renner, *Handbüchlein*, chapter 11.

174 Renner, *Handbüchlein*, fol. IIIr.

175 Knobloch, *De Lue Venerea*, pp. 39–40.

176 For this principle in Galenic medicine see Müller, *Humoralmedizin*, pp. 130–33.

177 For occult qualities see Keith Hutchison, 'What Happened to the Occult Qualities in the Scientific Revolution?', *Isis* 73 (1982), pp. 233–53; Nutton, 'Seeds', pp. 198–9;

our authors were agreed that the predominant qualities of the pox was cold-wet, sharp and acid or bitter, they recommended remedies that were believed to possess warming, drying and mollifying powers.

In the sixteenth century, two remedies promised the greatest chance of success: mercury, which had long been in use as a medication, and guaiacum wood, a new remedy imported from the Americas. The uses of mercury in treating ailments where the poisonous matter revealed itself on the skin had a long tradition stretching back to ancient times, though it has to be said that the ancient medical authorities had markedly different opinions on the subject.[178] For the most part mercury was used externally, either as an ointment cure or as a watery mercuric chloride solution.[179] Mercury could also be made into pills, which were administered to the sufferer orally. As we shall see in the Augsburg hospitals in more detail, fumigation was also popular, in which the sufferer spent a considerable amount of time inhaling the vapours of a mixture of mercury and various dried plants and spices heated over a fire.[180]

The well-known deleterious effects of a mercury cure – copious salivation, diarrhoea, excessive sweating, loss of teeth and all body hair – were explicitly desired by sixteenth-century medical practitioners and patients alike. It was believed that such effects were the excretion of the morbid matter of the pox and had to be endured. But since the ancient medical authorities had already warned against the dangers of too much mercury, rigorous attempts were made by sixteenth-century practitioners to keep its effects under control. 'The great goal was to extract its healing properties by force or cunning, while averting the effects of its poison.'[181] The form of mercury cure each author preferred – ointment, vapour or pills – depended on their own experiences with it. Renner considered

---

Maclean, *Logic, Signs, and Nature*, p. 242.

178 For an overview of the ancient discussion see Erna Lesky, 'Quecksilber und Quecksilberverbindungen im Wandel der Zeit', *Ciba-Zeitschrift* 8 (1959), pp. 3202–8; J. Rabisch-Bey, 'Zur Geschichte der Quecksilbertherapie', *Wiener medizinische Wochenschau* 47 (1898), pp. 487; 552; 599; Temkin, 'Mercurial Trends', p. 518; William Abramowitz, 'Historical Points of the Interest in the Mode of Action and Ill Effects of Mercury', *Bulletin of the New York Academy of Medicine* 56 (1978), pp. 695–705.

179 Karl Johann Proksch, *Die Quecksilbersublimatcuren gegen Syphilis: Eine literaturhistorische Studie* (Wien, 1876); Lesky, 'Schmier- und Rauchkuren', p. 3174.

180 Heinrich Paschkis, 'Über Quecksilberräucherungen, *Vierteljahrzeitschrift für Dermatologie und Syphilis*? (1878), pp. 415–32.

181 Lesky, 'Schmier- und Räucherkuren', p. 3175. One way to control the effects of the metal was to keep its dosage low. Moreover, the mercury could be '*gelöscht*' (extincto) or 'killed' (mortificatio). In these cases it was mixed with all kinds of other organic and non-organic substances such as fat and oil, pitch, vinegar or mustard but also lead, sulphur or arsenic. It was believed that this preparation would not only lower mercury's poisonous effect but also help to expel it easier from the body. For a contemporary description of which substances were mixed with mercury see von Hutten's description in Böcking, *Hutten*, p. 432.

salves and fumigation to be the most effective therapies, since 'where it is taken in, it drives such impure humours of the French Disease from the entire body'.[182] He personally rejected the use of mercury pills, since in his experience they could bring about dire, uncontrollable consequences for the patient:

> I have witnessed several times how the horrible cure consumes the stomach, tears apart the intestines, harms the brain and the white veins. Cholica, also apoplexia, epilepsia, apoplecia can follow. One can see how the mouth, the teeth and gums rot so that the teeth can be pulled out with the fingers. It also harms the tongue and turns the whole throat black and so stinking that absolutely nobody can bear to live with those people.[183]

Renner was not the only one who was concerned about the possible life-threatening consequences of a mercury cure. All the authors warned their readers to undergo such treatment only under the supervision of an experienced medical practitioner, who would be able to tell at what point the treatment should be immediately interrupted, so as not to gamble recklessly with the patient's life. Knobloch explained to his readers what physical signs would indicate that stage in a mercury cure:

> When a patient starts to sweat copiously or experiences strong diarrhoea it is time to stop anointing him because if one continues to do it, the patient's tongue will swell enormously, his throat will be become riddled with holes, he will lose one tooth after the other as well as all his hair. If the cure is not directed well he might even lose his life.[184]

Guaiacum was mercury's competition from the beginning of the sixteenth century, although the initial enthusiasm for it faded over the decades.[185] Finely grated, it was made into a decoction which was used in combination with a sweating cure. Heating the body, it was believed, would expel the morbid pox matter to the extent that it was 'completely consumed'.[186] After much debate there

182 Renner, *Artzneybüchlein*, p. 51.

183 Ibid.

184 Knobloch, *De Lue Venerea*, p. 134.

185 In the course of the sixteenth century other exotic drugs became 'fashionable' for treating the pox, such as Peruvian bark. See Vöttinger-Pletz, *Lignum Sanctum*, p. 57. For a sixteenth-century description of these drugs and their preparation see Wittich, *Ligno Guayacum*, fol. B2r–v; Knobloch, *De Lue Venerea*, pp. 117–19. For the new imported drugs from the Americas see also Carl Hartwich, *Die Bedeutung der Entdeckung Amerikas für die Drogenkunde* (Berlin, 1892); Antonello Gerbi, *Nature and the New World* (Pittsburg, 1985); Anthony Grafton, Nancy Siraisi and April Shelford, *New Worlds, Ancient Texts: The Power of Tradition and the Shock of the New* (Cambridge, MA, 1992), pp. 160–93); Raquel Alvarez-Pélaez, *La Conquista de la Naturaleza Americana* (Madrid, 1993).

186 Ukena, *Alexander Seitz*, p. 16.

was broad agreement about the wood's primary and secondary qualities, and its particular effectiveness in treating the pox.[187] Walter Ryff summarised opinion as follows: 'the Indian wood has a hot and dry nature in the second degree. It is therefore no miracle that those diseases and their victims are cured and healed [by it] which are of cold and moist nature'.[188]

Though our pox authors prized guaiacum as a cure for the pox on account of its supposed harmlessness to the patient, not one specifically rejected the use of mercury. Even von Hutten, stylised in most of secondary literature as an enthusiastic apologist for guaiacum and an implacable enemy of mercury, did not deny that mercury could be beneficial, despite his own painful experiences with it. Hutten thought mercury suitable for 'dissolving' the morbid matter in the body first to make it easier for nature to expel it later. Mercury treatment was only dangerous, he claimed, if it was applied by 'unlearned folk' and 'quacks' who, 'knowing nothing about medicine', neglected to adapt dosage and composition of the salve to the patient's individual complexion and the specific nature of the disease.[189] These 'ignorant anointers' had been known to use one ointment for all their patients, sometimes with often dramatic results. 'I have seen many die of such ointment cures', he told his readers, not sparing them the details:

> [t]hree or four times or more they smeared the limbs, arms and equally the legs. Some also smeared the spine and the crown; some also the temples and the navel, and some also the whole body. Some applied the salve once a day, some twice, the others three or four times. The patient was shut in a warm room that was continuously heated, and was laid on a bed in the room sometimes for twenty, sometimes for thirty whole days. He was swathed in blankets to compel him to sweat profusely. After receiving the salve the patient began to languish most wondrously. The salve was so powerful that it moved the disease from its location in the stomach to the brain and to the throat, and the mouth, from which the disease poured so greatly that the teeth fell out and one had to worry about the mouth in general. The throat and tongue began to fester … incessantly stinking saliva was pouring out of the mouth which polluted everything … The entire house was so full of stench that those waiting to be cured wished to die than to be cured in that way. Of one hundred sufferers hardly anybody recovered and many fell sick again, because such cure often does not last long.

187 How this agreement was reached is unknown. For one of the few studies that deals with the important question of how new imported drugs were 'tested' for their healing properties see Antonio Barrera-Osorio, 'Local Herbs, Global Medicine: Commerce, Knowledge, and Commodities in Spanish America', in Pamela Smith and Paula Findlen (eds), *Merchants & Marvels: Commerce, Science, and Art in Early Modern Europe* (New York and London, 2002), pp. 163–81.

188 Ryff, *New erfundne Artzney*, fol. DVv. See also Vöttinger-Pletz, *Lignum Sanctum*, pp. 56–9.

189 For this and the following quotations see Böcking, *Hutten*, p. 407.

Von Hutten preferred guaiacum because, after eleven painful and, in his case, ineffective treatments with mercury, it appeared to him far more effective (see Figure 1.1). In gratitude for his recovery and out of Christian brotherly love, he fervently recommended this heaven-sent miracle cure to other sufferers, while being careful to stress that his personal experiences were not necessarily applicable to all:

> So who follows me in this does so voluntary and is not forced to, because we do not speak of these things as a scholar, but warn and advise as someone who has experience, and therefore I wish to advise that whatever others consider from me I do not reveal wantonly, but what I learned and experienced with the disease I disclose, and what I had experienced differently I would not suppress.[190]

Among the other pox authors, only those behind the early anonymous pamphlets, *A Tried and Tested Prescription* (1518) and *A Clear Account* (1525), endorse von Hutten's unequivocal espousal of the New World miracle cure. Like Hutten's tract, these works were published at a stage when tales of the wood's alleged miraculous effects were just beginning to spread in Germany. Such undiluted enthusiasm is not evident in later publications. Magnus Hundt, who preferred mercury, observed maliciously in 1529 that the wood of a domestic apple or pear tree might be just as beneficial in treating the pox as the often praised wood of the foreign guaiacum tree.[191]

Hundt is the only one of our authors who calls the wood's effectiveness into question. Ryff, Renner, Wittich and Knobloch did not doubt its usefulness, though, unlike von Hutten and the two anonymous authors, they did not recommend exclusive reliance on it. They advised their readers to commence with a guaiacum-based pox cure. For sufferers of every complexion it was certainly less harmful and easier to administer than mercury, and especially where the disease was still 'fresh' and not yet 'firmly rooted' in the body, the treatment had already, in the unanimous view of these authors, been crowned many times with success. However, if the disease had raged in its victim's body for some time and was 'firmly rooted', it would be necessary to treat the morbid matter with mercury first, before one could expel it with guaiacum.

But when, according to our authors, could their readers regard themselves as 'cured'? Just as they were loath or unable to commit themselves on the question of the disease's duration, they were coy in expressing their views on this subject. Knobloch gave his readers one or two references. In his opinion, the pox in its early stages could sometimes be cured after twenty to thirty days using guaiacum, or in more stubborn cases of the disease, a mercury treatment.[192] Older, deep-rooted pox, however, often took far more than one hundred days.

190 Böcking, *Hutten*, pp. 408–9.

191 Hundt, *Nutzbarlichs Regiment*, fol. 20r.

192 Ibid., p. 23.

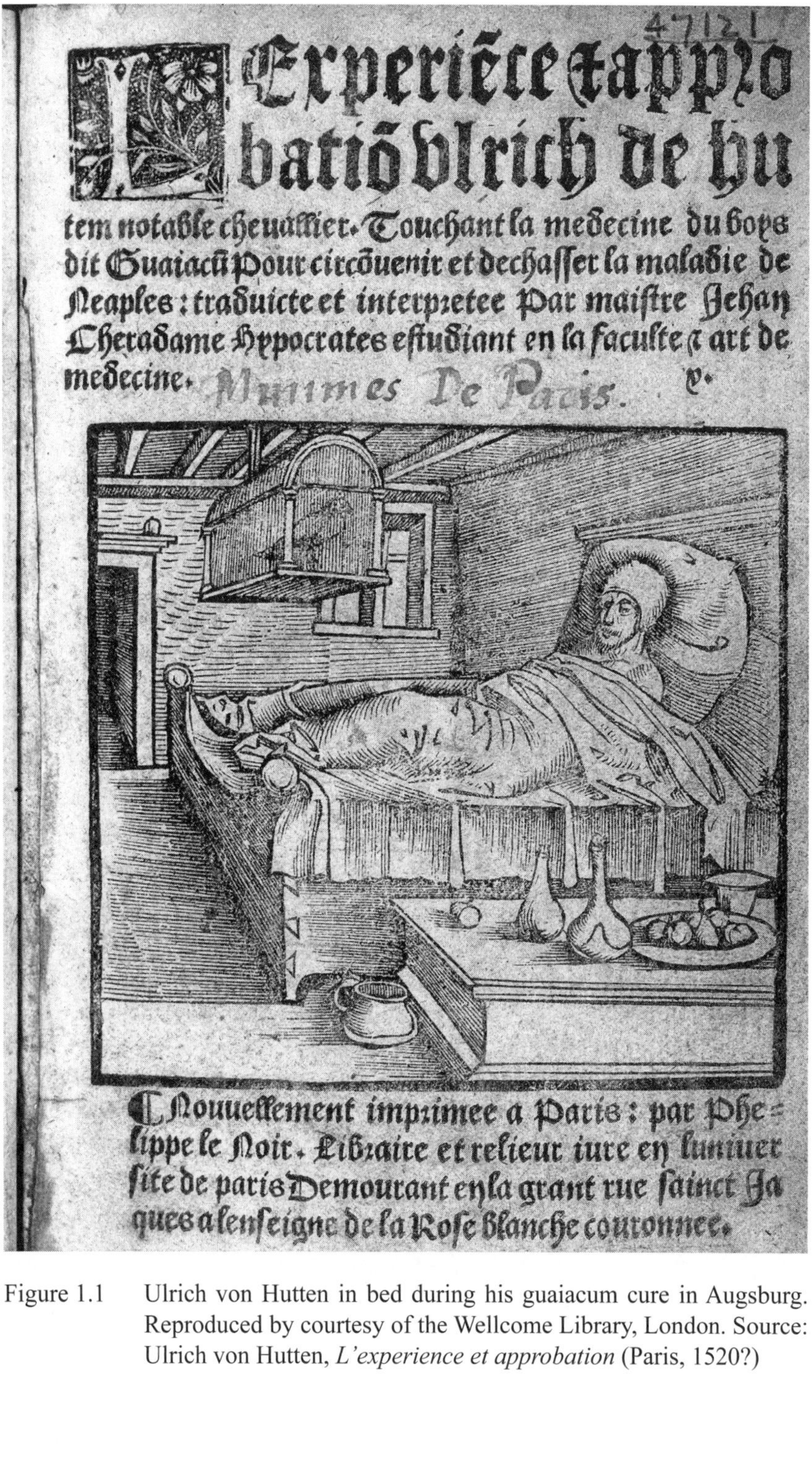
Lexperiēce et approbatiō Ulrich de Hutem notable cheuallier. Touchant la medecine du boys dit Guaiacū Pour circōuenir et dechasser la maladie de Neaples : traduicte et interpretee Par maistre Jehan Cheradame Hypocrates estudiant en la faculte et art de medecine. v.

Nouuellement imprimee a Paris : par Phelippe le Noir. Libraire et relieur iure en luniuersite de paris Demourant en la grant rue sainct Jaques a lenseigne de la Rose blanche couronnee.

Figure 1.1 Ulrich von Hutten in bed during his guaiacum cure in Augsburg. Reproduced by courtesy of the Wellcome Library, London. Source: Ulrich von Hutten, *L'experience et approbation* (Paris, 1520?)

In either case, the treatment was to continue until the last stubborn symptoms of the disease were banished. Even if only a single symptom remained, Knobloch warned, there was still a danger that the poison was concealed within it, and would redistribute itself in the body after a suitable interval.[193] Generally speaking, one could assume that a pox sufferer was cured when 'all symptoms or incidents such as pustules, boils and such with which the patient was afflicted have disappeared, the patient can once again taste food and drink, has no more pains in limbs or head, can sleep properly and naturally; in summary, all appears to be healthy and fresh'.[194] When this state was to be reached depended, very much like the moment of crisis, on the individual circumstances of the patient and on that none of the authors could logically predict.

All of them were well aware that their accounts of the pox were incomplete. Focusing on their own experiences as healers with the pox or as its victims, their descriptions presented only one facet of the multilayered experiences that generally made up each diagnostic act. What was absent was the voice of the individual pox sufferer, whose narrative was vital for fixing the meaning of any bodily sign. By way of compensation most pox authors offered their readers dense narrative accounts of the pox that claimed to comprise all its possible signs, causes, courses and cures. Moreover, they provided a number of different possible narratives to account for the various kinds of the pox, so that the disease in its physical dimension would emerge in front of the reader's inner eye.[195] One's own bodily symptoms and signs could be compared with the help of the descriptions in the text. However, for determining whether oneself really suffered from the pox, all readers knew that it was not sufficient to compare one's own symptoms with a description or a depiction in a book, as we might do today with the help of an anatomical atlas or the internet. The early modern understanding of physical signs made this simple analogy impossible. At that time, disease and its signs were bound together by a different code; crucially, they followed a different structure of visibility. It was accepted that the search for meaning of all immediate sensory perceptions had to be extended to a variety of extrasensory realms and had to take into account all manner of spiritual conceptions and ideologies as well as unlimited analogies and interdependencies between the two cosmos. Proper knowledge of

193 Ibid., p. 116.

194 Ibid., pp. 116–17.

195 Andrew Wear, *Knowledge and Practice*, pp. 133–4, observed the same phenomenon in many early modern English disease treatises. For the developing interest of Renaissance practitioners in recording narratives about individual patients and their diseases or injuries see Siraisi, *Clock and Mirror*, pp. 195–213. For an interesting analysis of narrative in modern medicine see Kathryn Montgomery Hunter, *Doctor's Stories: The Narrative Structure of Medical Knowledge* (Princeton, 1991); for comments on the status of patient narratives in the eighteenth century see Roy Porter, 'The Rise of Physical Examination', in Bynum/Porter (eds), *Five Senses*, pp. 179–97.

the pox was gained not by the mere act of 'sensing' the physical sign, but only by decoding its invisible meaning. Or, as Foucault has described it:

> to know must therefore be to interpret: to find a way from the visible mark to that which is being said by it and which, without that mark, would lie like unspoken speech, dormant within things. Divination is not a rival form of knowledge; it is part of the main body of knowledge itself.[196]

Although I do agree with Foucault that the role of philosophical-medical 'divination' played a vital role in the diagnosis of the pox, the following chapters go beyond his archaeological method of textual analysis loosely applied in this first chapter. The meaning of physical signs, I argue, was also shaped by the immediate socio-cultural context and the medical practices involved in the act of diagnosis at a given time and place. To bring us closer to what sixteenth-century contemporaries took to be the identity of the pox we need to investigate closely the setting of, and the practices involved in, its diagnosis. The following chapter will do exactly that by using the imperial city of Augsburg as a 'test-case'. Socio-cultural premises specific to the merchant city at the Lech, I suggest, shaped the epistemological understanding and the treatment of this new and previously unknown disease in significant ways. Thus, the identity of the pox was not only flexible and temporary, as argued in this chapter, but was also locally defined.

196 Foucault, *Order of Things*, p. 36.

Chapter 2
Sickness and Poverty in Sixteenth-Century Augsburg

In many ways the sixteenth century was Augsburg's golden age. Due to its favourable geographic location, at the meeting of both overland and water-borne trade routes from Italy to Northern Europe, the city became the economic and financial capital of the south of Germany by the 1490s. It reached the peak of its power during the first half of the sixteenth century, by then housing a population of around 45,000 within its walls.[1] Its merchants, above all the Fugger family, amassed fortunes of fantastic proportions through their control of an economic empire that included textile production, mining, international trade and banking. Close financial ties with the chronically cash-strapped Habsburg dynasty made the Fuggers important political players. Indeed, it was the wealth of Jakob Fugger (1459–1525, alias Jakob Fugger 'the Rich') that had permitted Charles V to 'buy' his election as Holy Roman Emperor in 1519.[2] Augsburg, the Fuggers' hometown, was one of the Emperor's favourite German haunts, a city of splendour, centre of the fine arts and book printing, as well as intellectual and political debate. Its impressive architecture, its lively squares and beautiful gardens attracted many visitors. A famous one was the French essayist Michel de Montaigne (1533–1592), who, in the spring of 1580, spent a couple of nights in a local inn before continuing his journey to the Italian spas where he hoped to find relief from kidney and bladder stone problems.[3] Judging Augsburg 'the fairest town of Germany', the French writer praised its outstanding cleanliness (rats and mice were nowhere to be seen, he noted with relief) and admired its sophisticated water supply system and ramparts. The latter had even attracted the interest of the Queen of England Elizabeth I (1533–1603) herself, Montaigne reported. By far the greatest impression on him, however, was made by the summer residences of the Fuggers. The French traveller was stunned by their lavishly-furnished interiors and extended gardens full of mechanical fountains and foreign plants and animals, including a pair of African ostriches. The Fuggers had acquired these animals for the Elector August

1 Barbara Rajkay, 'Die Bevölkerungsentwicklung (Augsburg) von 1500–1648', in Gunther Gottlieb et al., *Geschichte der Stadt Augsburg von der Römerzeit bis zur Gegenwart* (Stuttgart, 1984), p. 252.

2 On the Fuggers see Götz Freiherr von Pölnitz, *Die Fugger*, 2nd edn (Tübingen, 1970).

3 Michel de Montaigne, *The Journal of Montaigne's Travels in Italy by Way of Switzerland and Germany*, W. G. Waters (ed.) (3 vols, London, 1903), vol. 1, pp. 129–44.

of Saxony (1526–1586), a well-known collector of natural rarities, Montaigne informed his readers.

However, there was a less splendid side to Augsburg, which the writer might not have come across during his brief visit. Like any other German city in the sixteenth century, Augsburg also housed a great number of paupers, the majority of whom dwelled in the *Jakobervorstadt*, a walled suburb to the east of the inner city ring wall (see Figure 2.1). The number of the 'have-nots' – inhabitants with no taxable income – in this district sharply increased over the sixteenth century due to successive economic crises. Although all of the city's trades were affected, the weavers – the trade that had been the backbone of Augsburg's flourishing economy since the Middle Ages – were particularly badly hit. Weaver families therefore comprised a significant number of the *Jakobervorstadt* inhabitants, often living in unimaginably dire conditions.

Poverty has often been a fertile breeding ground for social unrest and new radical ideas and thus it comes as little surprise perhaps that it was in this eastern suburb of the city that the new evangelical ideas, articulated by Martin Luther and other religious reformers since the early 1500s, would find their first and most ardent supporters. Probably with great satisfaction these enthusiasts observed their hometown becoming the centre stage for some of the most pivotal events of the unfolding German Reformation. At several meetings of the *Reichstag* held at the city, German princes and free territories supporting the new Lutheran faith explained their religious convictions to the Catholic emperor, and discussed with him and their Catholic peers possible ways to keep up a politically unified empire, despite the religious differences. However, after the Diet of Augsburg in 1530, which had produced the first official document of the Lutheran faith, the Confession of Augsburg, these peaceful debates soon gave way to military confrontation between the Emperor and the Schmalkaldic League, an alliance of Lutheran princes and free cities (including Augsburg) formed in 1531. After sixteen years of smouldering conflict, the League was finally decisively demolished by Charles in the battle of Mühlberg (1547). Following the defeat, Charles proclaimed the Augsburg Interim, a declaration which (due to its overly ambiguous political-religious character) has been described by the late Bob Scribner as 'something of a politico-religious centaur, a theological statement worked out under diplomatic and political pressure to meet the demands of a particular political situation'.[4] Scribner was referring to the fact that the Interim's twenty-six articles primarily reflected a Catholic viewpoint, although it allowed clerical marriage and communion in both kinds for the laity. Charles insisted on its acceptance, but many evangelically-minded princes nevertheless resisted imperial pressure and rejected it, a decision which triggered more brutal military conflict. A resolution of the confessional tensions was only achieved at the Augsburg diet of 1555, when the Peace of Augsburg was concluded.

4 Robert W. Scribner, *The German Reformation* (Houndmills, 1986), pp. 3–4.

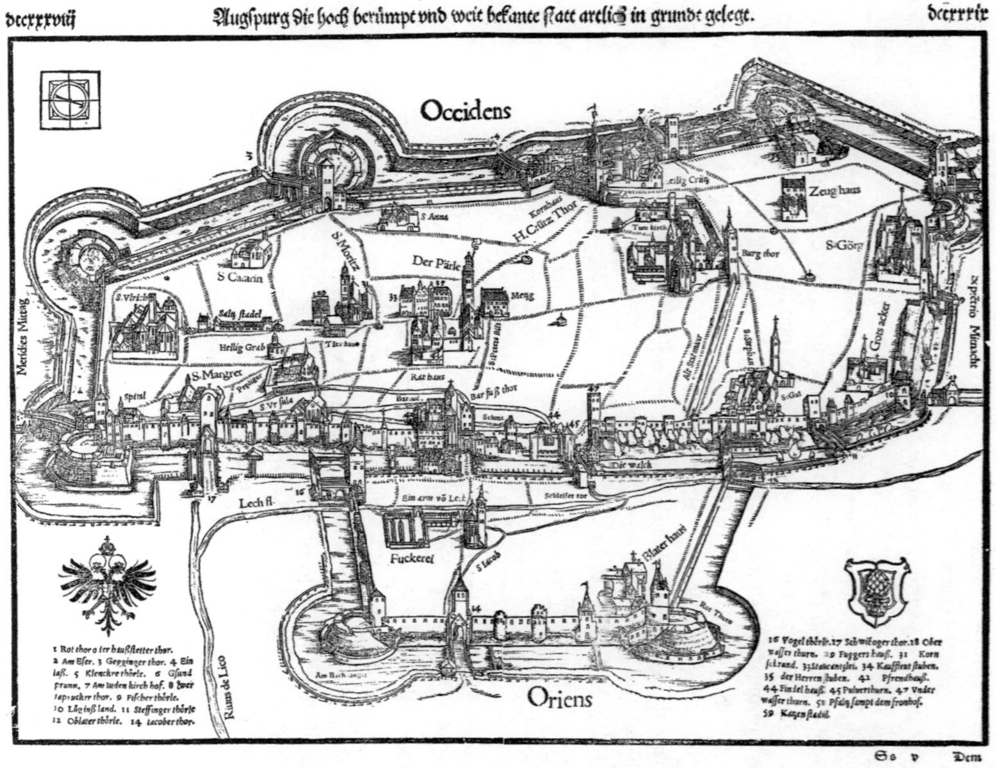

Figure 2.1 A view of Augsburg from above around 1550, after Sebastian Münster. The *Jakobervorstadtat* at the bottom of the map with the Fuggerei (here Fuckerei) and the *Blatterhaus*. Reproduced by courtesy of the Städtische Kunstammlungen Augsburg

This treaty acknowledged the Confession of Augsburg of 1530 and codified the 'cuius regio, eius religio' principle, which gave each prince the power to decide the religion of his subjects.

Augsburg's ill-fated affiliation with the Schmalkaldic League had triggered grave consequences. In 1548 Charles V reinstituted Catholicism in the city (abolished since 1537). He also changed its constitution: all higher political offices were to be filled by members of the Catholic patrician elite only. This created a difficult political situation as the majority of the city's population remained faithful to the new evangelical movement, and its ideas and practices continued to shape strongly all areas of the Augsburg's public life. Most prominently, these influences can be observed in the organisation of city's poor relief, which underwent significant changes over the course of the sixteenth century.[5]

This chapter investigates these changes, focusing on the organisation and administration of Augsburg's enclosed charity for the sick poor. A reconstruction of the institutional landscape of the city's public healthcare (and its historical roots) allows for a more rigorous evaluation of the role and significance of the three pox hospitals whose administration and organisation will be explored in detail towards the end of this chapter. Were they really the *only* charitable facilities in Augsburg providing fully-fledged medical care for a specific disease, as scholars have recently claimed?

Augsburg's Health Care Institutions

As in other cities of the Holy Roman Empire, the majority of Augsburg's institutions for the care and cure of the sick poor originated in an alliance of the Church with various lay initiatives during the Middle Ages.[6] The primary objective of these charitable foundations, in particular the Hospital of the Holy Ghost, three leper houses, and the Pilgrim House, was Christian charity to migrants, travellers, the elderly, and other infirm people as an act of hospitality.[7] The city's largest charitable institution was the Hospital of the Holy Ghost, founded in the thirteenth century by a local religious confraternity and located within the inner city walls

5 For Augsburg's poor relief see Max Bisle, *Die öffentliche Armenpflege der Reichsstadt Augsburg mit Berücksichtigung der einschlägigen Verhältnisse in anderen Reichsstädten Süddeutschlands* (Paderborn, 1904); Claus-Peter Clasen, 'Armenfürsorge im 16. Jahrhundert', in Gunther Gottlieb et al. (eds), *Stadt Augsburg*, pp. 363–85; ibid., 'Armenfürsorge in Augsburg vor dem Dreißigjährigen Krieg', *Zeitschrift des historischen Vereins für Schwaben* 78 (1984), pp. 65–115.

6 Rolf Kießling, *Bürgerliche Gesellschaft und Kirche in Augsburg im Spätmittelalter: Ein Beitrag zur Strukturanalyse der oberdeutschen Reichsstadt* (Augsburg, 1971).

7 For the most recent history of the hospital see Risse, *Mending Bodies*; indispensible still is Siegfried Reicke, *Das deutsche Spitalwesen und sein Recht im Mittelalter* [1932] (reprint, 2 vols, Amsterdam, 1970).

(see Figure 2.1).[8] It offered room for more than 250 elderly citizens. Also founded in the thirteenth century was the city's first leper house. Lepers – first mentioned in Augsburg's sources in 1264 – initially lived without proper accommodation as an 'extra muros' community, south-east of the city walls near the church of St Servatius.[9] A residence with eight rooms was made available to them later, thanks to charitable donations from pious Augsburg burghers. The St Servatius accommodation soon grew too small, and two further leprosaria, St Sebastian outside the Jakob Gate to the east, and St Wolfgang by the Wertach Bridge Gate to the northwest of the city, were established during the early fifteenth century.[10] While St Sebastian catered for about fifteen inmates, mostly women St Wolfgang housed the same number of both sexes. The Pilgrim House, also called the Almshouse or House of the Wretched, was founded in the fourteenth century by the bequest of a wealthy local merchant and offered more space to the infirm. Initially conceptualised as a shelter for only four poor sick vagrants and pilgrims, by the end of the sixteenth century it was able to accommodate about seventy patients of both sexes.[11]

Like the Pilgrim House, all facilities for the sick owed their existence to the private initiatives and generosity of pious citizens or to the Catholic Church. By the end of the sixteenth century this was no longer the case. While the number of private or church-run health care institutions plummeted during the sixteenth century (the two private pox hospitals of the Fugger family, opened in 1523/24 and 1572 were rare exceptions to this rule), the city magistrate became the most important benefactor. New health care institutions such as the *Blatterhaus*, established in 1495, were created at the behest of the council which also attempted to seize the administration of all such institutions.

Augsburg is not the only early-modern city where this phenomenon can be observed. Social historians explained this increasing centralisation of the care of the sick and poor in the hands of the cities' magistrates in terms of the culmination of an extended process of communalisation that began during the late thirteenth

8 Peter Lengle, 'Heilig-Geist-Spital', in Wolfram Baer (ed), *Augsburger Stadtlexikon* (Augsburg, 1985), p. 156; ibid., 'Spitäler, Stiftungen und Bruderschaften', in Gunther Gottlieb et al. (eds), *Stadt Augsburg*, pp. 202–8.

9 For some information on Augsburg's leper houses see Kießling, *Bürgerliche Gesellschaft*, pp. 169–73; Peter Rummel, *Katholisches Leben in der Reichsstadt Augsburg (1605–1806)* (Augsburg, 1984), p. 140; also Hammond, *Civic Health Care*, pp. 81–3. For a general overview on leper hospitals in Germany see Jürgen Mehl, *Aussatz in Rottweil: Das Leprosenhaus Allerheiligen der Siechen im Feld* (1298–1810) (Rottweil, 1993), pp. 34–45; for England see Carole Rawcliffe, *Leprosy in Medieval England* (Woodbridge, 2006).

10 StAA, Reichstadt, St Martinsstiftung, Karton VI, Nr. 47: Suppliken an die Stadtpfleger, Bürgermeister und den Rat um die Aufnahme ins Blatterhaus 1548–1804, Prod. 81: Bericht der Pfleger über St Servatius vom Dezember 1609. (Hereafter StAA, St Martin, VI, Prod.)

11 Johann Trometer, *Das Augsburger Pilgerhaus* (MA dissertation, Augsburg, 1997). See also Hammond, *Civic Health Care*, pp. 135–55.

century.[12] From then onwards, in most major Germany cities, burghers and residents of every status, from middling artisans to small shopkeepers to elite merchants and patricians, not only created new institutions for the sick and poor, but also began to exert more influence on the facilities already existing. Individuals who donated money or property placed the management of these bequests in the hands of lay administrators known as guardians.[13] This creeping encroachment on the Church's administration of its property was not necessarily an expression of anti-Church attitudes on the part of the donors. But even if not specifically intended, in the long run its effect did significantly diminish the influence of the Church, as the examples of the Hospital of the Holy Ghost and that of the leper house St Servatius in Augsburg show. The appointment of lay guardians in both institutions led to the supervision of the endowment capital and management of both institutions passing sooner or later into the hands of Augsburg citizens and their representative body, the city council.

The magistrate's efforts to reorganise the city's poor relief under its own auspices gained impetus in the early decades of the sixteenth century from the Reformation.[14] In accordance with reformed critique of traditional forms of Catholic charity, poor citizens were to be provided with relief only after careful examination and evaluation of their individual circumstances. The community and its representative body, the magistrate, felt it incumbent upon themselves as good Christians to take responsibility for the regulation and distribution of alms. They saw themselves as instruments of God, working in His name to provide 'fatherly' care for the poor and indigent 'children' and so duplicate God's spiritual family on earth.[15] The breadth of the council's charitable commitments was further intended to demonstrate before God that Augsburg's civic society was truly Christian and hence earned God's grace as insurance against the ever-present danger of His punishment in the form of catastrophes like war, plague or famine.

The poor relief ordinances issued by the council in 1522 and 1541 created a centralised system of poor relief, including a complete reorganisation of its financial resources.[16] The council aimed at channelling the total flow of charitable donations directly into the coffers of the newly established Alms Office. This was

12 For the process of communalisation see Jütte, *Armenfürsorge*; also Thomas Fischer, *Städtische Armut und Armenfürsorge im 15. und 16. Jahrhundert. Sozialgeschichtliche Untersuchungen am Beispiel der Städte Basel, Freiburg i. Br. und Straßburg* (Göttingen, 1979); Martin Dinges, *Stadtarmut in Bordeaux*, has shown that this trend was not unique to early modern German cities but a wider European phenomenon.

13 For this development in general see Reicke, *Spitalwesen*, vol. 1, pp. 196–8.

14 Jütte, *Armenfürsorge*, pp. 916–25.

15 Bernd Moeller, *Stadt und Kirche im 16. Jahrhundert* (Gütersloh, 1978); Thomas A. Brady, 'Göttliche Republiken: Die Domestizierung der Religion in der deutschen Stadtreformation', in Andreas Lindt and Alfred Schindler (eds), *Hoffnung der Kirche und Erneuerung der Welt: Beiträge zu den ökumenischen, sozialen und politischen Wirkungen des Pietismus* (Göttingen 1985), pp. 109–36.

16 For more information see Clasen, 'Armenfürsorge', p. 61.

run by six honorary Alms Lords, who administered the poor lists and supervised weekly distribution of alms in the city's three parishes. Four times a year, the Alms Lords and their deputies visited the registered homes of the alms-receiving poor to vet their individual circumstances. Management of the Pilgrim House was also delegated to the Alms Office, while the Hospital of the Holy Ghost, the leper houses, and pest houses, as well as the municipal *Blatterhaus*, continued to be run by council-appointed guardians.

This ongoing centralising process peaked with the official establishment of the Reformation in Augsburg in the 1530s. While the overwhelming majority of artisans sympathised with the evangelical movement as early as the 1520s, the majority of city's political leadership and patrician élite, most notably the Fuggers, remained loyal to the Catholic Church. The latter feared for their loss of trade relations and political influence with the Catholic Habsburg Emperor. However, after a series of riots the authorities bowed to popular pressure and gradually introduced the Reformation between 1534 and 1537. This meant, among other things, that Catholic clerics (including the Archbishop himself) were expelled from the city and the remaining independent monasteries and church foundations were dissolved. The responsibility for all the city's charitable institutions then passed into the hands of a new council, dominated now by the evangelical-minded members of the guilds.[17]

The council retained this control even after Charles V forced the re-Catholicisation of the city in 1548.[18] Charles punished the disloyalty of the Protestant council by abolishing the city's constitution.[19] The new one gave exclusive power to a small group of the Catholic patricians who had resisted the evangelical enthusiasm. They came to constitute the majority on the council, and all important government posts were exclusively reserved for them. Thus, as a result of the constitutional reform of 1548, a small minority of Catholic patrician families governed a predominantly Protestant population, a potentially explosive political situation. However, it is very interesting to note that with the exception of religious unrest associated with the introduction of the Georgian calendar in 1584, Catholics and Protestants managed to co-exist peacefully in Augsburg until the Thirty Year War (1618–1648). That confessional allegiance did not come to play a

17 Philip Broadhead, 'Popular Pressure for Reform in Augsburg 1524–1534', in Wolfgang J. Mommsen et al. (eds), *Stadtbürgertum und Adel in der Reformation* (Stuttgart, 1979), pp. 80–87; Friedrich Roth, *Augsburgs Reformationsgeschichte* (4 vols, Munich, 1901–1911), vol. 2, pp. 290–95.

18 Roth, *Reformationsgeschichte*, vol. IV, pp. 170–75; Paul Warmbrunn, *Zwei Konfessionen in einer Stadt: Das Zusammenleben von Katholiken und Protestanten in den paritätischen Reichsstädten Augsburg, Biberach, Ravensburg und Dinkelsbühl von 1548–1648* (Wiesbaden, 1983).

19 The constitution of 1368 resulted from the revolt of the city's rich merchants and artisans against the patrician elites. For a good summary of these developments see Stuart, *Defiled Trades*, pp. 34–9.

significant role in daily social life is most probably due to the council's successful strategy of religious tolerance.[20] At no point did the Catholic-dominated patrician council attempt to re-catholicise the city; instead it governed with discretion in order to minimise tensions with the Protestant community. This was particularly true when it came to the daily business of poor relief.[21] Favouring those of their own faith, the Catholic council members feared, could discourage the community's charitable generosity on which the city's Alms Office was dependent. Even worse, it might lead to riots and social unrest that could threaten their own precarious position.

The admission practices of all the city-run health care institutions reflected this strategy of confessional tolerance. Already before the Peace of Augsburg (1555), which introduced legal parity between Catholics and Protestants in the city, members of both denominations were equally entitled to admission and, once accepted, attention was paid to equal opportunities for, and the observance of, confessional rituals during their stay.[22] Thus, in 1620, the nurses' head matron of the Hospital of the Holy Ghost was instructed 'every day, after morning and evening prayers and whenever else it might be deemed necessary, to go from bed to bed and to enquire whether the patients are lacking anything in their care and comfort, whether they have enough food and drink, or whether indeed they require the attentions of a Catholic priest or Protestant pastor; and if this last be deemed necessary, such a visit is to be arranged forthwith by the father of the infirm'.[23] If a patient's physical condition indicated that they were not long for this world, it was the nurses' responsibility to ensure that they were prepared for death in the manner befitting his or her confessional beliefs.

> The Catholic shall be earnestly admonished to make confession and receive the Holy Sacrament and last rites and, as in ancient Catholic custom, be shown a crucifix next to a burning consecrated wax candle with sprinkling of holy water. Correspondingly, for the Protestant the minister shall be summoned to give Holy Communion and speak words of comfort, with nothing in preparation being neglected, but everything performed with diligence.

---

20 Martin Heckel, 'Autonomia and Pacis Compositio: Der Augsburger Religionsfrieden in der Deutung der Gegenreformation', *Zeitschrift der Savigny-Stiftung für Rechtsgeschichte, Kanonistische Abteilung* 76 (1959), pp. 141–248; also Roeck, *Krieg und Frieden*, vol. 2, pp. 654–97.

21 Roeck, *Krieg und Frieden*, vol. 1, pp. 123, 125; vol. 2, pp. 607, 867.

22 Roeck, *Krieg und Frieden*, vol. 2, pp. 607–8. For an interesting analysis of a contemporary account of the religious situation in sixteenth-century Augsburg see Benedikt Mauer, *'Gemeines Geschrey' und 'teglich Reden': Georg Kölderer – ein Augsburger Chronist des konfessionellen Zeitalters* (Augsburg, 2001).

23 For this and the following quotations see StAA, Heilig-Geist-Spital Tit III. Tom 254: Ordnungen und Receptionsignat. Von 1620.

Until the 1630s, the irrelevance of the patient's denomination applied also to the three leper houses where Catholics and Protestants were equally entitled to admission. The house rules specified that both confessions were to live in harmony with each other and avoid arguments.[24] The 'father of the infirm', who managed the facilities, was to ensure that all his 'house children' fulfilled their religious duties and that 'each may be permitted to practise his religion unimpeded, the one being forbidden to offend or insult, dispute with or quarrel with the other over his religion, and neither shall be provoked to such quarrels, but freely allowed to practise his beliefs'.[25] The Pilgrim House, originally a Catholic charitable foundation, was another institution that opened its doors to both denominations in the mid-sixteenth century, and continued to do so after 1578 when the Protestant Martin Zobel generously financed its expansion. In times of the plague, the ulcer-infested bodies of Catholic and Protestant victims would lie side by side in the city's plague houses. To provide spiritual comfort to them, so-called 'comfort women and men' of both denominations were employed by the council. Candidates for the job had to trust themselves to 'perform such a service without revulsion' and comfort the dying by hours of reading from the Scriptures.[26]

While the religious faith of an applicant was clearly not a matter of discrimination, the council devised other strategies to restrict beneficiaries as a reaction to the grave changes, which the city had to face in the second half of the sixteenth century. Migration from the surrounding rural areas and the economic recession that shook Augsburg's trades created an army of unemployed artisans (mainly weavers), servants and unskilled day-labourers. According to conservative estimates, the number of these residents without taxable income accounted for over 40 per cent of the entire city population.[27] The demographic and economic crisis reached its climax between 1570 and 1585, stretching the resources of the Alms Office to the limit and compelling the council to come up with measures for restricting welfare.[28] The distinction between *deserving* and *undeserving* poor

24 Whether the daily hospital life was as idyllic and harmonious as depicted in the normative house rules is perhaps questionable. Hammond, *Civic Health Care*, pp. 142–3 indicated that the cohabitation of Catholic and Protestant inmates was not always characterised by tolerance and mutual respect.

25 StAA, Ev. Wesensarchiv, Nr. 326, Acta Siechenhausordnung betr. 1595–1739: Verrichtungen des Hausmeister zu der St Servatii armen Hauß.

26 StAA, St Martinsstiftung, Kt. VII, Nr. 63–71: D. Lazarette, *Sanität und St Sebastianskapelle*, Prod. 68 (1–3).

27 Clasen, 'Armenfürsorge', p. 66; Rajkay, 'Bevölkerung', pp. 252–8; for demographic trends in early modern Europe see Jan de Vries, *European Urbanization* (London, 1984).

28 This crisis was intimately related to the shifting of the main trade routes from the south (Italy) to the north of Europe. Dutch cities increasingly challenged Augsburg's status as one of the most important trading centres in Europe. For Augsburg's economic development in the early modern period see Thomas Safley, *Charity and Economy in the Orphanages of Early Modern Augsburg* (Atlantic Highlands, NJ, 1996), pp. 19–57; Claus-Peter Clasen,

was introduced as a discriminating tool.[29] In the former category fell working individuals, however impoverished, who had resided for some time in Augsburg and whose family and/or friends could provide evidence of moral character and behaviour. Holding modest artisanal or service jobs, the authorities characterised them as modest and law-abiding and thus worthy of communal aid. Those paupers, however, who were neither citizens nor residents had little chance of being included in the existing charity schemes, particularly after 1550. Often without permanent residence, these were the 'undeserving' poor, all too readily identified by the authorities with social unrest, troublemaking and crime.[30]

This tendency to retrench and exclude was mirrored in the city's provision for the infirm: claims to free medical care or admission to one of the existing institutions was now dependent on proof of citizenship or residential status.[31] In practice this meant that vagrants and the itinerant paupers were no longer admitted either to the Pilgrim House, the leper houses or the municipal pox hospital (*Blatterhaus*). The exception was the Hospital of the Holy Ghost. The reason for its openness to foreigners was grounded in the fact that, unlike all other health care institutions, it owned substantial lands around Augsburg, from which it derived its income. As in the case of noble landowners, this was accompanied by paternalist responsibilities for those working its lands and residing there, such as the care of the elderly and sick.[32]

But while citizenship and residential status were important for admission, *the* decisive criterion for being accepted at one of the municipal hospitals (at least since the 1520s) was the physical condition of the applicant. As with the admission practices in the French hospitals investigated by Colin Jones, no one could be admitted without a previous examination by a learned physician and/or surgeon. Each candidate had to present him or herself to a committee of medical practitioners and council representatives, commonly called *Geschau*. According to

---

Die Augsburger Weber: Leistungen und Krisen des Textilgewerbes um 1600 (Augsburg, 1981).

29 Clasen, 'Armenfürsorge', pp. 363–85; more generally see Ole Peter Grell, 'The Protestant Imperative of Christian Care and Neighbourly Love', in ibid., and Andrew Cunningham, *Health Care and the Poor in Medieval and Renaissance Europe: Italy and England Compared* (London, 1997), pp. 43–65.

30 For a useful distinction between poverty and neediness see Dinges, *Bordeaux*, p. 19; for the manifold causes of early modern poverty see Jütte, *Armenfürsorge*, pp. 11–20.

31 For citizenship in Augsburg see Ingrid Bátori, *Die Reichsstadt Augsburg im 18. Jahrhundert: Verfassung, Finanzen und Reformversuche* (Göttingen, 1969), pp. 15–17; for a more general discussion see Otto Brunner, 'Zum Begriff des Bürgertums', in Th. Meyer (ed.), *Untersuchungen zur gesellschaftlichen Struktur der mittelalterlichen Städte in Europa* (Konstanz and Stuttgart, 1966), pp. 13–24; Heinz Schilling, 'Gab es in Deutschland im späten Mittelalter und in der frühen Neuzeit einen Stadt-Republikanismus? – Zur politischen Kultur des europäischen Stadtbürgertums', in H. G. Koenigsberger (ed.), *Republiken und Republikanismus, 15. bis frühes 17. Jahrhundert* (Munich, 1987), pp. 101–43.

32 Lengle, 'Heilig-Geist-Spital', p. 157.

the rules of civic hospitals, no patient could be admitted whose physical condition did not match that institution's specific criteria. What do the sources tell us about the physical admission criteria in these institutions?

Physical Admission Criteria

The entrance ticket for the Hospital of the Holy Ghost was the applicant's age, as the institutions had been founded 'for old and needy citizens'. Children were explicitly excluded from admission.[33] The Holy Ghost predominantly served as a kind of retirement home for elderly Augsburg citizens hospital subjects, and tenants from the surrounding countryside who lacked family or friends to take care of them. Often they brought their own endowment, which paid for their stay.[34] Moreover (but to a much lesser extent) the Holy Ghost also served as a hospital for the chronically infirm. The sixty-seven-year-old weaver Hans Klingenstein, for instance, having sustained an unspecified severe injury while working at his loom, had been nursed by his wife to whom he had been married for forty-four years and had reputedly fathered twelve children, 'of whom four are still living'.[35] After the death of his wife he could not provide for himself and feared, not without some justification, 'that I will have nothing to live on in my old age but must languish helplessly and die of hunger'. Citing his age, fragility and drawing attention to his great poverty and helplessness, he asked the hospital guardians and the city council to 'render him an act of mercy' and allocate him a free bed in the hospital. Like the weaver Klingenstein, most ailing applicants to Holy Ghost Hospital hoped that, once admitted, they could live there for the rest of their lives. They dreamed, like Klingenstein, of being allowed to 'see out my remaining days without too many burdens'.

However, by no means were all infirm and elderly citizens accepted. Only those applicants on whom the examining medical practitioners found no open lesions or 'infected matter' stood a chance of admission, as the case of Daniel Ziegler in 1618 demonstrates. On account of age and weakness, Ziegler had deteriorated into such fragility that he could 'not walk a single step' when he applied for admission. The examining doctor and barber-surgeon certified that 'his whole body is wasted or frostbitten, and shows other disabilities but nothing infected'.[36] Accordingly they authorised his admission to the hospital. A similar blessing also befell the former Hospital employee Katharina Meisch. Referring her case to the council, the

33 For the following see StAA, Heilig-Geist-Spital, Tit. III., Tom. 259, Nr. 35.

34 The prize for such a sinecure depended on the financial situation of the applicant see Reicke, *Spitalwesen* I, pp. 187–8; for the prebendiary regulations in Augsburg see StAA, Spital Archiv, Camera Kasten, Hospital Ordnungen: Ordnung des Spitals zum Heiligen Geist 1521, fol. Ir.

35 For Klingenstein's case see StAA, Heilig-Geist-Spital, Tit. III. Tom 259.

36 StAA, Reichsstädte, Zünfte, Kt. 5, Fasc. 3.

hospital authorities recorded that 'she has urgent need of hospital care. Since she has served here faithfully for twenty years, and has, we testify, no open wounds'. They recommended her admission as soon as a bed became available.[37]

Where supplicants or inmates were suffering from ailments believed to be infectious, the Hospital's authorities did everything in their power not to be burdened with these sufferers. This was especially so for those sick suffering from conditions in which other city hospitals were known to have specialised. This is illustrated in a mid-sixteenth-century case when physicians diagnosed some of the Hospital's inmates with the French pox.[38] In the view of the hospital authorities, such ailing persons belonged 'with respect, on account of their disability, in the *Blatterhaus* … and not the spital'. Out of fear for the health of their other patients – and almost certainly also to save costs – they appealed to the council and, after some negotiation with the *Blatterhaus* authorities and its medical practitioners, managed to have at least one female pox sufferer transferred. The Hospital of the Holy Ghost had its own sick ward in which ailing inmates could be treated: in 1620 it contained eleven beds.[39] Besides the beds in the infirmary, there were another eleven beds in the 'unsound ward' for the chronically mentally disturbed, for which the Hospital was also responsible. A further eleven patients suffering from the 'falling sickness' could be accommodated in the 'falling ward'.[40]

If, however, the appointed medical practitioners at the Holy Ghost Hospital diagnosed the ailment of an inmate as infectious, he or she would be immediately transferred to the Pilgrim House. Between 1573 and 1588, an average of 459 people per year were cared for in this institution. In 1588, for example, 486 of them were admitted, of whom 289 were discharged as cured in the course of the year, while 105 died.[41] Managed since the 1520s by the Alms Lords, this institution catered for poor citizens who were 'afflicted with open wounds and other vile diseases'.[42] But what exactly counted as an 'open' and 'vile' disease was further defined and restricted to those ailments which the appointed medical practitioners judged as 'curable'. Applicants diagnosed with 'incurable' diseases were refused admittance, and those whose conditions deteriorated dramatically during their stay, so that no hope of recovery remained, were immediately discharged. The decision to accept only curable illnesses was strongly influenced by financial considerations. The Alms Lords' greatest anxiety was that the institution might become a haven for the chronically ill, adding an extra financial burden for an administration that was already making regular complaints to the council about its empty coffers.

37 StAA, Heilig-Geist-Spital, Tit. III, Tom. 259, Nr. 34.

38 For following quotations see StAA, Heilig-Geist-Spital, Tit. III Tom. 256, Nr. 7.

39 For the following see ibid., Tom. 254.

40 For the care of the mad in early modern Germany see Kinzelbach, *Gesundbleiben*, pp. 342–4; Erik H. C. Midelfort, *A History of Madness in Early Modern Germany* (Stanford, 1999).

41 Clasen, 'Dreißigjähriger Krieg', p. 104.

42 For the following see Bisle, *Armenpflege*, p. 110.

The rigour with which the admission criteria were applied in the Pilgrim House is evidenced by the discharge in February 1587 of the goldsmith's apprentice Jakob Walther. At the request of his master, Tobias Klicker, Walther spent some time in the institution, but his condition deteriorated to the point where the medical practitioners and Alms Lords decided they could 'no longer suffer him in the hospital'.[43] His illness, they claimed, was not of the kind that could be cured at the Pilgrim House; it was 'so constituted that he is in much greater need of the medicines dispensed in the *Blatterhaus*'. Attempts by other institutions to 'unload' their patients to the Pilgrim House – as the authorities of the Hospital of the Holy Ghost tried to do at the close of the sixteenth century with some of the severely mentally disturbed inmates in their charge – were met with firm resistance by the Alms Lords.[44] To combat what they saw as a scandalous demand by the administration of the Holy Ghost, they enquired into how other imperial cities – Ulm, Nuremberg, Frankfurt and Strasbourg – dealt with their problem of those who were 'so possessed in body and soul by evil spirits' that it was feared they might take their own lives. The cities replied that the severely 'possessed' were detained in the city's Holy Ghost Hospital for their own safety. The Nuremberg authorities added in their report that such persons were secured, sitting or standing, to the foot of their beds by a thick leather strap to prevent them doing harm to themselves. On the strength of these reports the guardians of the Holy Ghost Hospital were forced to back down, and mentally distressed patients continued to be housed in the hospital's unsound ward.[45]

While the Hospital of the Holy Ghost was primarily responsible for caring for the frail and elderly, and the Pilgrim House admitted sufferers with infectious but curable diseases, both institutions refused to take in sick individuals who were 'afflicted with the terrible plague of leprosy'.[46] The care of these was in the hands of the three leper houses: St Servatius, St Sebastian and St Wolfgang. In sixteenth-century Augsburg, leprosy was no longer considered to be incurable.[47] Physicians and barber-surgeons in municipal employ were therefore contractually obliged to visit the leper hospitals at regular intervals to 'winkle out' those who

43 StAA, St Martin, VI, Prod. 52: Supplikation des Tobias Klicker vom 28. Februar 1587.

44 For the following see Bisle, *Armenpflege*, pp. 110–11.

45 Augsburg also had a special 'fools' house' (*Narrenhaus*) founded in 1553. But this was predominantly used as a prison for itinerant beggars. See Roeck, *Krieg und Frieden I*, p. 156.

46 StAA, St Martin, VI, Prod. 88: Supplikation der Anna Nidermair vom 19. December 1609.

47 For the widespread belief in the curability of leprosy in the early modern period see Karl Sudhoff, 'Was geschah mit den (nach erneuter Schau) als leprafrei erklärten und aus den Leprosorien wieder Freigelassenen von behördlicher Seite?', *Archiv für Geschichte der Medizin* 6 (1912), pp. 149–54; see also Luke Demaitre, *Leprosy in Premodern Medicine: A Disease of the Whole Body* (Baltimore, 2007).

had recovered.[48] According to the visitation report of the physician Gereon Sailer (?–1562) they were also asked to evict 'idle, work-shy people' who showed no visible signs of leprosy and who, in Sailer's view, were simply lounging around in the leper houses on account of the bad weather.[49] Not all doctors took these duties as seriously as Sailer, however, so that the leper houses were frequently filled to bursting. When three civic physicians, Leopold Trenklin (?–1570), Markus Wind (?–1596) and Jeremias Mertz (?–1585), paid a routine visit to the leper hospitals in April 1569, what they found most irksome about the serious overcrowding was that most of the 'lepers' they encountered there were no longer suffering from the 'harmful disfiguring hereditary disease'.[50] Many of them, they judged, were in the best of health and hardly represented an acute threat to the health of the rest of the urban population. However, on ordering those 'lepers' who they deemed to have recovered to leave the hospitals forthwith, the doctors reported stubborn resistance, with inmates claiming to have bought a sinecure in one of the leper hospitals for an agreed amount of money and insisting on their right to remain there for the rest of their lives, whether they were suffering from leprosy or not.[51] Without a detailed analysis of the inmates and organisation of the Augsburg leper hospitals, it is unclear how such claims should be regarded. In her study of the leper hospitals in the nearby cities of Überlingen and Ulm, Annemarie Kinzelbach has confirmed that prosperous citizens who suffered from the disease did indeed purchase a sinecure.[52] Whether the inmates of the Augsburg leper houses were residing there legally or not, their presence put the visiting doctors in 1569 in a tricky position. Where were they to house new leprosy sufferers who, shunned by everyone as soon as their affliction became known, lost their homes?[53] They earnestly requested the council to provide them with a second building as a temporary domicile for lepers, 'since such wretched persons should be conveyed there as soon as they are judged unclean, until such time as a place is made available elsewhere in the course of inspection'.[54]

48 For the leper instructions of Doctor Daniel Keller in 1568, who was also employed at the municipal *Blatterhaus*, see StAA, St Martin, VI, Nr. 50, Prod. 1.

49 StAA, Collegium Medicum, Ärzte, Ordnungen und Dekreta von 1526–1804: 2. Mai 1556, fol. 17r.

50 Ibid., fol. 25v.

51 Robert Jütte has shown that many early modern paupers considered a life in these institutions attractive because they were provided with food and shelter. Some would even go so far to simulate leprosy to gain access to one of the hospitals. Robert Jütte, 'LepraSimulanten De iis qui morbum simulant', in Martin Dinges and Thomas Schlich (eds), *Seuchengeschichte*, pp. 25–42.

52 Kinzelbach, *Gesundbleiben*, p. 357.

53 StAA, Collegium Medicum, Ärzte, Ordnungen und Dekreta von 1526–1804: November 1569, fol. 25v.

54 Evidence of an official examination of lepers in Augsburg, the so-called 'examen leprosorum', can be traced back to the end of the fourteenth century. During this examination the naked body of the sufferer was inspected 'a planta pedum usque ad

The chronic bed shortage in the leper houses led their chief guardians to refuse admission in cases where the examining medical practitioners were unable to reach a unanimous diagnosis, a rather common diagnostic verdict as we shall see further on in more detail. Such was the fate of 34-year-old Anna Nidermair from Oberhausen who, convinced she had been 'afflicted and infected by the grievous and repulsive plague and disease of leprosy', presented herself to a medical panel in December 1609.[55] As was customary, the learned doctors issued her with a sealed certificate recording the findings of their examination. It is clear from this document that the doctors could not agree on an interpretation of Nidermair's physical signs. At the time of her examination, she was, they wrote, 'afflicted with loathsome scabs' compatible with leprosy but which could also be related to the French pox. The practitioners were unable to arrive at a definitive verdict. They considered it advisable, however, to avoid endangering the healthy population and so segregated Nidermair for the time being, admitting her to one of the leper hospitals 'until there was persistent improvement' in her condition. Nidermair presented herself with this certificate at the doors of the leper house St Servatius, but was refused by its guardians on the grounds that her recommendation stated with certainty that she was not afflicted with leprosy, but suffering only from tenacious scabs and possibly the pox.[56] Furthermore, they submitted, for Nidermair to be accepted to their leper house would involve risks to herself. Since their institution contained patients suffering from a much more dangerous and loathsome disease than hers, her condition might worsen. They suggested therefore that she should be referred to the municipal *Blatterhaus*. The chief guardians of that institution, however, protested vehemently, citing once again the physicians' certificate, which clearly recommended that Nidermair should be admitted to one of the leper hospitals.[57] On 19 January 1610, finally, the council ruled that she should indeed be separated from the healthy population and admitted for observation to the *Blatterhaus* until a place was available in one of the leper hospitals.

This ruling, however, should not imply that all ambiguous diagnostic cases in the leper hospitals were automatically transferred to and treated in the *Blatterhaus*. If the appointed medical practitioners of the *Blatterhaus* believed in their examination, that the referred patient represented a danger to the health of their

capitis verticem', followed by an examination of blood and urine. For leprosy in Augsburg see Sudhoff, 'Leprafrei', pp. 150–52; for the act of diagnosis see Otto von Bremen, 'Die Lepra-Untersuchungen der Kölner Medizinischen Fakultät von 1491–1664', *Westdeutsche Zeitschrift für Geschichte und Kunst* 18 (1899), pp. 65–77; Hermann Keussen, 'Beiträge zur Geschichte der Kölner Lepra-Untersuchungen', *Lepra Bibliotheca Internationalis* 14 (1913), pp. 80–112; Karl Sudhoff, 'Lepraschaubriefe aus dem 15. Jahrhundert', *Sudhoffs Archiv* 4 (1910), pp. 370–78; 5 (1911), pp. 154–6, 434–5; 6 (1912), pp. 392–3.

55 For the following see StAA, St Martin, VI, Prod. 88: Supplikation der Anna Nidermair vom 19. Dezember 1609.

56 StAA, St Martin, VI, Prod. 88: Bericht der Pfleger des St Servatius Siechenhauses.

57 Ibid, Bericht der Oberpfleger über das Blatterhaus vom 16. Januar 1610.

inmates, he or she was either not admitted in the first place or, if already accepted, immediately discharged, as happened to Katharina Moltenrock in 1566.[58] Like Anna Nidermair, Katharina Moltenrock was admitted to the *Blatterhaus* for preliminary observation, as her symptoms suggested to the medical practitioners both leprosy *and* the pox. Despite treatment in the pox hospital, her condition did not improve, so the medical practitioners of the *Blatterhaus* asked the panel of civic doctors for an opinion. Doctors Leopold Trenklin (?–1570), Marcus Wind (?–1596) and Jeremias Mertz (?–1585) examined Moltenrock on 3 September 1566 and ruled that some of her bodily signs indeed indicated leprosy. Until her condition improved with God's help, they stated, she should be discharged from the *Blatterhaus* to protect the other inmates from being further 'contaminated'. Moreover, so that 'the healthy be not made unclean by her', they thought it best to accommodate her in the leper hospital of St Servatius.

If the leper houses of Augsburg had shed much of their stigma by the sixteenth century, in that healthy Augsburg citizens were trying to gain admittance, the same cannot be said of the city's two plague houses, established in 1521 and in the 1570s: they only opened their doors when the most dreaded of all diseases made a visit. Both were designed for victims who had no domicile in the city (travellers, soldiers or itinerant beggars) or who did not possess the financial resources to remain quarantined at home for what might be several weeks. Referral to one of the plague houses (also referred to as *Lazarethe*) was decreed as soon as the civic doctors or barber-surgeons diagnosed the boils and pustules as the feared symptoms of plague. Those who contracted the disease, it was believed, had to be immediately sectioned off from the healthy population.[59] Sixteenth-century eye-witness accounts indicate that this segregation process was executed in a far more orderly fashion than might be supposed.[60] A recent study on Augsburg submits that official and public reaction was marked neither by knee-jerk responses on the part of the authorities, nor blind terror and panic on the part of the population, let alone any kind of collective madness.[61]

---

58 For the following see StAA, Collegium Medicum. Wundärzte, Bader u. Barbire, in specie betr. von 1570–1804; c) Siechen von 1555–1649: Supplikation von Leopold Trenklin, Marcus Wind und Jeremias Martius vom 3. September 1566.

59 For the plague in Augsburg see Karl Fries, *Die Pest in Augsburg im Dreissigjährigen Krieg: Ein Beitrag zur Geschichte der Pest* (dissertation, Munich 1886). The current doctoral research undertaken by Mariusz Horanin into the social-cultural responses to the plague in early modern Augsburg will shed further light on this neglected issue.

60 Jean Delumeau, *Angst im Abendland: Die Geschichte kollektiver Ängste im Europa des 14. bis 18. Jahrhunderts* (Hamburg, 1989) is only one example of the many works which depict medieval and early modern plague as provoking a complete breakdown of society.

61 Mauer, *Augsburger Chronist*, p. 304. Mauer's recent findings echoes earlier claims made by the medical historian Paul Slack, 'Responses to Plague in Early Modern Europe: The Implications of Public Health', *Social Research* 55 (1988), p. 117.

Moreover, although its high mortality led many contemporaries to view the plague as the worst of divine punishments, its victims in the Augsburg plague houses were by no means abandoned to their fate. To be 'touched by the plague' – as many sources term it – was not synonymous with death. The city's medical practitioners were joined in their efforts by maids, servants and male and female comforters, who attended not just to the physical needs of the victims, but also to their spiritual comfort. Remarkably, many carers appear to have been unmindful of their own physical safety. During the plague of 1563/1564, for example, the plague house barber-surgeon Peter Willig succumbed to the disease and could not carry out his duties for several weeks. But as soon as he felt better, he returned voluntarily to his post.[62] In the same outbreak the plague house caretaker, the plague father Bastian Staffer and his wife, were stricken for several weeks, with the doctors and surgeons giving up all hope. When the couple defied expectations by recovering, they seem to have given no thought to quitting their posts. This is not the place to discuss the possible reasons for such 'fearless' behaviour among practitioners and staff, but it is worth referring to the Augsburg barber-surgeon Joseph Schmid (1603–1667), who treated the plague in his hometown over a number of years and recorded his experiences in print.[63] In one of his publications, Schmid wondered why he had never succumbed to the plague himself, positing, first, that medical practitioners as well as ministers of the church 'are watched over and protected above all others by Almighty God because such is their profession and chosen vocation'.[64] Second, he believed that a plague sufferer could only infect a healthy person when the composition of their bodily fluids and its qualities was similar. In the third place, he reasoned, daily contact with plague victims was the norm for any medical practitioner, pastor or priest, 'and what we are accustomed to daily cannot hurt or injure us so freely'. In Schmid's experience the best precautions were 'if healthy people [who] have much and frequent contact with infected sick, [should] always have God in their thoughts, pray fervently, be moderate in eating and drinking, and do not live in fear … for it is said: Where a thousand fall to your left, and ten thousand to your right, it shall not afflict you. And I have thanked God many times for it that I have willingly served in the plague and never been harmed in my body but remained healthy'.

---

62 For the following see the original report by the guardian Michael Reischlin in StAA, Collegium Medicorum, Acta, die Stadt- und Pestphysicos betreffend von 1548–1789, Fasc. 5: Bericht über die Vorgänge in den Brechhäusern 1563/64.

63 For Schmid see the Ute Ecker-Offenhäußer, 'Pest, Franzosen, Scharbock' – *Krankheitserfahrung und medizinischer Alltag des 17. Jahrhunderts im Spiegel der Werke des Augsburger Wundarztes Joseph Schmid* (MA thesis, Augsburg, 1994); ibid., 'Joseph Schmid. Handwerkschirurg und Schriftsteller in Augsburg im 17. Jahrhundert', *Medizin, Gesellschaft und Geschichte* 15 (1997), pp. 117–39.

64 For the following see Joseph Schmid, *Kurzter iedoch Gewisser bericht, dreyer Erblicher kranckheiten, alß da sein, die Pest, Frantzosen, und Scharbock, wie sie mögen curiert werden ...* (Augsburg, 1667), pp. 29–31.

Schmid not only offered his services to the city's two plagues house but also worked, for a while, in the municipal *Blatterhaus*, which was located immediately adjacent to the small plague house in the *Jacobervorstadt*. Together with the two private institutions established by the Fuggers (*Holzhäuser*), all three pox hospitals directed their services exclusively towards pox victims. The particularities of their organisation and administration and admission practices will be investigated in the following section.

The Civic *Blatterhaus*

In 1495, as soon as the French pox reached Augsburg, the city council provided a special house for the diseased.[65] The building had been purchased the previous year for the sum of 306 fl. from the knight Caspar Stunz, the council originally planning to use it as a shelter for plague victims.[66] The decision to turn it into a French pox hospital instead made Augsburg the first city in the German-speaking territories to provide such a facility.[67] As mentioned above, the first civic plague house was not established until 1521, more than twenty years later.

Like the other municipal facilities for the sick in Augsburg, the *Blatterhaus* was for the less prosperous. It was situated at the southwest limit of the predominant Protestant and poor suburb of the *Jakobervorstadt*, near the Jakob Gate and the Red Tower (see Figure 2.1).[68] Early references to the *Blatterhaus*, such as 'the hospice of the wretched' and the 'paupers' spital', indicate that from the outset the council intended it to benefit the city's poor.[69] Very little is known about the architecture of the house or how it was furnished. A map of the city from 1550 shows it to be a simple, two-storey building with a saddle roof. The cross on the roof suggests there was a chapel attached to it (see Figure 2.1).[70] Patients were accommodated in two rooms on the first floor of the building, segregated by gender.[71] The number

65 The German situation differs from that in Italy where most of the pox hospitals were privately founded. For a detailed analysis of the Italian pox hospitals see Arrizabalaga/French/Henderson, *The Great Pox*, chapters 7 and 8.

66 Von Stetten, *Geschichte Augsburg*, I, p. 247.

67 Kinzelbach, *Gesundbleiben*, p. 364.

68 For the geographical coordinates of the *Blatterhaus* see von Stetten, *Geschichte Augsburg* I, p. 247 and StAA, St Martin, VII, Nr. 61, Prod. 1–2: Blatterhaus-Baussachen 1513, 1576.

69 These terms can be found in the first surviving house rules dating from 1494. In my view, however, the date is wrong and was most probably added later to the document. The date given in the document itself is unfortunately illegible. Considering that all other surviving archival sources report 1495 as the founding date of the hospital I decided to follow them. However, whenever I quote from this document I shall refer to it as to be found in the town archive's *Findbuch*.

70 Kießling, *Bürgerliche Gesellschaft*, p. 232.

71 StAA, Blatterhaus, Inventar nach 1671.

of inmates treated at one time varied over the century, ranging between forty and over 120.[72] A room adjoining the two wards was for a nurse. The first floor also had a women's room, perhaps for pregnant women or mothers with children. The caretaker of the hospital, the so-called 'pox father' (*Blattervater*) and his wife, 'the pox mother' (*Blattermutter*), lived on the ground floor. On this floor we also find the hospital kitchen and adjoining dining room, a flour vault, and a separate 'boiling' kitchen, in which one of the medications, the guaiacum wood potion, was prepared. The barber-surgeon had an extra ointment room, in which he cooked his salves, plasters and potions, and where, once a month, the official public examination took place. Various house regulations from the sixteenth century indicate that there were two other smaller rooms on the ground floor. These were isolation wards for those undergoing treatment (such as mercury fumigation), which was considered injurious to the health of other inmates.

Admissions to the *Blatterhaus* did not differ from those at other municipal health care institutions. As sufferers from outside the city were generally unwelcome, every applicant needed to provide proof of citizen or residential status. The first house rules, dating from 1495, stipulate that 'no one may be taken in who is not a citizen or resident of the city'.[73] If the applicants were maids and servants living outside the city walls but employed by Augsburg burghers and thus entitled to admittance, they had to prove that they 'have served here … and contracted the disease while in service here'. The regulations of 1535 narrowed the admissions criteria further: servants from outside had to have served in the city for at least two years to be accepted.[74] This tightening of the restrictions was designed to prevent victims of the pox being covertly 'brought in from the countryside, cities, market towns and villages outside Augsburg' and hence from enjoying benefits to which they were not entitled.[75] Only in exceptional cases were strangers sometimes accepted, but they had to pay over the odds for the compulsory entrance examination. Until 1581, except in cases where the Alms Office agreed to defray the costs, burghers and residents were charged 1 fl. for the examination. Strangers, however, paid double that until 1581. Thereafter, the

72 See StAA, Blatterhaus, Ordnung von 1581, pag. 38; and StAA, Baumeisteramt, Baumeisterbücher Nr. 153, fol. 124b; StAA, St Martinsstiftung, Karton VII, Nr. 55, Prod. 1–13: Blatterhausrechnungen 1549–1589, 1702–1721, Prod. 55 (3): Zahlungen ins Blatterhaus 1555–1560: 5 Januar 1560. Several sixteenth-century Augsburg chroniclers – such as Hector Mülich quoted in the introduction – talk about even greater numbers of patients. However, Bernd Roeck has drawn attention to unreliability of their accounts when it comes to numbers. See Roeck, *Krieg und Frieden*, pp. 302; 304–5, and in relation to the reliability of Hector Mülich see Mauer, *Augsburger Chronist*, p. 302.

73 For the following see StAA, Blatterhaus, Ordnung von 1494.

74 StAA, Blatterhaus, Ordnung von 1535.

75 There is no evidence that Augburg's gate keepers had specific orders to prevent pox victims from accessing the city as was obviously the case in other towns. These orders existed, however, for times of plague.

cost for outsiders rose to 3 fl.[76] As in other municipal institutions, Catholics and members of the new faiths were equally entitled to admittance.

The sources provide only a fragmentary picture of how the *Blatterhaus* was administered and managed in the first half of the sixteenth century. Until 1581, the year in which it became a financially independent foundation, the *Blatterhaus* had no capital of its own, and in this respect was entirely unlike the private institutions endowed by the Fugger families, as we shall see. Its finances and administration were under the control of various municipal departments and their responsibilities seemed to have changed several times over the decades. From 1496 until 1581 there are records of payments (sometimes substantial) to the *Blatterhaus* from the Public Work Office, the municipal authority that was entrusted with all the city's expenditure.[77] Smaller amounts for the running of the institution sometimes came from private donors, and, after the dissolution of all Church property in the city during the Reformation (after 1537), from the revenues of the dissolved convents of St Martin (Franciscan), St Margretha (Dominican) and St Nikolaus (Benedictine).[78] The council exercised *de facto* supervision, and the Public Work Office provided the lion's share of the necessary funds. But the question of who actually bore responsibility for what went on within its walls is difficult to determine, as it probably was for contemporaries as well. For a time, at least, the guardians of the Hospital of the Holy Ghost seemed to have assumed its management.[79] The lack of transparency in the *Blatterhaus*' finances and administration eventually led to massive confusion, causing not only ongoing disputes among the different civic departments, but also an explosion in running costs.[80] To end these disputes and put the hospital's finances back on an even keel, the council decreed on 22 May 1581 that the entire income of the dissolved convents of St Martin, St Margretha and St Nikolaus 'be handed over to the appointed chief guardians of the plague and *Blatterhaus*, so that from now on the same shall administer and account for

76 StAA, Ordnung von 1581, pag. 38.

77 The city budget and its distribution during the sixteenth century is extremely opaque and confusing. For some details see Ingrid Bátori, *Reichsstadt Augsburg*, pp. 63–4; and Roeck, *Krieg und Frieden* I, pp. 270–99, who tried to reconstruct the city's budget for the year 1606/7.

78 The confiscation of Church property engendered an ongoing struggle between the council and Augsburg's bishop Otto Truchsess von Waldburg, which was only settled in 1551 when the bishop finally agreed to abandon all his earlier demands in return for annual payments from the city. See StAA, Literalien Sammlung, 21. September 1551; see also Roth, *Augsburgs Reformationsgeschichte* II, pp. 19–27. For the role of the bishop and cardinal Otto von Truchsess von Waldburg during the Reformation see Friedrich Zoepfl, *Das Bistum Augsburg und seine Bischöfe im Reformationsjahrhundert* (Augsburg and Munich 1969), pp. 173–463.

79 StAA, Baumeisteramt, Baumeisterbücher 160 (1567), fol. 8a; Nr. 163 (1570, fol. 8a; Nr. 171 (1578), fol. 126b; Nr. 166 (1573), fol. 8a.

80 The exact figure is unknown. StAA, Blatterhaus, Urkunde betreffend die Aufsicht über die Klöster St. Martin, St. Margarethen und St. Nikolaus vom 22. Mai 1581.

them'.[81] As stated in the decree, the two chief guardians were to use the convents' revenues to finance not just the *Blatterhaus*, but also the two municipal plague hospitals. The latter hitherto had always been managed by *Blatterhaus* staff in times of plague, but the costs of caring for plague victims – three or four times as much as in plague-free years – had then been borne entirely by the Public Work Office. Not surprisingly, in times of plague the convent revenues were nowhere near sufficient.[82] Financially overstretched by the upkeep of all three facilities, the chief guardians tried continually to hand back responsibility for the plague hospitals to the Public Work Office, but without success.[83]

Despite the dearth of information on the day-to-day running of the *Blatterhaus*, three management levels can be reconstructed, at least from the 1530s. The highest level was the city council, which ultimately took all decisions relating to the hospital at its weekly council meetings.[84] It bore the overall administrative and legal responsibility, appointing the two guardians, hiring or discharging in-house medical practitioners, the pox father and his wife and other employees. It defined the roles, powers and duties of the individual officials, and laid down behavioural guidelines.[85] From the institution's beginning in 1495, the two council-appointed guardians functioned as an intermediate authority between the city council and the *Blatterhaus* staff. At least until the forced abolition of the city's constitution in 1548 by Charles V, they seem to have been mostly recruited from the guilds, which (until then) dominated the council.[86] They received 3 fl. a year for their service.[87] The earliest insight into their duties is provided by the house rules of 1535, which stipulate that the two in-house medical practitioners and the pox father were directly answerable to the guardians.[88] The pox father settled accounts with them once a week, and once a month he, the physician and the barber-surgeon were required to deliver a report to the guardians on the hospital's finances, 'since it is at the

81 Ibid. As part of this arrangement, the chief guardians were charged with repaying the hospital's debts and those of the three convents.

82 An example for the explosion of costs is the plague of 1563/1564. While the annual costs for the pox house in 1561 and 1562 amounted to 1,442 fl. and 1,475 fl., respectively, they rose steeply to 5,892 fl. in 1563. It was only in 1566 that the expenditures sunk to the pre-plague level. See StAA, Baumeisteramt, Baumeisterbücher, 154 (1561), fol. 126a–b; 155 (1562), fol. 126a–b; 156 (1563), 157 (1564), fol. 126a–b; 158 (1565), fol. 126a–b; 159 (1566), fol. 126a–b; 160 (1567), fol. 126a–b; 161 (1568), fol. 126a–b.

83 For such an unsuccessful attempt see StAA, Blatterhaus, Streit zwischen den Oberpflegern über das Blatter- und Brechhaus und dem Baumeisteramt. For the plague of 1627/28 see Roeck, *Krieg und Frieden* II, pp. 630–52.

84 The meetings took place on Tuesdays, Thursdays and Saturdays at 10 o'clock at the town hall.

85 For the set-up of the city council see Roeck, *Krieg und Frieden*, pp. 239–300.

86 StAA, Reichsstadt, Baumeisteramt, Baumeisterbücher Nr. 97 (1503), fol. 63r; Nr. 98 (1504), fol. 66r.

87 Ibid., Nr. 99 (1505), fol. 80r.

88 For the following see StAA, Blatterhaus, Ordnung von 1535.

pleasure of the guardians that the monies be increased or reduced'. In the first few decades of the *Blatterhaus* the guardians seem to have been directly answerable to the city council for its expenditure, submitting accounts every quarter and getting reimbursed weekly by the Public Work Office.[89] Besides financial administration, the two guardians were responsible for maintaining peace and order.[90] Once a month, in their presence, the pox father read out the house rules in all the wards. Employees and inmates alike could present themselves to the guardians 'free of all fear' and voice any complaints they might have. However, if it was revealed that an inmate made a complaint 'untruthfully', for instance about a hospital employee, the guardians could immediately discharge him or her, or they could be banned from ever returning.

After the establishment of the new constitution in 1548, the responsibility of the two guardians changed. Although they continued to be recruited from the guilds, they were no longer directly accountable to the council for the hospital's affairs, but reported to two chief guardians. The latter were now recruited from the Small Council, which from 1548 was made up exclusively of Augsburg patricians of the Catholic faith. The chief guardians' duties were honorary, and from this point on they took on the mediating role between the council and the *Blatterhaus*. They managed the hospital's income from the dissolved convents' estates, oversaw the collection of taxes and rents, and ruled on matters of jurisprudence.[91] With the deputy guardians now answerable to the chief guardian, the formers' responsibility was reduced to managing the hospital's accounts and internal organisation *in situ*. For these services they continued to receive 3 fl. per annum. This payment remained fixed over decades despite regular requests for an increase from the respective office holders, who claimed that, since it was not enough to live on, they had to continue practising the trades they had pursued before assuming their civic responsibilities.[92]

The burden of practising their profession at the same time as carrying out their civic responsibilities could indeed become a major problem for the two deputy guardians, particularly whenever the plague struck their hometown. The increased workload in the plague hospitals, which they also supervised, often led them to neglect their own trades and get into financial difficulties. In October 1592 the deputy guardians Endriss Fischer and Paul Balthas, the one a tinsmith, the other a leather tailor, complained that after twelve weeks of unremitting labour in the plague houses, they were 'so burdened with work and care that our proper trades

89 StAA, Baumeisteramt, Baumeisterbücher, Nr. 106 (1512), fol. 66r; Nr. 111 (1517), fol. 88r.

90 For the following see StAA, Blatterhaus, Ordnung von 1535.

91 See for example StAA, Blatterhaus, Unvollständige Jahresrechnungen von 1613–1629 der Herrschaft Oberhausen.

92 For one of these complaints see the case of the two deputy guardians Georg Bützel and Jacob Kummer in 1613 see StAA, St Martin, VII, Prod. 8: Supplikation der Unterpfleger Georg Bützel und Jakob Kummer vom 21. Mai 1613.

have been abandoned'. Their guardian salaries, being their only income, could not begin to compensate them either for the extra workload, or for the lurking danger to their health.[93] Balthas stressed that he had often had to call upon his family for help, and that 'my two sons are overtaxed with reckoning and writing'.[94] Fischer and Balthas asked the council for an increase in their pay until the plague died down, and threatened that they would otherwise give up their jobs. To satisfy them and to avoid exacerbating an already hopeless situation, one of the two chief guardians, the patrician Christoph Rehlinger, took up their case with the council. In the end they were granted an additional gulden per week until the plague was over, but no increase in their annual remuneration was contemplated.

The most important requirements for the position were the ability to read, write and do sums – assets that candidates were prone to emphasise 'not without pride' in their application letters.[95] The applicant's denomination was not a consideration for the municipal employers; none of the candidates during our period ever mentioned their faith. The council attached great value, however, to the applicant's lifestyle, which in cases of doubt would be more deeply researched by the chief guardians. A 'perfect' candidate was, for example, the weaver Georg Kaut in 1592. In his application he stressed that he had 'conducted [himself] so well all the days of my life, both in my bachelor and married status, in all honesty and propriety, that I hope none who might wish to complain of me would receive a hearing'.[96] Despite extensive enquiries, the chief guardians seem to have found nothing untoward with the weaver and much to recommend, as he also stressed in his application that he was at ease with calculating and writing, so much so that 'I believe I can, with God's help, fulfil my deputy guardian's duties while continuing to exercise my trade'. Once accepted, generally speaking, a deputy guardian remained in office for life. Those who wished to quit the service prematurely applied to the council for discharge. Georg Kaut, for example, resigned from his office in September 1610, believing he had found a better source of income as a cellar master in the weavers' guildhall.[97]

Everyday tasks in the hospital were not performed by the deputy guardians in person, but by employees specifically engaged for the purpose. Medical treatment and patient care were in the hands of a learned physician and a barber-surgeon

93 For the following case see StAA, St Martin, VII, Prod. 2: Supplikation der Unterpfleger Endris Vischer und Paul Balthas vom Oktober 1592.

94 A couple of years later, in 1602, his son Jeremias applied for his father's position. Ibid., Prod. 5: Supplikation des Säcklers Jeremias Balthas vom 7. Februar 1602.

95 Ibid., Prod. 5: Supplikationen um die Stelle des verstorbenen Unterpflegers Andreas Vischer vom Februar 1602.

96 Ibid., Prod. 5: Supplikation des Webers Georg Kaut um die Stelle des Unterpflegers Andreas Vischer vom Februar 1592.

97 Ibid., Prod. 7: Supplikationen um die Stelle des Unterpflegers Georg Kaut vom Januar 1610.

who were each paid, in 1568, for example, 120 fl. per year.[98] The caretakers, the pox father and his wife, organised the purchase of provisions and allocated daily tasks to the male servant and two maids in his employ.[99] Their expenses were settled with the deputy guardian once a week. To keep the peace in the household and remind the inmates of their rights as well as their responsibilities, the pox father read the house rules in both wards every Sunday. Once a month this was done in the presence of the two deputy guardians. The pox mother supervised the care of the sick, the preparation of meals and the dispensing of the various medicines. In this she was obliged to strictly follow the medical practitioners' instructions. Without their knowledge, she was not allowed to make any alterations to the patients' diet or to the ingredients for the guaiacum potion. Good skills at reading, writing, and calculating were also required by the pox father, together with experience in patient care. Ideally, the couple were to be childless, or of an age where their children had left home, so they might not be distracted by family matters. As with the deputy guardians, the couple's denomination was not considered relevant: at least it is never recorded in applications for the post. The weaver Martin Schlecht, who applied for the position of the pox father in 1558, met all the required criteria: not only had he considerable experience in patient's care but he was also (he claimed) very skilled at reading and writing. Furthermore, 'I and my wife get on well with each other, and have no children other than a son who is married and lives separately'.[100] Another applicant for the same post, Mathes Walz, emphasised that his wife had spent five years nursing patients in the hospital of the city of Nördlingen. Assuring the council that his four children would not present a problem, he notified them of his intention to send out all four to other towns 'where they shall learn a trade, as I have already apprenticed the two eldest, so that none of my children shall hinder or distract me'.[101] A candidate, Lienhart Hieber, claimed that he and his wife Katharina had nursed so many sick and infirm people over the course of more than twenty years that his house could almost be dubbed 'an open hospital'.[102] A few decades later, the bath master Georg Mair, of the local Wall Bath, highlighted his experience in attending and treating the sick when applying to succeed the late Andreas Röckenbach as pox father in 1586. Recommending his wife as an excellent cook, Mair emphasised that 'as a bath master, I know how to be of service to the appointed doctor with surgical dexterity and good advice'.[103] His fellow candidate, Georg Jerer, having no pertinent medical

98 StAA, St Martin, VI, Karton 1, pag. 3, and StAA, St Martin,VIII, Prod. 1, pag. 2: Bestallung des Doctor Daniel Zeller von 1568. His servant received 24 kr. und the apprentice of the barber-surgeon 1 fl. StAA, St Martin, VII, Nr. 55, Prod. 1.

99 For the following see StAA, Blatterhaus, Ordnung von 1535.

100 StAA, St Martin, VII, Nr. 53, Prod. 1: Supplikation des Webers Martin Schlecht von 1558.

101 Ibid., Prod. 1: Supplikation des Mathes Walz.

102 Ibid., Prod. 1: Supplikation des Lienhart Hieber.

103 Ibid., Prod. 2: Supplikation Georg Mair von 1586.

experience to offer, took pains to stress his culinary skills, having worked as a cook for 34 years in the homes of two of the wealthiest men in town, Christoph and Hans Fugger who appended their signatures to his application. However, 'the continuous heat from the fire', explained Jerer, had with time so ruined his eyes that the Fuggers, 'to spare my face, have released me from their service as cook with good will and grace'.[104] Such service in the homes of the socially prominent could boost a candidate's chances. Balthasar Wilden in his application in December 1586, for example, emphasised that he had 'served since my youth those of noble birth and have fulfilled several offices there, and, kind and gracious gentlemen, have no child, but am only married, … especially as regards housekeeping my wife is very competent'.[105] In recommending Balthasar's candidacy the chief guardians underlined that he was not only 'unencumbered with children, and his wife an experienced cook', but that he had sufficient 'experience of accounting, administration and dealings on behalf of aristocratic persons elsewhere'.

Having served members of the Fugger family, the above mentioned Georg Jerer was most probably aware of the family's support of pox victims. At the time of his application for the position of the deputy guardian at the civic *Blatterhaus*, in 1586, the *Holzhaus* at the Fuggerei had been treating pox sufferers for over sixty years.

The *Holzhaus* at the Fuggerei

The years 1523–1524 provide the first evidence of the existence of a French pox hospital in the housing estate built for poor and Catholic Augsburg residents by Jakob Fugger, the so-called Fuggerei (see Figure 2.2).[106] During those years, three houses on the Fuggerei's main street, *Herrengasse* no. 40–41, were extensively refurbished to accommodate pox victims.[107] The name of this institution, the *Holzhaus* (wood house), referred to one of the drugs used there for treatment, the guaiacum wood, introduce to Europe from the New World in the last decade of the fifteenth century.

104 Ibid., Supplikation Georg Jerer vom Dezember 1586.

105 Ibid., Supplikation Balthasar Wilden vom Dezember 1586.

106 The Fuggerei complex with 52 houses was finished in 1523. For details on the Fuggerei see Marion Tietz-Strödel, *Die Fuggerei in Augsburg. Studien zur Entwicklung des sozialen Stiftungsbaus im 15. und 16. Jahrhundert* (Tübingen, 1982); most of the archival documents are reprinted in Josef Weidenbacher, *Die Fuggerei in Augsburg. Die erste deutsche Kleinhausstiftung: Ein Beitrag zur Geschichte des deutschen Kleinhauses* (Augsburg, 1926). For a reprint of the foundation charter from 1521 see Hermann Kellenbenz und Maria von Preysing (eds), 'Jakob Fuggers Stiftungsbrief von 1521', *Zeitschrift des historischen Vereins für Schwaben* 68 (1974), pp. 95–116.

107 For a report by the Fuggerei administrator Georg Handschücher from 11 March 1624 see F.A. 5.2.11., fol. 20v; for the ground plan of the *Fuggerei* Tietz-Strödel, *Fuggerei*, p. 42.

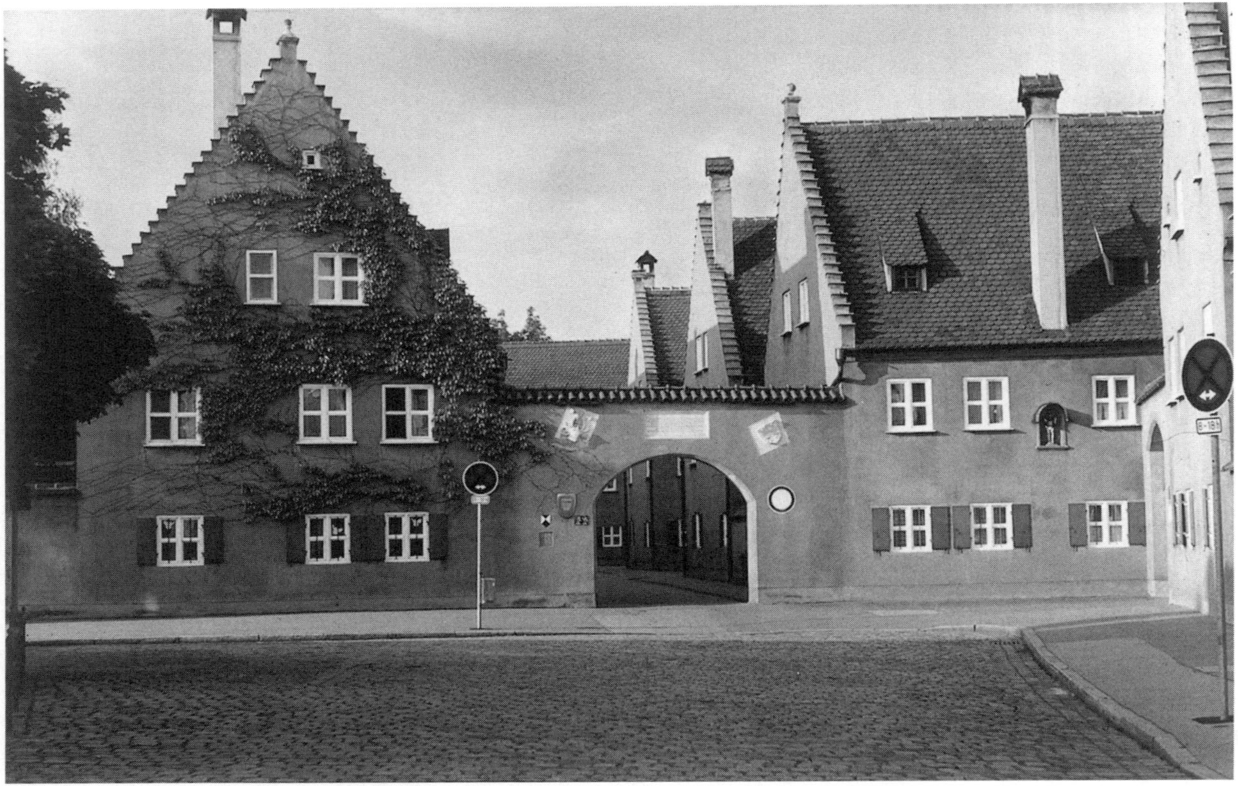

Figure 2.2 The entrance gate of the Fuggerei today. Source: Author

Dividing walls were removed on the first floor to create two large wards with nine beds each, one for male and one for female patients. As in the civic *Blatterhaus*, there were two smaller wards on the ground floor equipped with two beds each in which patients undergoing dangerous mercury cures could be isolated.[108] On the ground floor lived the wood father and his wife. Next to their room was that of the barber-surgeon, where the official entrance examinations took place. On the ground floor we also find the laundry, the kitchen and a bathroom for the patients. The *Holzhaus* garden grew vegetables, herbs and flowers used both in the preparation of ointments and plasters by the barber-surgeon, and the preparation of meals by the caretaker's wife, the wood mother.[109] Unlike other buildings in the Fuggerei, the *Holzhaus* could also be entered by the rear via the garden and the yard. This additional access was probably created out of concern for the healthy residents of the rest of the Fuggerei complex.[110] Although, as shown above, the isolation of pox sufferers was not as strictly observed as that of plague victims, it was still deemed advisable to limit contact with them to a minimum.

We can only speculate as to Jakob Fugger's reasons for founding a French pox hospital, since no letter of endowment has survived. The first surviving house regulations of 1525 indicate that he trusted it would be viewed by contemporaries as an act of Christian charity to take into the *Holzhaus* 'poor folk from other parts who are afflicted with the evil disease of French pox so that they cannot perform their trade or service, nor in any other way earn their livelihood'.[111] Such acts of mercy would serve, the house regulations state, 'to praise the Almighty and help those who are sick to recover their health'. Other considerations have been advanced by the historian Marion Tietz-Strödel. According to her, Jakob Fugger's charitable motivation included the assurance of personal salvation and of continuity of the Catholic faith in an increasingly Protestant environment. Furthermore, she suggested that this charitable deed towards his less successful fellow citizens might have helped to justify to his conscience the enormous financial success of his merchant-banking empire, achieved through and based on new 'capitalist' economic methods. Jakob Fugger applied fierce and for his own time unusual economic strategies, which included money lending as well as the creation of trade monopolies. These activities were deemed unchristian by many of his pious contemporaries, who did not refrain from publicly chastising him.[112] One motivating force, however (not specifically mentioned by Tietz-Strödel, but

108 The sources refer to these rooms as 'F-rooms' (*F Stöblins* = F(rench pox)-rooms). See F.A. 66.2.4. (n), fol. 14v; F.A. 66.2.1., fol. 50v. For the mentioning of the French pox rooms see F.A. 66.2.5. (d), fol. 9r u. 11v (1572).

109 F.A. 66.2.8. (k), pag. 8.(1624). See for a list of plants and herbs bought by the gardener and their use during the year 1581, F.A. 66.2.4. (h), fol. 25r.

110 Weidenbacher, *Fuggerei*, p. 64.

111 Ibid., p. 112.

112 Tietz-Strödel, *Fuggerei*, pp. 29–30; see also Götz von Pölnitz, *Jakob Fugger: Kaiser, Kirche und Kapital in der oberdeutschen Renaissance* (2 vols, Tübingen, 1951),

reiterated in almost all the scholarly literature on early modern Germany), can be safely excluded. I am referring here to the widely known 'fact' that Jakob Fugger founded the pox hospital only to make a profit out of the guaiacum wood on which he allegedly held the trade monopoly. We shall see later on in this chapter that this claim is unsupported by any archival evidence.

Although these different reasons should not necessarily be distinguished from each other, the setting-up of a clearly visible sign or 'bulwark' of the Roman Catholic faith in an increasingly Protestant city was certainly of primary importance for the deeply-devoted Catholic Jakob Fugger.[113] It is significant (given that the Fuggerei was built in what at that time was a predominantly Protestant part of Augsburg) that Jakob Fugger insisted that only Catholic 'women, poor day-labourers and craftsmen and citizens, and inhabitants of this city of Augsburg' should find care and cure in the Fuggerei.[114] Foreign paupers were not explicitly excluded, but only those of Catholic faith could be admitted. All candidates had to prove their denomination and bring written evidence of their last confession from their local priest.

In contrast to the municipal *Blatterhaus*, which accepted patients all year, the private Fuggerei *Holzhaus* was only open during the warmer months of the year (end of March to early November). Therapeutic and financial considerations were among the main reasons for these restricted opening times. As we shall see in Chapter 4, from a medical perspective the warmer months of the year were considered most favourable for the pox cure which included long periods of sweating in heated wards. Firewood became extremely expensive during the course of the sixteenth century. As the *Holzhaus* only had a limited yearly budget at its disposal it thus made not only therapeutic but also economic sense to run it during the spring and summer months in which less heating was required.

The *Holzhaus* was initially financed by funds from the Fuggerei residential endowment. This changed in 1548 due to the separation of property between Anton Fugger (Jakob's nephew and heir), and the sons of his late brother Raymond (1489–1535). It resulted in a restructuring of the joint endowments by the two separate branches of the family, which also affected the legal status and financing of the Fuggerei *Holzhaus*.[115] Anton Fugger and his nephews decided on 31 July 1548 that 17,444 fl. and 21 kr. from the endowment funds of the family church, Sepulchre of St Anna and the Fuggerei, plus a further 2,555 fl. 39 kr. from the Fuggers' general trading and banking business, should be invested in a separate, independent pox

---

vol. 1, pp. 264–6; Hermann Kellenbenz, 'Die sozialgeschichtliche Bedeutung der Fuggerei', *Schwäbische Blätter* 22 (1971), pp. 105–17.

113 Pölnitz, 'Stiftungen', p. 13.

114 Weidenbacher, *Fuggerei*, p. 112.

115 After that date the oldest son of the two family branches, the so-called *Senioren* (seniors), officially lead the various foundations of the family. For the organisation of these foundations see in detail Götz von Pölnitz, Anton Fugger (Tübingen, 1957/71), vol. 2.2, pp. 586–92; p. 814 fn. 203.

hospital foundation. The endowment capital for the *Holzhaus* thus amounted to 20,000 fl.[116] At first – as with all the Fuggers' other endowments – it was a capital endowment with funds being reinvested in the Fuggers' commercial businesses at a fixed interest rate of 5 per cent. In the case of the *Holzhaus*, an annual interest thus accrued of 1,000 fl.[117] Anton and his nephews decided that this sum was to be spent annually on the care and medical treatment of eighteen inmates.[118]

The date of 31 July 1548 also marks an additional endowment by the Fuggers for the Holzhaus consisting of funds from the so-called Veil Hörl foundation. Veit Hörl had worked as the Fuggers' agent in Antwerp. When he died childless on 15 July 1546, it transpired that in his will he had left his entire fortune (17,403 fl. 12 kr.) to his employers, 'to set up a foundation in Augsburg or elsewhere for the support, now and in perpetuity, of the frail and elderly'.[119] Anton Fugger and his nephews agreed to invest 2,000 fl. of this trust's capital 'in the endowment of our common *Holzhaus*', in order to finance the care of two additional patients with the interest.[120] In 1548 the *Holzhaus* Trust's capital thus stood at 22,000 fl. generating annual interest of 1,100 fl. This financed the care of twenty patients. In 1554 the Trust's capital received a further 2,000 fl. from the Veit Hörl fund, although this time the hospital's bed capacity was not extended.[121] The additional capital was needed because after six years the annual interest no longer covered the hospital's running costs. With the extra 2,000 fl., the *Holzhaus* could now dispose of 1,200 fl. per annum.[122]

With the establishment of a separate endowment for the pox hospital, which turned it into a legal entity with its own source of funding, came a change in the stipulations as to who was entitled to the hospital's benefits. In the endowment deed of 31 July 1548, Anton Fugger and his nephews reiterated that Jakob Fugger had established a *Holzhaus* from the proceeds of the Fuggers' banking and merchant business, with the intention of 'allowing to be cured each year a number

116 Weidenbacher, *Fuggerei*, p. 116.

117 F.A. 5.1.1., p. 65. For the changes in the Fuggers' investment strategies see Franz Karg, 'Emersacker im 17. Jahrhundert: Zur Erwerbung durch die Fuggerschen Stiftungen', *Jahrbuch des Historischen Vereins Dillingen* 93 (1991), pp. 391–403.

118 Weidenbacher, *Fuggerei*, p. 116.

119 The Fuggers used the money for various charitable projects such as endowments for poor girls or care for pregnant women. See Hans Liermann, 'Zur Rechtsgeschichte der Fuggerschen Stiftungen', in *Zeitschrift für bayerische Landesgeschichte* 19 (1955), p. 401; Weidenbacher, *Fuggerei*, Anh. 9, p. 116.

120 Weidenbacher, *Fuggerei*, p. 116.

121 Weidenbacher, *Fuggerei*, p. 60, suggested that the hospital accepted 22 patients after that date. According to the account books of the *Holzhaus*, which I consulted, his number is wrong.

122 In the following years the hospital received further endowments from various family members. However, it is difficult to establish the exact amount of money available each year due to peculiar accounting practice. For these see F.A. 66.1.3, fol. 20a–25b; and see Karg, *Fugger*, fn.77.

of strangers, poor sick folk, afflicted with the evil pox'.[123] Anton and his nephews now overrode their uncle's original intention with a request that 'predominantly our, the Fuggers' subjects and tenants and own people in the countryside' be preferred in the admissions process, 'and as long as any of our or our descendants' subjects or villains be in need of such treatment', other French pox sufferers from outside the city should be turned away. In addition, Augsburg citizens afflicted with the pox who had not been specifically excluded by Jakob Fugger were now explicitly barred: 'of the burghers and inhabitants of the city of Augsburg none shall be admitted to this cure'.

The Fuggers' motives in 1548 in excluding the Augsburg citizenry from admission to the Fuggerei *Holzhaus* and allowing only their subjects or those in their employ on their estates preferential access to medical services has been often associated with a supposed shift in the family's self-perception. It has been argued that by the mid-sixteenth century the Fuggers no longer considered themselves as belonging to the Augsburg's patrician elite, but rather as noble landowners.[124] However, Olaf Mörke has suggested that such a clear-cut division between prosperous citizens on the one hand, and land-owning nobility on the other, fails to do justice to the complex social status of the Fuggers. In his view, they represented a *Sonderstruktur* that transcended all the conventional social hierarchies of the period.[125] The lifestyle of a family that originally stemmed from poor artisanal weavers violated the conventions and self-imposed regulations of the traditional society of estates. In the eyes of many of their contemporaries the Fuggers, as internationally operating entrepreneurs and personal bankers of the emperor Charles V, were the personification of the infringement of then widely accepted social hierarchies.[126] The Fuggers were members of the guilds and citizens of an imperial city, yet they completely ignored the many civic and moral codes of behaviour, for instance, the limitations on conspicuous consumption issued by the council for its wealthy burghers. At the same time, as Imperial nobility their

123 For the following see Weidenbacher, *Fuggerei*, p. 115.

124 See von Pölnitz, *Anton Fugger*, vol. 2.2, p. 587; also Liermann, 'Stiftungen', p. 403; and Peter Kriedte, *Spätfeudalismus und Handelskapital: Grundlinien der europäischen Wirtschaftsgeschichte vom 16. bis zum Ausgang des 18. Jahrhunderts* (Göttingen, 1980), p. 76.

125 Olaf Mörke, 'Die Fugger im 16. Jahrhundert: Städtische Elite oder Sonderstruktur?' *Archiv für Refomationsgeschichte* 174 (1983), pp. 141–62.

126 Dana Koutná-Karg, 'Die Ehre der Fugger', in Johannes Burckhard (ed.), *Augsburger Handelshäuser im Wandel des historischen Urteils* (Berlin, 1996), pp. 87–106; Barbara Stollberg-Rilinger, 'Gut vor Ehre oder Ehre vor Gut? Zur sozialen Distinktion zwischen Adels- und Kaufmannsstand in der Ständeliteratur', in Johannes Burkhardt (ed.), *Handelshäuser*, pp. 31–45. For the territories of the Fugger see Robert Mandrou, *Die Fugger als Grundbesitzer in Schwaben, 1560–1618* (Göttingen, 1997), p. 60, map 1; for their aristocratic lifestyle see Klaus Mertens, 'Die Landschlösser der Familie Fugger im 16. Jahrhundert', in *Welt im Umbruch. Augsburg zwischen Renaissance und Barock*, exhibition catalogue (3 vols, Augsburg, 1981) vol. 3, pp. 66–81.

business activities violated and infringed traditional understanding of appropriate sources of aristocratic income. Their immense wealth and political influence overshadowed the Augsburg elites *and* the landowning aristocracy. This peculiar mixture of civic and aristocratic lifestyles matches the Fuggers' dual legal status as 'burghers of Augsburg and estate of the Roman Empire'.[127]

The history of the Fuggerei and the *Holzhaus* trust admission rules reflects, I submit, the Fuggers' increasing awareness of significant changes in their social status as the sixteenth century progressed. Jakob Fugger, himself the offspring of poor rural weavers near Augsburg, donated the Fuggerei and the *Holzhaus* to his less fortunate Catholic 'fellow-citizens', as the stone tablet above the gates of the Fuggerei has testified since 1519 (see Figure 2.2).[128] His nephew and heir Anton, by then in possession of vast territories all over Europe, preferred to play down the 'fellow-citizen' element of his uncle's social identity and to stress instead his patriarchical duty of care as a noble landlord. Nevertheless, the Fuggerei continued to cater to the poor citizens of Augsburg: the public spirit of the burgher and the aristocratic duty of care of one's subjects co-existed peacefully in the Fuggerei and its *Holzhaus*.

The administrative structure of the Fuggerei *Holzhaus* after 1548 was much clearer than that of the municipal *Blatterhaus*. Overall authority was in the hands of the oldest male heirs of each branch of the family, referred to as the two chief trustees, or chief guardians, sometimes also called chief administrators.[129] They were assisted by 'two honourable men', respected members of the ruling elite of the community. This double insurance – of family heirs on the one hand, and burghers connected with the family on the other – was designed, so the charter claimed, to 'sustain the foundation for eternity'. The two trustees appointed an administrator to oversee the *Holzhaus*, 'who shall be present in the house, attend to all needs, and be present at the visits of the doctors, so that the patients' requirements shall be heeded and well served'. The administrator at the same time managed the entire Fuggerei complex. The Fuggers' official on-site representative, he was responsible for good housekeeping and supervised the hospital staff. His letters of appointment committed him to keeping the building in good order and providing 'the poor people in the pox house … with the care and treatment they deserve'.[130] Whenever he 'observed or sensed disorder', for example, if the medical practitioners neglected their duties, he was 'to instruct them accordingly, or otherwise point it out to them without delay, so that through his foresight it can

127 For chronicle see Meyer, *Chronik*, p. 68.

128 Ropertz, *Kleinbürgerlicher Wohnungsbau*, p. 223.

129 For this and the following quotations see Weidenbacher, *Fuggerei*, pp. 115–17. For description of these duties from 1620 see F.A.5.1.10, fol. 110v.

130 F.A. 5.2.1, Bestallung des Verwalters Georg Handschücher vom 30. Mai 1617, fol. 3r.

be averted'.[131] For these duties the first administrator known to us by name, Moritz Kronegger, received 80 fl. in 1549.[132] By 1555 this salary had been increased to 100 fl., by 1619 p.a. to 125 fl. This later sum remained constant until the closure of the *Holzhaus* in 1632, during Swedish occupation of the city in the Thirty Year War.[133] In addition to his salary, the administrator received food, clothing and an annual firewood supply, and lived rent free with his family in a designated house right next to the main entrance of the Fuggerei.[134]

For the day-to-day running of the *Holzhaus*, the administrator appointed a caretaker, the so-called wood father, who (very much like the pox father in the municipal *Blatterhaus*) was required to be married but childless.[135] The duties of the wood father and his wife were also similar to those of the municipal pox father and his spouse, comprising general household and medical tasks such as buying provisions, preparing and administering medicines prescribed by the medical practitioners, and nursing the patients. Two maids and a laundress assisted them. Fortunately, unlike the municipally employed pox father, information about what the wood father was paid has survived.[136] In 1555, for his eight month service during the opening period of the *Holzhaus*, he and his wife received 2 fl. a week, a small portion of which went on food for the maids. When the hospital was closed, as it always was during the colder months of the year, he was allowed to continue to live there and received ½ fl. a week, plus a supply of firewood. As remuneration for their services during the cure period, the maids received 4½ fl. between them and either a pair of shoes or an additional ½ fl. each. Whereas the maids were released during the winter closure and had to find other work in the city, the laundress was employed all year round, being paid 48 kr. a week during the treatment period and 15 kr. a week during the closing period of the hospital.

The administrator paid the salaries of the wood father and the menial staff, as well as those of the in-house physician and barber-surgeon. The appointment of the learned doctor Adolph Occo III (1524–1606) – a prominent member of the new faith who was deeply involved in the city's confessional politics until his

131 F.A. 5.1.2, p. 4, Bestallung des Fuggereiverwalters Moritz Kroneggers vom 1. Oktober 1549, reprinted in parts in Weidenbacher, *Fuggerei*, pp. 117–18. Kronegger was adminstrator from 1537–1580.

132 For the administration of the Fuggerei and its chapel St Anna he received an extra 70 fl. See Weidenbacher, *Fuggerei*, p. 118; for further details on duties and payment see F.A.66.1.1, fol. 47b; F.A.66.1.5, fol. 115r.

133 Weidenbacher, *Fuggerei*, p. 117.

134 Weidenbacher, *Fuggerei*, p. 118. For the location of the custodian's house see Tietz-Strödel, *Fuggerei*, p. 53.

135 For their names see Weidebacher, *Fuggerei*, p. 126. A few names can be added to his list: Michael Gigl (from 1520), Bernhard Hörmann (from 1540), Hans Mair (from 1560), Hans Steger (from 1570), Achaius Kramer (between 1580–1590), Michael Bair (1600), Georg Scheiner (between 1610–1620), Melchior Köllin (between 1630–1647), Hans Neher (after 1647–?), although the Holzhaus was closed since 1632.

136 For the following see StAA, Fuggerei, Ordnung von 1555.

death – indicates that although the Fuggers considered the denominational aspect important in the selection of patients, such factors were of little concern in the choice of their medical staff.[137] Until 1584 the doctor received a total of 100 gold fl. In 1585 his salary was increased to 120 fl., which, considering that he only served during the summer months, was a better salary than that of his colleagues in the *Blatterhaus*.[138] While the doctor received a fixed annual sum, which was paid in full even when – as in 1579 – the treatment period ended earlier than usual, the barber-surgeon was only paid per visit. Strangely, the amount was not listed in the hospital records. We do know that his apprentice was paid 3 fl. a year. Bills for the medicines the barber-surgeon bought for his salves and plasters from the city's apothecaries were settled separately.[139]

The *Holzhaus* on the Goosehill

The Fuggerei *Holzhaus* did not remain the only institution for the treatment of the French pox in Augsburg financed by the Fugger family. In his will, dated 26 July 1560, Anton Fugger set up another 'endowment for poor folk and children' with 28,000 fl. original capital from his own private fortune.[140] From the 5 per cent interest they generated, two hospitals in the *Jakobervorstadt* were financed: the *Holzhaus* on the Goosehill (Gänsbühl), not far from the Fuggerei, and a surgical facility at the Horse Market. These personal foundations were managed exclusively by Anton's branch of the family. Legally the *Holzhaus* and the surgery were regarded as one 'corpius' and never opened at the same time for financial reasons.[141] The surgery at the Horse Market, in which an in-house barber-surgeon treated patients with bladder and kidney stones, hernia, or broken bones, was

137 See StAA, Baumeisterbücher 171 (1578), fol. 136b. On the Occo family see Martz, *Gesundheitswesen*, pp. 16–17; p. 22; and Hans Viktor Bühler, 'Das Ärztegeschlecht der Occo', *Sudhoffs Archiv für Geschichte der Medizin und Naturwissenschaften* 28 (1935), pp. 14–42.

138 Appointed doctors were: 1524–1573 Adolph Occo (F.A. 66.1.1, fol. 47 b; F.A. 66. 1.1, fol. 53b); 1573–1580 Christoph Herberger (F.A. 66.1.1, fol. 54b; F.A. 66.2.4 (g), fol. 43v); 1581–1584 Hieronimus Martius (Mertz) (F.A. 66.1.2, fol. 47b; F.A. 66.2.4 (p), fol. 22v); 1585–1601; Tobias Kneulin (Cneulin) (F.A. 66.2.4 (r), fol. 17v; F.A. 66.2.6(c), fol. 23b); 1602–1621 Johann Ulrich Rummler (F.A. 66.2.6 (e); F.A. 66.1.5, fol. 129a); 1622–1632 Urban Schlegel (F.A. 66.1.5, fol. 138a; 66.2.6 (ii), fol. 24a).

139 Barber-surgeons were: 1563–1573 Hans Tannmiller (F.A. 66.1.1, fol. 49r; F.A. 66.1.1., fol. 54b); 1573–1594 Georg Brendler (F.A. 66.1.1, fol. 53b; F.A. 66.2.5 (n), fol. 27b); 1595–1598 Leonhard Österreicher (F.A. 66.2.5 (p), fol. 29b; F.A. 66.2.5 (u), fol. 28b); 1599–1607 Hans Mendler (F.A. 66.2.5 (w), fol. 28a; F.A. 66.2.6 (o), fol. 35a); 1608–1632 Johannes Brendler (F.A. 66.1.5, fol. 27a; F.A. 66.2.8 (ii)).

140 Preysing/Simnacher, *Fugger Testamente*, pp. 159–61.

141 See F.A.5.3.3, fol. 124a; F.A.5.3.3, fol. 204r; fol. 207v; and F.A.5.1.10.

open from mid-November to Whitsuntide.[142] As soon as the surgery closed, the *Holzhaus* on the Goosehill opened its doors to French pox sufferers.[143] During each hospital's periods of closure, necessary repairs were undertaken to the interior and exterior of the building along with fixtures and fittings.

On 28 May 1586, Anton's son Marx Fugger (1529–1597) added a further 4,000 fl. from his private fortune, raising the share capital to 32,000 fl. As the letter of endowment makes clear, Marx Fugger felt obliged to take this step because 'so many poor diseased people come forward, daily increasing in numbers, that the revenues and interest from the foundation are not sufficient to offer them all help and advice'.[144] Although Anton Fugger had set up the endowment in 1560, and his son Marx had drawn up the first plans for the administration of the institution on 1 September 1568, the *Holzhaus* project did not materialise until 1571, when Marx Fugger bought a house with garden on the Goosehill, close to the Barfüsser gate.[145] Once the remains of earlier building works had been cleared, the construction of this *Holzhaus* finally commenced on 25 June 1571 and was completed by the end of October 1572. The costs of the two-storey stone building came to 2,620 fl.[146] For the interior furnishings, 'with linen, pots, crockery made out of pewter, and copper and wood, also with the tools and equipment of the barber, with kitchen shopping, and also with firewood', the Fuggerei administrator Georg Stegmann, who had supervised the construction work, paid 319 fl.[147] It is more or less possible to reconstruct the room lay-out from three separate sources: a contract of 26 October 1571 between Marx Fugger and the Augsburg carpenter Caspar Hag relating to the interior development of the building; an inventory from 1584; and some of the annual accounts.[148] The entire living area of the house amounted to some 125 square meters. The first floor housed a male and female ward. Next to these two large rooms was a smaller chamber reserved for sick servants and employees of Anton Fugger's family, in accordance with the founders' wishes that such dependents should have a ward of their own and not have to lie with the other patients. On the ground floor was the barber-surgeon's ointment room, which sometimes also catered for male patients undergoing mercury vapour treatment. A mercury treatment room for women on the ground floor was called the women's closet. The wood mother or wood father and her or his spouse lived in a room on

142 F.A.81.1.

143 It did happen, however, that one of the facilities stayed open beyond the fixed closure date due to a high demand for its services. In those years the twin institutions remained closed. See F.A.10, fol. 113v (1639).

144 F.A.88.1.

145 It was purchased from the fisher Hans Ortel (or Oertel) for 600 fl. F.A.88.1; also F.A.5.3.2. (b), fol. 4r.

146 F.A.5.3.2 (b), fol. 1r; fol. 11v.

147 Ibid.

148 For the following see F.A. 88.1.; for the inventory see F.A. 5.3.2. (c), Holz- und Schneidhaus Inventare 1572–1669.

the ground floor next to the kitchen, and there was a small room for a maid. In the garden was a wooden washing bench for the laundress, a bath and a wooden toilet shed, the so-called 'secret place'.

The admission practices of the *Holzhaus* on the Goosehill also mirrored the Fuggers' consciousness of their dual role as 'burghers of Augsburg and estates of the Roman Empire': ten of the eleven beds were available to Augsburg citizens. The eleventh, at the express wish of the founder Anton Fugger, remained exclusively reserved for Fugger family servants and subjects.[149] Last but not least, with these admission rules Anton Fugger (very much like his uncle Jakob) made a clear statement about Catholic resistance to the pace of evangelical reform in Augsburg. Like in *Holzhaus* at the Fuggerei, and, *unlike* in the municipal *Blatterhaus*, Protestants were rejected without exception.

Excursus: Dispelling a Myth

What has been said so far provides the basis to refute one of the most persistent myths in the history of early modern Germany: the monopoly of the Fuggers on guaiacum wood. There is hardly a study that fails at least to mention the hypothesis that the internationally-operating Fuggers, in their unscrupulous pursuit of profit, not only introduced guaiacum to Europe, but secured for themselves a monopoly of the wood's import and sale.[150] This myth originates in the sixteenth century but the early modern story of Fugger's allegedly aggressive promotion of the 'Holy Wood' from the New World remained a tenacious slow-burner throughout the centuries and still haunts today's scholarship.[151] The claim of the medical historian Karl Sudhoff made at the turn of this century is still extremely popular. Sudhoff had argued that the two *Holzhäuser* founded by the Fuggers served a purely promotional purpose: they were designed first and foremost to raise awareness of the New World wonder drug among the citizens of Augsburg and so help to boost sales.[152]

Such claims have persisted in historical scholarship not least because they fit so well with the image of the family that many of the Fuggers' contemporaries

149 F.A.5.3.2 (c), fol.11v.

150 For a recent example see Quétel, *Syphilis*, p. 63, and Grell/Cunningham, *Four Horses*, pp. 260; 261; 268.

151 For a summary of early modern opinions on this topic see Richard Toellner, 'Mattäus Kardinal Lang von Wellenburg und Paracelsus: Zur Polemik des Paracelsus gegen Kardinal Lang und die Fugger', in R. Blaser and H. Buens (eds), *Aktuelle Probleme der Geschichte der Medizin. Verhandlungen des XIC. Internationalen Kongresses zur Geschichte der Medizin* (Basel, 1966), pp. 489–97.

152 Sudhoff, 'Augsburg', pp. 1443–4. He also claims that the early modern literature on guaiacum (much of it was printed in Augsburg) merely served to advertise the Fuggers' monopoly. See Toellner, 'Polemik', pp. 489–97.

held, and which is mirrored in their writing on them.[153] The Fuggers' introduction of new economic practices and methods, not to mention their credit business, monopoly and cartel agreements, hardly made them popular with their pious contemporaries. What is more, the family's share of the papal trade in indulgences and its strict adherence to Catholic doctrine turned them into easy and favourable targets for Protestant critics. Protestant polemics of the time lead to the inescapable conclusion that in godlessness and unscrupulousness no one outdid the Fuggers. Nor were such black-and-white polemics only from the mouths of Protestant theologians. Paracelsus, who dismissed guaiacum as ineffective (and believed mercury a better cure for the pox) joined in the howls of derision, claiming that the family's monopoly of the guaiacum import trade made them directly culpable for the deaths of countless innocent French pox sufferers.[154] To many of his contemporaries, Protestant and Catholics alike, Paracelsus's tirades against the Fuggers had the ring of truth, and many of today's historians are still loath to doubt his assertions. The Fuggers' alleged monopoly of the guaiacum trade is seen as just another instance of the family's legendary opportunism and ruthless exploitation of the hopes, fears and agonies of their contemporaries.

The persistence of these allegations is interesting as it is already some years since this 'myth' was subjected to well-researched critique. Two of the most intimate connoisseurs of the Fuggers' commercial businesses in the sixteenth century, the Fugger archivist Jakob Strieder and the economic historian Hermann Kellenbenz, pointed out that there was no evidence of the Fuggers actually being significantly involved in the trading of the wood, let alone of holding a monopoly of its import and distribution.[155] Admittedly, entries relating to the import of various goods from the Spanish colonies contained occasional references to guaiacum.[156] One of these rare entries is an invoice dated 8 December 1518 for a few pounds of the wood acquired by the Fuggers on behalf of Holy Roman Emperor

153 For the often tense relations between the Fuggers and their contemporaries see Koutná-Karg, 'Ehre der Fugger', pp. 87–106; Stollberg-Rilinger, 'Gut vor Ehre', pp. 31–45.

154 Toellner, 'Polemik', pp. 489–97.

155 Jakob Strieder, 'Die Fugger und die Guajakholzkur', *Dermatologische Wochenschrift* 99 (1934), pp. 888–90; Hermann Kellenbenz, 'Fuggersche Sozialpolitik', in Hans Pol (ed.), *Staatliche, städtische, betriebliche und kirchliche Sozialpolitik vom Mittelalter bis zu Gegenwart* (Stuttgart, 1991), pp. 65–88.

156 For the trade of the Fuggers with the new world see Karl Heinz Panhorst, *Deutschland und Amerika. Ein Rückblick auf das Zeitalter der Entdeckungen und die ersten deutsch-amerikanischen Verbindungen unter besonderer Beachtung der Fugger und Welser* (Munich, 1928); Hermann Kellenbenz, *Die Fugger in Spanien und Portugal: Ein Großunternehmen des 16. Jahrhunderts* (2 vols, Augsburg, 1990); also useful is Mark Meadow, 'Merchants and Marvels: Hans Jacob Fugger and the Origins of the Wunderkammer', in Pamela Smith and Paula Findlen (eds), *Merchants and Marvels: Commerce, Science, and Art in Early Modern Europe* (London, 2002), pp. 182–200.

Maximilian I (1459–1519).[157] However, according to Strieder and Kellenbenz, these purchases, surfacing here and there in surviving invoices and commercial correspondence, represent an utterly insignificant portion of the Fuggers' total volume of trade.[158]

However, what the Fuggers did have an interest in was the sale of mercury: from the mid-1520s they held the lease of estates in the Spanish Maestrazgo region.[159] Charles V had transferred these lands to them as security for the huge sums that Jakob Fugger had invested in his election as Emperor in 1519. Besides grain from these estates, the Fuggers traded in mercury and cinnabar from the Spanish mines of Almaden. Little is known about this import business but one thing is clear: the trade in mercury and cinnabar (products much in demand in various branches of the early modern economy) was much more profitable for the Fuggers than buying and selling guaiacum wood which, at that time, had almost entirely medical uses. Karl Sudhoff's claim that the Fuggers founded their pox hospitals only to advertise the wood and boost its sales is thus hardly convincing.

Moreover, it was shown earlier in this study that the 'miracle drug' from the New World was already well known in Augsburg several years before the first Fugger *Holzhaus* was opened in 1523/24. Treatises on the pox, such as that of Ulrich von Hutten, and various anonymous broadsheets printed in Augsburg and sold for little money on its streets and marketplaces, extolled the benefits of the wood as early as 1518. My research supports Jakob Strieder who, many years ago, challenged Sudhoff's claims.[160] Not only is there no source material to support Sudhoff's thesis, as Strieder argued, but one should also refrain from applying modern criteria when judging the family's motives in establishing their charitable foundations. Above all, the religious convictions of the devoutly Catholic Fuggers need to be weighed as seriously as – and not as subservient to – their supposed economic interests. Both Götz von Pölnitz, biographer of Jakob and Anton Fugger, and Hermann Kellenbenz have argued that one cannot overstate the importance

157 See the invoice dating from 8 December 1518, quoted in Wiesflecker, *Kaiser Maximilian I.* vol. IV, p. 617, fn. 27: '167 fl. rh. für 58 Pfund indianischholtz für die platern ... so die Fugger für ... K[aiserliche] M[ajestät] bezalt hat'. For Maximilian's suffering from the pox see also Arrizabalaga/Henderson/French, *The Great Pox*, p. 225.

158 Some of these occasional purchases are mentioned in Pölnitz, *Anton Fugger*, vol. 1, p. 576, fn. 116, and also in Kellenbenz, *Fugger in Spanien und Portugal*, vol. 1, p. 393, Anm. 731; see also Pölnitz, *Anton Fugger* II, p. 434. In none of the yearly inventories a trade with guaiacum is mentioned. For this see Strieder, 'Guajakholzkur', p. 888; also Kellenbenz, *Fugger in Spanien und Portugal*, vol. 1, p. 393. A phone conversation on 3 December 1995 with the late historian Helmut Driesche, who was then working on the Fugger trade after 1560, confirmed this view. He did not find any documentation in the Fugger trade records that suggested a significant trade in, much less a monopoly of guaiacum either before or after 1560s.

159 For the history of the Spanish Maestrazgos territories and their exploitation by the Fuggers see Kellenbenz, *Maestrazgopacht*, pp. 90–110.

160 Strieder, 'Guajakholzkur', p. 888.

of religious conviction and, deriving from that, a sense of social responsibility to their fellow citizens and subjects as motivating factors in the Fuggers' charitable activities.[161] Though credited with introducing advanced economic methods, the family remained, with regard to their charitable endowments, firmly entrenched in the medieval Catholic tradition of almsgiving. In that context, building hospitals for purely capitalist profit-driven motives would have been unthinkable. Jakob Fugger, in particular, did perceive the increasing marginalisation of the Catholic faith in Augsburg due to the Reformation as a genuine threat to his immortal soul. Towards the end of his life he even felt compelled to abandon the political neutrality which he had tried to uphold throughout his life in order to do all he could to counter the spread of Protestant reform in the city. As previously stated, the construction of the Fuggerei almshouses and the opening of the two *Holzhäuser*, to which only impoverished Catholic pox victims were admitted, should be considered as serious attempts to erect a visible 'bulwark'[162] of the Catholic faith in a predominantly Protestant environment.[163]

The following chapter, which reconstructs the early decades of the civic *Blatterhaus*, will provide further evidence that Sudhoff's claims were unsubstantiated. Guaiacum wood was being administered in the wards of the *Blatterhaus* at least as early as 1522, two years *before* the Fugger's *Holzhaus* in the Fuggerei admitted its first patient. Nor is there anything in the archival records to suggest that the Fuggers were involved in introducing guaiacum into the *Blatterhaus*, or that the wood administered there had been obtained by or from them.[164] As to the Fuggers' guaiacum connection, Götz von Pölnitz's final conclusion drawn from his forty years of archival research remains valid: '[c]ontrary to a more general belief, the Fuggers did not trade in guaiacum wood, but used their worldwide commercial network to meet the requirements of their *Holzhäuser* and supply the wood to the needy free of charge.'[165]

Conclusions

The overview of the institutional landscape of early modern Augsburg has shown that since the turn of the sixteenth century almost all of the city's health care institutions (private- or municipal-run) were specialised in the treatment of

161 Pölnitz, 'Stiftungen', pp. 3–21; Kellenbenz, 'Fuggersche Sozialpolitik', pp. 65–88.

162 Pölnitz, 'Stiftungen', p. 13.

163 For Jakob Fugger's charitable activities see Immenkötter, *Reformation und Parität*, pp. 392–5; also Konrad Häbler, 'Die Stellung der Fugger im Kirchenstreit des 16. Jahrhunderts', *Historische Vierteljahrszeitschrift* 1 (1898), pp. 473–510.

164 There is, however, the possibility that archival evidence of a Fugger trade with guaiacum may be discovered in Archivo General de Indias in Seville. I was unable to check the holdings of this archive for this study.

165 Pölnitz, 'Stiftungen', p. 13.

particular diseases. Thus, contrary to what some historians of medicine have claimed, Augsburg's institutions for pox sufferers were neither exceptional in their strong focus on treatment and cure, nor were they the only ones which specialised in curing a specific physical condition. On the contrary, all three pox hospitals (recent facilities compared to most of the city's other health care institutions) were part and parcel of what one may label an elaborate 'disease-specific' network of hospitals whose administration revealed striking similarities.

The distribution of responsibility for the treatment and care of the human body was the outcome of a long process of negotiation between the different parties involved in the organisation of Augsburg's poor relief system. In these negotiations financial considerations always played an important part. However, Augsburg's institutional landscape would have looked very different without the dramatic changes to its overall structure due to the Reformation, particularly its new radical ideas about charity and almsgiving. The official introduction of the Reformation in 1537 put an end to almost all private or Church-funded health care activities (the Fugger pox hospitals being one of the few exceptions) and led to a concentration of all responsibility for these institutions in the hands of the city council. But not all changes to the city's poor relief can be attributed to reformed ideas. As this chapter has shown, the process of communalisation of poor relief had already begun much earlier, in the mid-thirteenth century.

The foundation of the city's pox hospitals, their specific organisational and administrative structure as well as their medical responsibilities were couched within and shaped by these wider and long-term socio-cultural changes. One result can be stated for certain: although the appearance of the new disease in the city by the end of the fifteenth century was certainly unexpected, it did not account for the many (and often dramatic) changes in the city's public health organisation during the sixteenth century.

Chapter 3
Negotiating the Pox

Identifying the Pox

When the pox reached Augsburg in 1495, the city council responded immediately with the opening of a special hospital for its victims, the *Blatterhaus*. This instant reaction might suggest that the authorities were well acquainted with the disease phenomenon they were trying to contain. However, according to the earliest archival records offering insights into the medical organisation of the new pox hospital, this was not at all the case. In fact, it took over two decades to negotiate the pox's nature and treatment. It was only in the early 1520s that the medical practitioners working in the hospital wards and the municipal authorities in charge of the institution reached an agreement over what the pox was and how it should best be treated. This chapter reconstructs these negotiations over the identity of the pox. By doing so it will link the discussions in the *Blatterhaus* to wider debates over professional duties and hierarchies between two important groups of Augsburg's official healer community, the academic physicians and the city's barber-surgeons. I argue that the agreement reached in 1522 over the nature and treatment of the pox has to be understood in close relationship to the struggles between these two healer groups over the official right and authority to define the human body and control its treatment.

At the first encounter with the disease in 1495, confusion reigned among Augsburg's licensed healers (particularly the city's academic physicians) as to the pox's specific essence and matter.[1] This at least is the gist of a Latin pamphlet published in 1497/98 by two Augsburg doctors, Johann Jung (?–1515) and his son Ambrosius Jung (1471–1534).[2] Both stressed, however, that they were not alone in their predicament. Even for their most eminent German and Italian colleagues, they claimed, the nature of the 'Mal de francoß' was a total mystery,

---

1 For the debate in Germany see Roger French, 'The Arrival of the French Disease in Leipzig', in Neithard Bulst and Robert Delort (eds), *Maladies et société XIIe–XVIIIe siècle: Actes du colloque de Bielefeld, novembre 1986* (Paris, 1979), pp. 133–41; Stein, 'Leipziger Ärztestreit, pp. 215–33.

2 For the reprint of the memorandum see Karl Sudhoff, 'Syphiliserfahrung zweier Augsburger beamteter Ärzte, Johannes und Ambrosius Jung in den Jahren 1497 und 1498', *Pharmazeutische Monatshefte* 4 (1923), pp. 142–3. Both men were members of Augsburg's ruling and social elite due to their marriage to local patrician women. For more information see Martz, *Gesundheitswesen*, pp. 18–20; Josef Fleischmann, 'Die Ärztefamilie Jung', *Lebensbilder aus dem bayerischen Schwaben* 4 (1955), pp. 14–25.

although its signs and symptoms – nasty suppurating sores and fetid exhalations – were similar to those of scabies and leprosy. But as no one could pronounce on it with certainty, academic physicians everywhere erred on the side of caution when it came to suggesting treatment. Sadly, however, the Jungs reported, the prudent treatment they advised did not go down well with those suffering from the pox. In Augsburg, as elsewhere, pox victims were desperate for a cure and, instead of waiting patiently until doctors had agreed on one, the Jungs continued, many sought relief in the mercury salve from Italy that was touted by unqualified quacks.[3] These 'empirici', as the two learned doctors disparagingly labelled the itinerant healers, knew absolutely nothing about the internal workings of the body and were therefore totally unable to decipher the invisible 'universalia' behind the sensible and outwardly signs of the disease. They distributed their expensive ointment without considering the age, sex, or complexion of the sufferer and how his or her individual lifestyle might affect the course and outcome of the disease. This ignorance 'of course' triggered dire and often fatal consequences: Drs Jung claimed to have witnessed a great number of pox victims dying miserable deaths as a direct consequence of unprofessionally administered mercury cures.

The Jungs's colourful description of the alleged therapeutic chaos after the arrival of the pox in their hometown was not simply convenience to gloss over their own indecision and professional impotence. As we have seen in Chapter 1, learned physicians such as them perceived their healing task primarily as an intellectual activity. Despite the growing importance of hands-on subjects, such as anatomy in medical faculties all over Europe, the study of medicine was still predominantly a matter of books and intellectual debate. With a comprehensive knowledge of the relevant ancient medical texts, and training in Aristotelian logic, rhetoric and natural philosophy, university-educated physicians believed themselves equipped to interpret the inner secrets of the human body and to unveil the complicated relationship between physical signs, disease, and its causes. Moreover, archival sources reveal that their Augsburg customers expected them to take into account the manifold interrelations between their bodies and the wider surrounding macrocosm, especially the astrological influences on disease causation and its possible outcome. Hence academic medical practitioners, such as the Jungs, seriously believed that not knowing the invisible and hidden causes of disease would put their patients at risk. In the case of the pox, this fear was even more acute given the absence of ancient medical texts on which to fall back. Johann and Ambrosius Jung firmly understood that without such ancient knowledge and guidance they were gambling recklessly with lives. Their efforts to discredit the mercury cures of their 'empirical' competitors were thus, at least to a degree, well intentioned, and not simply driven by professional competition.

Dire warnings about the use of mercury were scarcely news to their readers, however. As Chapter 1 has shown, since classical times the metal's pernicious side-affects were well-known and feared by practitioners and patients alike.

3 For the ingredients of the salve see ibid., p. 143.

Nevertheless, mercury treatment was extremely widespread in sixteenth-century medical practice. It was used for all kinds of disorders manifesting themselves on the skin by university-trained and artisanal healers alike. Thus, when Drs Johannes and Ambrosius Jung concluded their treatise by trumpeting their own 'tried and tested' therapy, it probably surprised no one to discover that it was none other than a mercury ointment, albeit, however, one that could *only* be administered under the strict supervision of a university-trained physician.

In any case, the Jungs's attempts to discourage Augsburg pox victims from using the services of allegedly dangerous 'empirici' were doomed to failure. In 1495, when the *Blatterhaus* admitted its first patients, the authority of the academic physician in the matter of the pox was by no means established. Indeed, when the council opened the hospital that year, it did so without the benefit of any 'learned advice'.[4] The first *Blatterhaus* inmates were treated by a 'doctor' (*arzet*), but the archival sources suggest that he was a practitioner with an artisanal background.[5] In any case his influence on the daily running of the hospital in 1495 was slight compared to the caretaker of the institution, the so-called master of the infirm (later referred to as the pox father).[6] As the direct representative of the civic authorities, he had full authority over the daily running of the institution, its staff and inmates.[7] His influence extended even to the control of the patients' diets, which two decades later would fall to the medical practitioners. The master collected payment for board of 1 fl. from each new inmate, and asked them what they 'desired to eat or drink'. As long as their wishes remained within the budget, the master's wife would prepare their meals. It seems that in the early years of the hospital no one thought of even consulting a medical practitioner as to whether the foodstuffs chosen by a patient were compatible with his or her individual diseased state. While it is unknown if the inmates were examined by the medical practitioner before admission, he had at least some say in their discharge. The rules of the *Blatterhaus* stipulated that a patient was to stay in the hospital 'for as long as the doctor and the master of this house allow'.[8]

It may have been the prevailing confusion about the nature and causes of the pox that initially discouraged the council from engaging a full-time in-house

---

4 In sixteenth-century Spanish pox hospitals it was common to first appoint academic doctors and only later barber-surgeons. See María Luz López Terrada, 'El Tratamiento de la sífilis en un Hospital renacentista: La sala del mal de siment del Hospital General de Valencia', *Asclepio* XLI 2 (1989), pp. 19–51.

5 For this see Karl Sudhoff, 'Vorsorge für die Syphiliskranken in Würzburg und Augsburg zu Ende des 15. und bis ins zweite Viertel des 16. Jahrhunderts', *Dermatologische Wochenschrift* 97 (1933), p. 1436.

6 The following is based on StAA, Blatterhaus, Ordnung von 1494.

7 He was, for instance, allowed to expel disobedient patients from the hospital without permission from the council.

8 StAA, Blatterhaus, Ordnung 1494.

medical practitioner at the *Blatterhaus*.[9] Instead, they employed several healers at any one time and paid for each successful individual treatment. A cure was considered a 'success' if the patient recovered health sufficiently to leave the hospital unaided, and was able to take up an occupation to provide for his or her living. The healer Bernhart Mayr, who was hired in 1499, built up a particularly impressive 'track record' and received ½ fl. for every such 'cure and discharge'. The council also reimbursed him for medication he produced by himself, such as an unspecified 'ointment' (which probably contained mercury) and some kind of 'dab water'.[10] French pox specialists like Mayr kept only a loose connection with the *Blatterhaus* and were by no means obliged to devote their energies and expertise exclusively to its inmates: they were allowed (and even encouraged by the council) to treat pox sufferers all over the city, sometimes even at the council's expense. And the authorities had every reason to rely on Mayr's expertise: in the course of only six months he restored the health of 143 people (43 of them outside the *Blatterhaus* at their private homes) to the extent that they could rise from their sickbed as 'cured'.[11]

But it is not only men who appear in the hospital records as successful pox healers. On 11 November 1499 the hospital guardian Hans Pfefferlin paid an unspecified female healer who had cured twenty people and, like her male colleague Mayr, received ½ fl. per cure, e.g. a total of 10 fl.[12] Moreover, Pfefferlin's own sister specialised in the treatment of the pox. On 8 February 1500 he paid her 15 fl. for curing thirty patients and a further advance payment of 16 fl. 'for treating all those who, God willing, may soon be discharged'.[13] But the engagement of independent female healers in the municipal pox house was to be short lived; by 1500 they had all disappeared from the records.

It was also in the spring of 1500 that the Public Work Office's accounts records indicate for the first time learned physicians and barber-surgeons in full-time municipal employment. The council then also engaged its first full-time pox specialist for the *Blatterhaus*.[14] Their choice was Johannes Wurzel from Friesland, a practitioner with an artisan background who was paid 26 fl. per quarter.[15] Wurzel's influence on the hospital's running was still rather limited, for although he was now the only healer with a yearly salary, the council did not rely exclusively on

9 The following is based on Karl Sudhoff, 'Augsburg', pp. 1431–45. He reported in this article that the archival material describing the early years of the *Blatterhaus* was kept in two folders in the Augsburg town archive. These folders are now lost.

10 Sudhoff, 'Augsburg', p. 1435.

11 Ibid., p. 1436.

12 Female healers were also employed in the pox hospitals of Ansbach and Munich. See Karl Sudhoff, 'Syphilis und Pest in München am Ende des 15. und zu Anfang des 16. Jahrhunderts: Eine Urkundenstudie', *Münchner Medizinische Wochenschrift* 60 (1913), p. 1339.

13 Sudhoff, 'Augsburg', p. 1437.

14 StAA, Baumeisteramt, Baumeisterbücher, Nr. 95 (1500/1), fol. 54r.

15 Sudhoff, 'Augsburg', p. 1437.

his abilities. It continued to call on the service of a number of other non-academic practitioners.[16] When exactly, and why, the town council began to officially employ physicians with a university degree in the *Blatterhaus*, in addition to local barber-surgeons and itinerant practitioners like Mayr or Wurzel, is unknown. But the archival records make reference to two academic doctors and three barber-surgeons who worked there sometime before the hospital's reorganisation in the early 1520s.[17] However, as the continuous disputes over authority and suitable treatment indicate, the two learned physicians did not exercise any dominant influence on the way their artisanal colleagues went about their work. No agreement on how to cure the patients was reached, and the arguments usually resulted in each practitioner simply following his own experiences and preferences. They each purchased their own medicines and administered them in the way they wished without consulting the other.[18]

In an attempt to resolve the simmering disputes and, above all, to reduce the costs of medication, the council canvassed the opinion of four learned physicians in 1521. The request is connected with the more general discussions in the council about reorganising the city's poor relief at this time. The four physicians, who included Ambrosius Jung (1471–1534), his brother Ulrich Jung (1478–1539),[19] along with Johann Trenklin (?–1533)[20] and Sigmund Grimm (c. 1480–1532),[21] were already in the full-time employ of the city as physicians and worked in various health care institutions. Grimm and Trenklin also treated patients in the *Blatterhaus*.[22] Who were these men and what were they suggesting?

Through marriage, all four doctors were members of the city's social and political elite. This was by no means unusual. Marriages between learned physicians (many of whom were not born in Augsburg and did not come from prosperous backgrounds) and daughters of patrician families became increasingly common during the sixteenth century.[23] They are indicative of the respect and social status accorded to academically-trained physicians among the city's elite and simultaneously served to strengthen the doctors' prestige and influence in the

16 Ibid., p. 1438.

17 StAA, Blatterhaus, Ordnung von 1522.

18 Ibid.

19 For Ulrich Jung see Reinhard, *Augsburger Eliten*, p. 400.

20 He held this position until his death in 1533. See StAA, Baumeisteramt, Baumeisterbücher, Nr. 111 (1517), fol. 113r; Nr. 127 (1533), fol. 103r. See also Martz, *Gesundheitswesen*, p. 21.

21 For more information on this interesting character see Ernst Theodor Nauck, 'Dr. Sigmund Grimm – Arzt und Buchdrucker zu Augsburg', *Zeitschrift des Historischen Vereins für Schwaben und Neuburg* 60 (1969), pp. 311–19; Martz, *Gesundheitswesen*, p. 21. For Grimm's publishing activities see Künast, *Buchdruck*, pp. 66–70; also StAA, Baumeisteramt, Baumeisterbücher, Nr. 101–24 (1507–1530).

22 For the full list of medical practitioners in city employ see StAA, Baumeisteramt, Baumeisterbücher, Nr. 115 (1521), fol. 93r–v.

23 See the list of doctor's wives in Martz, *Gesundheitswesen*, p. 62.

city. The social network and marriage strategies of Augsburg's physicians have not been fully researched, but it is safe to assume that marrying into politically influential families enhanced their impact on the city council's decision-making in all areas of public health.

The four doctors' written reply to the council bears some similarities to the memorandum of Ambrosius Jung and his father from 1497/8. It contained dire warnings about the improper use of mercury salves, advising that its use would be unlikely to bring about a cure. In fact, they warned, incidences in the municipal *Blatterhaus* proved all too clearly that it did harm the patients: 'It is also our opinion in regard to the *Blatterhaus* that so many people there are dying and that their illnesses prolonged through the salve. We have considered and taken into account all this and came to the conclusion that this salve is a great destruction for the sick people.'[24] Whether the scenario of pox victims dying agonising deaths from mercury poisoning matched the reality in the hospital wards is open to question. What is significant, however, is that, unlike Johann and Ambrosius Jung two decades earlier, the foursome now appeared to have knowledge of an alternative to mercury treatment. Where this sudden certitude came from is unknown. It is likely that Johann Trenklin's experience in treating the pox, which he had gained during his studies at various Italian universities, was helpful when composing their response. Italy, particularly the medical faculties of Ferrara and Bologna (both cities in which Trenklin had studied), were important centres of the early debates on the new disease and also established specialised hospitals for its treatment.[25] The four physicians informed the city council that they knew a 'safe, effective and less harmful method' to treat the pox. This, they promised, would not only help patients 'being restored to health without violence to their natures', but, moreover, would cost the council much less than other cures. As to the details of this wondrous alternative therapy, the physicians kept their counsel in their written reply: but should the authorities be interested, they would of course be ready to reveal further details. The council took the bait. Always concerned to find ways of reducing costs in one of the civic institutions, it was quick to show interest in the so-called 'miracle cure'.

What was revealed by the four doctors obviously persuaded the council; according to the *Blatterhaus* rules from 1522 the 'miracle cure' was introduced. In the rules the council also lifted the veil of mystery in which the four physicians had shrouded their alternative cure. For some time, the rules state, 'with the aid and involvement of the physicians and some barber-surgeons', guaiacum wood had been used with positive results in the *Blatterhaus*, convincing the resident medical staff of its effectiveness.[26] In the unanimous opinion of the learned physicians, the rules continue, the 'wood had been fruitful and effective', far surpassing the

24 Quote in Hoffmann, 'Bäder', p. 28; also in Gensthaler, *Medizinalwesen*, p. 51.

25 For the Italian debate see Arrizabalaga/Henderson/French, *The Great Pox*, pp. 56–87.

26 StAA, Blatterhaus, Ordnung von 1522.

results achieved by all other medicines to date.[27] This apparent success, the rules conclude, convinced the council that henceforth all *Blatterhaus* inmates were to be treated first and foremost with guaiacum wood.[28]

But the council's interference in the running of the hospital did not end there. The standardisation of treatment had an immediate bearing on the number of practitioners employed in the hospital: why continue to pay so many of them for their individual favourite therapies when it was now proven that a miracle cure was available which 'could help the poor patients more effectively than any cure before'?[29] Since purchasing the wood had added considerable costs to the hospital's expenditure, it seemed only prudent to the council that the number of healers be reduced from five to two – a learned physician and a barber-surgeon – employed full-time. Although there were fewer practitioners working on the pox wards, their influence on the daily routine was now significantly enhanced. For the first time, the house rules of 1522 installed them at the head of the staff hierarchy. The entire hospital routine was strictly tailored around the two daily visits of the appointed 'medical 'team'. Also regulated for the first time was the relationship between the practitioners and their areas of expertise. Each was expected to perform different, if complementary, tasks.[30] The visible outer body of the pox victim was the exclusive domain of the barber-surgeon: he examined lesions and ulcers, and cleaned and dressed them; he also purged, applied leeches, administered enemas, and drew blood. He administered the dangerous mercury ointment, and, if necessary, amputated pox-infested body parts. The university-trained physician focused only on the inner body. With his knowledge of ancient medical authors and Aristotelian natural philosophy he was to decipher the hidden, invisible 'universalia' of the sick body.[31] Employment contracts at the *Blatterhaus* also show that the physicians' learned knowledge and university degrees put them in charge of the rest of the staff. The far less-well-paid barber-surgeon was, for example, not allowed to perform any of his services without the explicit consent and under the supervision of the learned physician.[32] But it was not only the barber-surgeon whose activities were controlled by the much better paid physician. In

27 For the 'testing' of new drugs from the Americas in sixteenth-century Spain see Barrera, 'Global Medicine', pp. 163–81.

28 Since 1522/23 the *Blatthaus* account registers the purchase of substantial amounts of the wood. StAA, Baumeisteramt, Baumeisterbücher, Nr. 118 (1523), fol. 92r.

29 For following see StAA, Blatterhaus, Ordnung von 1522.

30 Gianna Pomata and Hal Cook observed a similar division of labour in regard to the human body among the healer communities of early modern Bologna and London. See Pomata, *Contracting a Cure*, p. 128; Harold J. Cook, 'Good Advice and Little Medicine: The Professional Authority of Early Modern English Physicians', *Journal for British Studies* 33 (1994), pp. 1–31

31 See, for instance, StAA, St Martin, VII, Nr. 50, Prod. 1: Vertrag Daniel Zeller vom 19. November 1562.

32 See, for instance, StAA, St Martin, VII, Nr. 50, Prod. 1: Vertrag Meister Hans Gablinger vom 14. August 1562.

fact, from the 1520s, the entire daily organisation of the *Blatterhaus* was arranged and closely monitored by the learned physician. He did not only preside over the physical examination but also determined the treatment as well as the daily dietary intake allocated to each inmate. Absolutely nothing, not even the opening times of the ward windows to let in fresh air, could be altered by anyone *without* the doctor's explicit knowledge and consent.

Negotiating Professional Boundaries

Administrative and particularly financial considerations were certainly important factors that influenced the council in 1522 to reorganise the daily affairs of the *Blatterhaus*. However, these interests alone, I argue, do not adequately explain why the council suddenly decided to rely almost exclusively on the judgement of the appointed learned physician in all questions concerning the institution's organisation. In the following section, I show that the increasing power of the learned physician over treatment in the *Blatterhaus* parallels a wider development on Augsburg's medical marketplace, namely the attempt of the group of academic physicians to gain control over all the other healer groups. In fact, I argue, the reorganisation of the *Blatterhaus* in 1522 represents the first visible success of the Augsburg's learned physicians in this regard. Their aim was fully achieved in 1582, when the city council founded the board of health, the *Collegium Medicum*, over which they presided.

The first initiatives of Augsburg's doctors in gaining control over all other licensed and un-licensed healer groups can be detected as early as the beginning of the sixteenth century. After then, they began drawing the council's attention to alleged failings in the city's health care organisation, while at the same time putting forward proposals of their own suggestion how to remedy it. Although at that time the learned doctors, as yet, had no official representation, they never acted as individuals, but always promoted their interests as a unified body. The professional unity they exhibited to the outside world was, as we shall see, a crucial aspect of their future success. Probably it was also one of the reasons why the council increasingly relied on them as equal and competent partners in all questions related to public health, illustrated by the growing employment of learned doctors in municipal posts from 1500 onwards. Whenever a question arose about the health of the city population, the magistrate sought learned medical advice, and was increasingly inclined to act upon it.[33] The discussions over the organisation of the *Blatterhaus* are an early example of this cooperation between

33 But the council did not follow them blindly. There are many examples in which the magistrate played off all the different healer groups (licensed and unlicensed) against each other. See Claudia Stein, 'The Function of the Quack as a Means of Group Distinction in the Medical Community of Sixteenth-Century Augsburg – Preliminary Thoughts', *Ludica, annli di storia del gioco*, 5–6 (2000), pp. 192–200.

the city authorities and the learned physicians. Another was their joint effort in the struggle to control the plague in 1521–1522. This scourge reached Augsburg in spring 1521 and was one of the worst outbreaks the city was ever to experience. The official figure for the dead was 2,698 in the summer of 1521 alone. It was largely due to the efforts of Ambrosius and Johann Jung, Leopold Trenklin and Sigmund Grimm that the plague houses inside and outside the city walls were erected by the end of that year. In a joint letter in which the four doctors laid out in detail their medical opinions on and how to best treat and prevent the plague from spreading further, they urged upon the council the necessity of housing the victims outside the walls to prevent its spread among the healthy population.[34]

All the official petitions reflect the authors' strong solidarity and conformity with the principles of ancient Hippocratic-Galenic medicine. Preserving the classical medical canon was one of their declared aims throughout the sixteenth century and stood at the core of their official representation, the *Collegium Medicum*, in 1582. Less orthodox, and more controversial medical and natural-philosophical ideas and practices, such as those advanced by Paracelsus, were firmly rejected by the majority of Augsburg's learned doctors. Paracelsus's questioning of some of the basic tenets of ancient medicine, such as the doctrine of the four humours, found little acceptance, and deliberate attempts were made to obstruct the dissemination of his ideas.[35] One of the victims of these efforts was the civic physician Wolfgang Thalhauser (?–1546). Thalhauser knew Paracelsus personally and was very receptive to his ideas.[36] When Paracelsus's *Die Grosse Wundarzney* was published in Augsburg in 1536, Thalhauser wrote a favourable foreword, aligning himself with Paracelsus's warnings of the decline of medicine and welcoming his efforts to bring about a general reform of medical practice.[37] Thalhauser's colleagues, however, took this as a personal and professional attack and forced him to publish an official apology. His foreword was omitted from later editions.[38] The treatise, *Conclusiones et Propositiones Universam medicinam*, published in 1538 by the civic physicians Ambrosius Jung, Adolf Occo II (1494–1572), Johann Tieffenbach (?–1548), Gereon Sailer, Damian Behem, Bernhard Schludi (?–1566) and Johann Vogt, left no room for doubt how little foothold Paracelsian ideas found among Augsburg's

---

34 See StAA, Collegium Medicum, Ordnungen und Decreta, 1525–1804, Nr. 2.

35 Hammond, *Civic Health Care*, pp. 105–9. For the spread of Paracelsian ideas in Augsburg see ibid., 'Paracelsus and the Boundaries of Medicine In Early Modern Augsburg', in Gerhild Scholz Williams and Charles Gunnoe (eds), *Paracelsian Moments* (Kirksville, 2002), pp. 19–33

36 For the Thalhauser affair see Joachim Telle, 'Wolfgang Thalhauser: Zu Leben und Werk eines Augsburger Stadtarztes und seinen Beziehungen zu Paracelsus und Schwenkfeld', *Medizinhistorisches Journal* 7 (1972), pp. 1–30.

37 For the foreword see Sudhoff, *Hohhenheim*, vol. 10, pp. 12–14.

38 Telle, *Thalhauser*, pp. 8–10.

academic healers. The authors assured their readers that they would never deviate from the teachings of Hippocrates and Galen, and they explicitly warned against the use of all chemical remedies (favoured by Paracelsus), describing them as extremely reckless and life-threatening for every patient.[39]

The increasingly close professional cooperation between council and learned physicians allowed the latter ample opportunity to display their medical opinions and beliefs in public. This was no doubt aided by the doctors' intimacy with the city's social and political elite. The dexterity with which academic physicians like Gereon Sailer took advantage of their family ties to pursue their own professional objectives can be observed in the regulation of midwifery. During the early 1520s, through intensive lobbying, the doctors had already acquired the right to be consulted in the midwives' examinations process. Their influence was indirectly extended when, in 1531, the municipal midwives were brought under the control of four patrician women who supervised the midwives' work, informing the council of any malpractice and other punishable offenses. The social profile of these women is revealing: not only were they members of the Augsburg patrician elite, but many of them were married, as in the case of Gereon Sailer's wife Felicia, to learned physicians.[40] That Sailer authored several petitions regarding the effective reorganisation of midwifery – of course under his own and his colleagues' auspices – hardly comes as a surprise.

However, the physicians' increasing control over other official healer groups in the city was not only helped by their family relations: they were also quick to exploit the ongoing disunity among their most serious competitors, the bath masters (*Bader*) and barbers (*Barbiere*) (the city's licensed practitioners of external surgery). In Augsburg, in contrast to other cities, barbers and bath masters were organised in one craft, and not in a guild. This particularity excluded them from government representation and made it thus difficult for them to exert influence on the council's decision-making in questions concerning the organisation of the city's health care. Over the course of the sixteenth century they were joined by a new group of practitioner, the barber-surgeons (*Wundärzte*). Unlike the bath masters and barbers, who managed the city's bathhouses, cut hair, shaved, performed bloodletting, and treated minor external injuries, the barber-surgeons went through a longer training process and dealt with more serious surgical cases, such as broken bones, bladder and kidney stone problems, hernia operations or amputations. The lack of a clear distinction between all these different groups triggered bitter disputes throughout the sixteenth century. While these internecine rivalries crippled concerted effort to secure common goals, they were more than welcomed by the learned physicians who immediately exploited this power vacuum and attempted to increase their influence over this branch of

39 Gensthaler, *Medizinalwesen*, pp. 95–7; also Künast, *Buchdruck*, p. 206.

40 Since 1524 the candidates for municipal office were examined by two midwives and an academic doctor. For more detail on Augsburg's midwives see Hammond, *Civic Health Care*, pp. 98–101.

medical services in the Augsburg.[41] Their particular focus was the group of barber-surgeons whose activities the physicians' aimed at defining and regulating. The overall aim was to clearly separate the barber-surgeon's medical activities from their own. The ancient distinction of the human body into an inner and outer sphere was the guideline learned physicians followed in seeking to reserve all treatments of the inner body for themselves. The barber-surgeons, so the doctors wished and were never wearied of stating in public, should only be allowed to deal with treatments related to the outer body.

In daily medical practices a neat distinction between the inner and outer body was of course difficult, if not impossible, to maintain. The body's blurred boundary gave rise to continuous disputes between the two groups as the hundreds of official complaints to the city council surviving in the archive reveal. Were, for instance, barber-surgeons permitted to administer inner purgatives, or even bleed in emergency situations without the supervision of a learned physician? These questions of professional responsibility and authority over the human body were, in the long run, resolved in favour of the academic physicians. Though the barber-surgeons had hitherto performed inner medicine under their own auspices, from 1532 they were forbidden to do so by council decree.[42] Further edicts during the following decades confirmed that barber-surgeons could only administer such medicines 'as are necessary to cure falls, stabs, gangrene, gunshot and in summa all which are necessary to cure other external injuries such as open sores, ulcers, boils belonging to the domain of surgery'.[43] But even these activities could only be performed in the presence of a learned physician. The grounds for this injunction – which, needless to say, was enforced on the initiative of the learned physicians[44] – were that the barber-surgeons, having had only practical training, allegedly understood nothing of the hidden causes and manifestations of many diseases and 'even less of the nature of the human temperament and the operations and qualities of many medicines'.[45] Only the learned physicians, on account of their many years of university training, possessed the requisite knowledge of the secret, invisible processes in the microcosm of the body. Only they, therefore, were in a position to recognise and interpret the eternal 'universalia' that lay behind the mere physical symptoms and signs, hidden in the body. And it was solely on the basis of that

41 For this see Hoffmann, 'Bäder', pp. 21–3; also Ecker-Offenhäuser, *Franzosen*, pp. 50–55. Hammond, *Civic Health Care*, 74–5; pp. 166–80.

42 StAA, Collegium Medicum, Ordnungen und Decreta, 1625–1804, 4. Juni 1532; Hoffmann, 'Bäder', 29.

43 StAA Reichsstadt, Zünfte, Akten, Kt. 4, Fasc. 1, Supplikation der Barbierer und Bader vom 8. April 1568.

44 StAA, Collegium Medicum, Ordnungen und Decreta, 1525–1804, 4. Juni 1532; Hoffmann, Bäder, 29; Gensthaler, *Medizinalwesen*, pp. 78–80.

45 StAA Reichsstadt, Zünfte, Akten, Kt. 4, Fasc. 1, darin: Gegenbericht vom 22. April 1568 der Doktoren Adolph Occo II., Achilles Pirmin Gassner, Leopold Drinkel, Lucas Stenglein, Christopf Heuberger, Marcus Wind, Jeremias Martius und Adolph Occo III. auf die vorangegangene Supplikation der geschworenen Wundärzte vom 8. April 1568.

knowledge, the physicians concluded, that a suitable treatment could be devised for a patient, which did no harm but corresponded to his or her individual nature. In response to the barber-surgeons' appeal against the extension of the ban in 1568, the physicians fulminated that it was heinous in the extreme that these artisanal practitioners claimed to have as much knowledge of the workings of the body as they.[46] And it was downright 'impudent' of the barber-surgeons to borrow academic usage in calling their ridiculous practical tests 'examinations', like those that the doctors underwent at university, when all that these 'examinations' consisted of was 'cupping, bleeding, and concocting plasters and ointments'.[47]

The learned physicians were exaggerating on this point. The barber-surgeons' day-to-day practical dealings with the human body, and their surgical interventions in particular, required a solid knowledge of human anatomy and the body's humoral economy. Nor were the 'examinations' that barber-surgeon apprentices had to pass (in front of the committee of local masters) restricted to concocting ointments. They were not only required to demonstrate delicate surgical skills, but also had to answer questions about the use and effects of mineral and plant-based medicines, as well as on the nature and workings of the four humours and other vital bodily fluids and spirits. Furthermore, as the *Examen Chirurgicum* (a practice manual and exam guide for budding barber-surgeons) by Joseph Schmid reveals, 'knowledge and experience' of the various influences of the seasons on the body was required. In the view of Schmid and many of his colleagues, young barber-surgeons also needed basic knowledge of astrology for determining favourable dates for beginning treatment and prognosticating its outcome.[48]

The limits on the activity of the city's barber-surgeons, prompted by the learned physicians and sanctioned by the council, seriously compromised the way they went about their business. The barber-surgeons complained in 1568, for instance, that in emergencies, to which they were called first, it was often imperative to administer the victim a purgative inner medicine upon arrival.[49] If they always had to wait for the arrival of the learned physician, there would inevitably be victims for whom the remedy would come too late. Furthermore, many of their patients lacked the financial resources to pay for the advice of a learned doctor in addition to theirs. It was well-known, the barber-surgeons claimed, that their clients were generally among the poor of the city, while the wealthy sought out the services of university physicians. This subtle imputation of greed, the learned doctors

46 StAA, Reichsstadt, Zünfte, Akten, Kt. 4, Fasc. 1, Supplikation der sechs geschworenen Meister der Wundärzte vom 8. April 1568.

47 Ibid., Gegenbericht der Doktoren auf die Supplikation der Wundärzte vom 22. April 1568.

48 Schmid, *Examen Chirurgicum*, pp. 3–6. For the examinations of Augsburg's barber-surgeons see also StAA, Reichsstadt, Zünfte, Akten, Kt. 16; Fasc. 1, Ordnung der Bader und Barbiere von 1549.

49 For the following StAA, Reichsstadt, Zünfte, Kt. 4: Fasc. 1: Supplikation der sechs geschworenen Meister der Wundärzte vom 8. April 1568.

Adolph Occo II, Achilles Pirmin Gasser (1505–1577), Leopold Trenklin , Lucas Stenglein (1523–1587), Christoph Heuberger (?–1582), Marcus Wind (?–1596), Jeremias Martius (?–1585) and Adolph Occo III (1524–1606) took as a serious insult to their professional integrity.[50] In repost, they claimed that the barber-surgeons never charged their patients a 'just' price, but always doubled or tripled their fees. Even worse, it was they who generally refused to treat poor patients, instead sending them to the municipal institutions, such as the *Blatthaus*, to save trouble and expense.

The disputes and accusations between these two official healers groups were often aggressive and polemical, and expressed in deeply offensive rhetoric. However, I argue that despite the abundance of archival documents testifying to their animosities and rivalries, neither party seriously wished to deny the other competence in treating the human body. Both ultimately accepted as given the dichotomy of the human body, which on one hand provided the basis for their disputes, but was, on the other hand, responsible for their inextricable professional interdependence. Each group, after all, had frequently to rely on the other's knowledge, experience and practical know-how in daily medical practices. The physicians, for all their theoretical knowledge, needed the barber-surgeons to help them access the mysterious, invisible processes inside the body; they were largely reliant on the barber-surgeon's first-hand information about the body's actual physical condition.[51] Moreover, they needed their artisanal colleagues to translate learned diagnosis and proposed cures into actual practice. Thus, Augsburg's learned doctors had no interest in eradicating their surgical colleagues from the Augsburg medical marketplace. That the physicians, in fact, only sought to control the barber-surgeons not to destroy them is obvious from their frequently expressed support of the latter's efforts to drive unlicensed itinerant healers out of town. In this respect, the two groups were pursuing a common interest, as a petition in the early 1530s from the learned doctors Johann Trenklin, Gereon Sailer, Adolph Occo II and Johann Tieffenbach demonstrates.[52] This petition warned the council that many poor pox sufferers in the city had been completely ruined by the unprofessional cures of itinerant pox 'specialists'. But as the city's paupers could often not afford other medicines – or so at least the learned physicians claimed – they often had no alternative but to purchase the often cheaper but damaging mercury ointments sold by the many unlicensed itinerant healers. The physicians asked the council nonetheless to

50 Ibid., Fasc. 1, Gegenbericht der Doktoren auf die Supplikation der sechs geschworenen Meister der Wundärzte vom 8. April 1568 vom 22. April 1568. The imputation of the greedy medical practitioner is a topos that can be already found in the classical medical literature. See Barbara Elkeles, *Aussagen zu ärztlichen Leitwerten, Pflichten und Verhaltensweisen in berufsvorbereitender Literatur* (dissertation, Hannover 1979), pp. 137–43.

51 For the diagnostic tools of learned physicians see Jütte, *Ärzte*, pp. 108–18.

52 StAA, Collegium Medicum, Ordnungen und Decreta, 1525–1804, 4. Juni 1532.

ensure that outside the city's pox hospital mercury-containing remedies could only be prepared, sold and applied by licensed journeymen residing in the city, and by citizen barbers-surgeons with the requisite skill, whose craft (claimed the doctors) was already being damaged by the large number of foreign healers hawking their wares in Augsburg's streets and marketplaces. By banning itinerant healers from selling and applying such ointments, the council would help ensure the livelihood of local official healers so that they would be better able to 'carry the burdens of citizenship'. In this way the physicians tactfully reminded the council of its obligation as a benevolent authority appointed by God whose 'fatherly' task it was to ensure the livelihood of all its citizenry. However, whenever the physicians aligned with their artisanal colleagues their actions were never entirely altruistic. Not surprisingly, in this case as in many others, they also used the opportunity to advance their own cause. In a seemingly disinterested fashion, ostensibly 'for the sake of the poor', they offered to support their artisanal colleagues in treating the French pox outside the *Blatterhaus* by supervising their work and offering 'assistance to ensure that only correct, harmless ointments are used'.

Although relations with physicians were frequently very tense, Augsburg's barber-surgeons too accepted, in principle, that when it came to treating the human body the different licensed healer communities in the city were mutually dependent on each other. With regard to their own medical capabilities, they were hardly lacking in self-confidence. Years of practical experience in dealing with the human body made them, in their own eyes as well as those of the authorities, at least as important in treating illness as the learned physicians.[53] 'For who or where is the young medicus', the Augsburg barber-surgeon Joseph Schmid asked the readers of his *Examen Chirurgicum*, 'who can cure all kinds of inner and outer illnesses which from head to sole can daily or hourly appear, such as wounds, stab wounds, gunshot wounds, broken, dislocated and rotting limbs, tumours, ulcers, gangrene, and other diseases and infirmities of the body, without the aid of surgery?'[54] 'True, honest and perfect medicine cannot exist without surgery', claimed Schmid. Their professional confidence made the Augsburg barber-surgeons not averse to recognising the learned physicians' competence in other areas of medicine and using it to support their own practice. At their own request, for example, they met with the municipally-employed physicians at the start of each year to learn which dates the latter deemed astrologically propitious for bloodletting or purging. They were happy to declare that, as long as the doctors kept away from the field of external medicine, they for their part would refrain from meddling in internal medicine.[55]

53 For more details on how the authorities regarded the barber-surgeons and their skills see Hammond, *Civic Health Care*, pp. 168–80.

54 Schmid, *Examen Chirurgicum*, Foreword. Schmid is an excellent example of such a self-confident physician who also expressed his opinions in print.

55 Hofmann, *Bäder*, p. 29.

Redefining the Body

This general acceptance of each others' healing competences in regard to the two-sphered human body allowed for relatively conflict-free cooperation between the barber-surgeons and doctors appointed to the civic *Blatterhaus* throughout the entire sixteenth century. The learned doctors' privileged authority over the definition of the pox (which was reflected in the official institutional hierarchy) was considered by everybody involved in the organisation and administration of the *Blatterhaus* a guarantee for peace and order as well as a warrant for correct and efficient treatment.

However, this chapter has shown that this specific distribution of power in regard to the pox-infested body (in place in the *Blatterhaus* after 1522) was only the result of decades of negotiations between the various healer groups working in the hospital and the civic authorities. The archival records revealed that in the early years of this institution the group of academic doctors exerted, no, or rather limited, control over the definition of the human body in general and the treatment of the pox in particular. Although it can be assumed that the understanding of the body as divided into an inner and an outer sphere was widespread among Augsburg's general population and its healers, neither were the internal workings of the body assigned greater importance in the definition of disease, nor were the academic doctors considered the only competent guardians of the body's inner sanctum. In the first decade of the *Blatterhaus*'s existence inmates were cared for by non-academic healers, whose mercury treatments for external and internal conditions had the approval both of the authorities and the inmates themselves. Thus, in the *Blatterhaus*'s early institutional history, the dominance of the learned physicians is no more evident than is the pre-eminence of the inner body over the outer.

It was not until the early sixteenth century, when the learned physicians as a group began to demand publicly greater authority over questions of the city's health care provisions, that the body's dualism was increasingly expressed in the *Blatterhaus* records, as well as in archival material depicting the situation on the wider medical marketplace. By demanding exclusive rights to the internal body and propagating its greater significance for the definition of disease and medical treatment, the physicians gradually succeeded in relegating the city's barber-surgeons (and other healer groups) to an inferior position concerning the official control over the treatment of the sick body: by the 1530s the latter were officially denied any authority over definition of the inner body, so much so that their medical practice (restricted to the treatment of the body's surface) had to be guided and supervised by their learned colleagues. The endless public disputes, often involving patients, which resulted from this official distinction of the body were important to further implement this dualistic body image and the distribution of healing authority in the wider public's mind. Archival material reveals that by the 1530s patients expected from a learned physician that he deciphered the inner secrets of their diseased bodies, while they turned to barber-surgeons, barbers and bath masters for the more practical procedures relating to their body's hygiene and health. And, interestingly, they were happy to pay substantially more for such academic advice.

This chapter has ultimately argued that the growing influence of academic physicians over all questions of public health (supported by their close ties with the city's ruling elites) re-shaped the wider local perceptions and understandings of the human body in Augsburg from the beginning of the sixteenth century. The strategies they applied to make internal medicine appear more significant for the diagnosis and treatment of disease were more successful than those of their artisan colleagues who, although they claimed to be able to treat both, were increasingly restricted to the care of the outer body.

The doctors' attempts to deepen the distinction between the inner and the outer body may help explain why they were so dismissive of Paracelsian ideas as evident in the 'Thalhauser-affair', mentioned earlier in this chapter. Paracelsus was generally in agreement with the division of the body into internal and external, but often he deplored the fact that so many academic physicians confined themselves to practising internal medicine from books and had little idea how to actually physically treat the body. A 'knowledgeable physician', he thundered, should never restrict himself to one area of the dualistic body and rely exclusively, as so many of the learned doctors did, on knowledge gleaned from university textbooks to diagnose disease and determine a course of treatment. Paracelsus argued that the physician also needed to acquire practical knowledge of external surgery and should use it in his daily practice.[56] For Augsburg's physicians these suggestions were too radical and utterly impossible even to contemplate. Not only were they convinced that their academic studies were epistemologically superior to the practical work of the barber-surgeons, but also their elevated social status as members of the city's ruling elite made it impossible for them to seriously consider training in an artisanal craft, or to envisage its practice, which was reserved for the lower echelons of Augsburg society. Augsburg's doctors owed their dominant position among the local healer community as much to their theoretical knowledge acquired at university (and the esteem in which such knowledge was held by Augsburg's elites) as to their actual social connections to the city's political decision-makers, which made is easy for them to influence public health decisions. However, another significant factor in the physicians' rise to power should not be overlooked and that is the continuous disunity among barber-surgeons, bath masters and the barber-surgeons. Their learned colleagues knew very well how to exploit these conflicts for their own ends.[57]

56 Ernst Kaiser, *Paracelsus. In Selbstzeugnissen und Bilddokumenten* (Hamburg, 1969).

57 A good example for this is the initiative of Doctor Gereon Sailer to reform all pharmacies from July 1557, which at the same time aimed at restructuring the craft of barbers, barber-surgeons and bath masters. Sailer's reform suggestions are reprinted in Gensthaler, *Medizinalwesen*, pp. 180–83.

It has been suggested that the disputes between the learned physicians and their artisanal colleagues over the diagnosis and the treatment of the French pox in the municipal *Blatterhaus* were related to more than concerns about professional hierarchy and economic interest. Also at stake for each group was the official right and authority to define the human body and control its treatment. The territory on which the battles between Augsburg's two official healing groups were fought was the human body, and the divisions of that territory, as we have seen, were redefined in the course of the sixteenth century.

The Sufferer's Story

So far this chapter has investigated the emergence of a specific power relationship between the medical practitioners at the municipal *Blatterhaus*. It has claimed that the hierarchical order between the appointed academic physician and the barber-surgeon (in place since 1522) reflected the authority each of them held over the definition of the pox and its treatment. This distribution of medical authority in regard to the poxed body in the *Blatterhaus* became the model for the two Fugger hospitals (est. 1523/24; 1572); indeed, in this respect, the house rules and employment contracts in all three institutions were identical.

Although the verdict of the two medical practitioners was vital, it was only one component of the diagnostic act. Equally important was the opinion of the pox sufferer and his or her disease narrative. To be able to identify the invisible essence of the pox and its causes, and to predict its future manifestations, the two healers required detailed, first-hand information from the sick about daily habits and the exact circumstances of how they fell ill. This chapter reconstructs the pox sufferer's story in the diagnostic act.

It has often been deplored that the reconstruction of the 'patient's narrative' is particularly challenging for the early modern period due to a general lack of sources.[58] The clinical encounter in the Augsburg pox hospitals presents no exception: the information that was exchanged between the candidate and the medical practitioners during the actual physical examination has not survived the centuries. However, at least for the *Blatterhaus*, we are lucky to be able to investigate roughly one hundred petition letters, written by the applicants to the council prior to their examination.

Although these petitions offer rare and fascinating insights into the lives of Augsburg's pox sufferers and their understanding of their illness, they also have limitations. First of all, they do not represent the entire social spectrum of pox victims in the city. The municipal *Blatterhaus* catered exclusively for the poorer strata of Augsburg's society; only those residents and citizens who 'cannot be

58 Porter, 'Physical Examination', pp. 170–97.

properly treated at home' were to benefit from such free hospital treatment.[59] Pox sufferers 'wealthy enough to be restored to health in their homes' were discouraged from seeking to burden the authorities with their care.[60] If they did not wish to undergo treatment at home, the prosperous could call on the services of small private hospitals run by local barber-surgeons. Ulrich von Hutten, who underwent a guaiacum treatment in Augsburg, most probably booked himself into such a facility. The barber-surgeon Joseph Schmid, for example, operated a private clinic in one of the spare rooms of his residence, in which, so he boasted, the pox-infested bodies of many rich and influential Augsburg citizens were nursed back to health. However, aside from Schmid's 'success stories' (which have to approached with caution), no further archival material survives to illuminate the experiences of Augsburg's better-off poxed population.

All of the *Blatterhaus*'s petitioners came from pauper backgrounds; most of them were artisans, predominantly weavers.[61] This is not particularly surprising, since, as mentioned earlier, the trade underwent several severe economic crises during the sixteenth century, leaving the majority of its practitioners and their families in a state of destitution and often entirely dependent on municipal handouts. The second largest group of applicants was single men and women who had recently migrated from the neighbouring countryside or other German towns, attracted by the employment possibilities in the city's service industry. Most of these were in their teens or early twenties; the older ones were often widowed. Another group frequently applying for admission at the *Blatterhaus* were soldiers who were temporarily stationed at Augsburg, or who fell ill when passing through. The fact that the pox caused severe physical impairment, often rendering its victims immobile and confining them to their beds for weeks or even months, was particularly disastrous for all of them. To be diagnosed with the pox often cost them their jobs and meagre incomes, and all lacked the reserves necessary to support themselves through periods of unemployment, let alone to pay for medication. Moreover, single servants or apprentices would often lose their lodgings.[62] Their employers, whose dwellings they usually shared, were not prepared to accommodate them any longer once they had been diagnosed with the pox, whether from fear of infection or unwillingness to cover the costs of medical care. Since most of these migrant workers (this also includes soldiers) had not been in Augsburg long enough to accumulate reliable social capital – networks

59 For this and the following quotations see StAA, Blatterhaus, Ordnung 1576, p. 1.

60 For private treatments in sixteenth-century Cologne see Jütte, *Patienten*, pp. 351–81. For the treatment of the pox among sixteenth-century élites see Walter Uhlig, *Ein Beitrag zur Geschichte der Holzkur in der zweiten Hälfte des 16. Jahrhunderts* (dissertation, Leipzig 1913).

61 The sources also mention bakers, millers, hatters, cutlers, tanners, tailors, carpenters, joiners, shoemakers, goldsmiths.

62 For the background to Augsburg's journeymen see Roeck, *Krieg und Frieden* I, pp. 406–25.

of neighbours and friends – to assist them while they were sick, the municipal *Blatterhaus* was often their only option.

Although the petition letters often reveal detailed and personal information on the lives and the ordeals of pox sufferers, they do not provide unmediated access to the 'pox experience' of Augsburg's poor. The majority of the petitioners were, in all likelihood, illiterate and asked friends, relatives or their employers to write the petitions for them. Some even hired professional letter-writers to help. These writers-for-hire were well versed in the rhetoric of civic administration and were able to offer their clients valuable advice on how effectively to 'construct' the narrative so as to evoke pity and compassion from the authorities. They also drew the client's attention to those details best to avoid if one did not wish to risk rejection.

These 'narrative strategies', however, were well known to the council. In order to prevent fraud, the *Blatterhaus* admission panel (the pox father, two deputy guardians, and the medical practitioners who met every first Saturday of each month in the hospital's consulting room) were strictly advised to double-check the information provided in the application letters *before* proceededing to the applicant's physical examination. Was the petitioner eligible according to the institution's own admission rules (e.g. the applicant's financial situation and legal status)? Would they be able to afford the entrance examination fee, which (as shown in Chapter 2) depended on the applicant's status as citizen, resident or foreigner? And was there any further information available, particularly concerning the petitioner's moral conduct, which might hinder admission? If the panel discovered that an applicant had deliberately provided false information in his petition on any of these issues, it was instructed to reject the application of the candidate.[63]

What, with these caveats in mind, do these the petitioners' 'stories' tell us about those believed to be suffering from the pox and hoping for admission? Philipp Jakob, who applied in 1552, was a native of Lorraine, but at the time of his petition he had already been working for several years as a journeyman for different masters in the city.[64] Like all the applicants to the *Blatterhaus*, Jakob regarded the pox as a curable illness and was convinced that a brief stint in the hospital would restore his capacity for physical work. He felt certain that the Almighty would support his recovery as He had done a year ago, when Jakob had been admitted to the *Blatterhaus* for the first time. After that recovery,

63 Applicants who had 'forgotten' to send in this preliminary letter could be examined on the day of the official examination but they could not be admitted. See the case of Simon Wöbely, StAA, St Martin, VI, Prod. 67: Supplikation des Simon Wöbely vom 3. November 1594. Admissions in between these official examination days were impossible. See for instance StAA, St Martin, VI, Prod. 41: Supplikation der Agatha Knöll vom 14. Februar 1581.

64 For the following see StAA, St Martin, VI, Prod. 10: Supplikation des Philipp Jakob aus Lothringen 1552.

he had immediately found another position in the hatter's trade. Unfortunately, Jakob reported in his petition, he had recently suffered a relapse, and 'now that discharges (*fliß*) have again appeared on my head and face, I can no longer do my work and earn my bread'. As he was not born in Augsburg, he claimed to have 'no friend and no one to whom I might turn for help'. Addressing the city authorities in flattering terms as 'fathers, protectors and patrons of poor strangers' like himself, he asked them, once more, for admission. A stay of a month or two would cure him sufficiently, Jakob believed, so that he would no longer require municipal support but could 'resume my work and feed and look after myself'. To emphasise his willingness to work and ensure the council that he harboured no intention to become a long term or even permanent *Blatterhaus* resident at their expense, Jakob enclosed with his petition a letter from three master milliners. These expressed complete and utter satisfaction with his work, praising his exemplary moral and social conduct in his dealings with them, and concluded with the hope that his cure would be rapid so that he could resume work as soon as possible.[65]

Philipp Jakob's case (which is fairly typical) shows, first of all, that pox sufferers were firmly convinced that the right course of treatment would help them overcome the disease in a relatively short period of time. Secondly, his case suggests that it was apparently not difficult for those recovered from the pox to find new employment in a respectable profession. In fact, there is little in the hospital sources to suggest that a successful cure in the *Blatterhaus* triggered any discrimination and stigmatisation for pox sufferers after their release from the hospital. After their recovery, Augsburg ex-pox victims were generally able to resume their old way of life without difficulty.[66] However, that does not mean that all employers of workers and journeymen were as understanding and supportive as those of Philipp Jakob when their employees fell ill. The case of Caspar Mauterer shows this clearly. Mauterer had worked as a menial in the civic mills for eighteen years when he suddenly fell ill in the summer of 1549 with 'the French pox in my throat' and was consequently admitted to the *Blatterhaus*.[67] Just when his condition began to show signs of improvement in response to the guaiacum treatment, his employer informed him that his absence could no longer be tolerated, threatening

65 Most guilds and journeymen cooperations offered help to their members in case of illness. Whether Philipp Jakob had sought their support is unknown. For these support systems see Sigrid Fröhlich, *Die soziale Sicherung bei Zünften und Gesellenverbänden. Darstellung, Analyse, Vergleich* (Berlin, 1976), pp. 61–2; 74–85; 156–8. For the coexistence of cooperatively organised self-help and centralised civic poor relief since the early Middle Ages see Otto Gerhard Oexle, 'Armut, Armutsbegriff und Armenfürsorge im Mittelalter', in *Soziale Sicherheit und soziale Disziplinierung. Beiträge zu einer historischen Theorie der Sozialpolitik*, in Christoph Sachße and Florian Tennstedt (eds) (Frankfurt a. M., 1986), pp. 73–100. For masters who petitioned for an employee see StAA, St Martin, VI, Prod. 58; Prod. 24; Prod. 52.

66 See also Robert Jütte, *Ärzte*, pp. 320–28.

67 See StAA, St Martin, VI, Prod. 2: Supplikation des Caspar Mauterer von 1549. This case is also mentioned in Kinzelbach, 'Böse Blatter', p. 51.

to dismiss him outright if he did not return to his post forthwith. This ultimatum, combined with Mauterer's own alleged dislike of idleness, convinced him to leave hospital prematurely against the strict advice of the medical practitioners. Alas, he would soon regret having so 'freely returned to work', as his condition deteriorated rapidly. A repentant Mauterer confessed in his petition that 'I broke off treatment myself, and obstructed my own recovery', and humbly beseeched the council to readmit him, 'lest my throat be completely eaten away … and so that I may be restored to good health'.

Mauterer was not the only one to encounter indifference or even hostility at his workplace when the pox first manifested itself on his body. Few employers, however, forced their pox-stricken employees to continue to work. On the contrary, due to fear of infection, most in fact were eager to get rid of a pox-infested maid, servant or labourer, particularly when the latter was lodging in the employer's own home. While journeymen and apprentices could expect some degree of support from their guilds or apprentices' associations, domestic maids and servants had no claims at all to assistance in the event of illness. Their fate was in the hands of their masters, not all of whom showed sympathy and understanding for their subordinates' plight. For example, in petitioning on behalf of his maid Ursula Aichlin on 16 February 1551, the weaver Hans Heckel explained that he could not tolerate the girl in his house any longer, since she might infect his own 'children, wife and members of my household'.[68] Disclaiming all responsibility for her care, Heckel underlined that the maid had not fallen ill in his service, but had 'brought her disease into my house'.

The brickmaker Veit Schuster showed rather more sympathy and responsibility for his maid when he petitioned for her to be admitted to the *Blatterhaus* just before Christmas in 1584.[69] Although the girl had only been with the family for a year looking after the children 'in return for bread and clothing', Schuster and his wife had taken the 'poor orphan' into their hearts. Nevertheless, she could not, he wrote, remain in the house any longer. The danger that she might infect 'my wife and child, making the misery even greater', could not be overlooked. Explaining that the girl had suddenly 'complained of great pains in all her limbs', and that the disease had become 'visible upon her', Schuster and his wife immediately suspected the pox without even consulting a medical practitioner. However, to be absolutely certain, his wife took the girl to the official examination at the *Blatterhaus* and paid the examination fee on her behalf. The presiding medical practitioners having confirmed his opinion, Schuster now hoped the council would share his concerns and admit the orphan to the *Blatterhaus*.

68 For the following see StAA, St Martin, VI, Prod. 4: Supplikation des Webers Hans Heckel vom 16. Februar 1551.

69 For the following see StAA, St Martin, VI, Prod. 48: Supplikation des Veyt Schuster vom 22. Dezember 1584.

Fear of infection did not only impact on employers and their sick employees, it also placed emotional burdens on the victims' own families.[70] In extreme cases this could lead to a family rejecting a loved one who had contracted the pox. This is illustrated in the case of Philipp Eß. After a couple of weeks in the *Blatterhaus*, Eß was discharged by the medical practitioners in January 1618, as the treatment had failed to effect an improvement in his condition.[71] His wife Anna was appalled, fearing for the health and safety of her newborn child. She tried everything in her power to prevent her husband returning home, but to no avail.

Anna Eß's behaviour, however, does not appear to have been typical. Most of the petitions submitted by family members of pox victims clearly suggest that efforts had been made to nurse the sick at home *before* applying for admissions to the *Blatterhaus*.[72] What exactly families did is difficult to reconstruct. While the petitions mention prior recourse to medical advice, there is neither information concerning the kind of therapies that had been tried nor the cost. In the case of Philip Eß, for example, it seems that he had undergone two unsuccessful private cures with Augsburg barber-surgeons before his wife Anna applied to the council for his admission to the *Blatterhaus*.[73] Similarly, a weaver's wife, Appolonia Wetzl, whose husband Baltasar suffered from 'cold discharges (*Flüsse*) all over his body', had already sought the advice of friends as well as learned physicians and barber-surgeons before applying to the council in February 1551.[74] To pay for these private treatments Appolonia Wetzl had borrowed substantial sums. None of the costly therapies, however, had proven effective. Indeed, Wetzl humbly submitted that her husband's cold discharges, 'may develop into the evil pox' if not treated with a preventative guaiacum wood cure. As her savings were exhausted by Baltasar's long illness, she hoped that the council would allow him to undergo the treatment free of charge in the *Blatterhaus*.

Many parents, in particular, spared no effort or expense in attempting to restore the health of their pox-infected offspring. For example, the prolonged illness of Onophorius Pfefferlin (the Younger) drove his father, Onophorius Pfefferlin (the

70 For cases in which family members petitioned for other members see StAA, St Martin, VI, Prod. 2; Prod. 1; Prod. 36; Prod. 63; Prod. 66; Prod. 70; Prod. 77; Prod. 78; Prod. 79.

71 StAA, St Martin, VI, Prod. 7a; Prod. 86: Supplikation der Anna Eß, ihres Bruders und einiger Nachbarn vom 13. Januar 1618.

72 For this see also Kinzelbach, *Gesundbleiben*, pp. 300–304. For various forms of neighbourly support in case of sickness in early modern Cologne see Jütte, *Ärzte*, pp. 202–4.

73 Unfortunately the sources do not reveal further details about these cures. See StAA, St Martin, VI, Prod. 86: Supplikation der Anna Eß, ihres Bruders und einiger Nachbarn vom 13. Januar 1618.

74 StAA, St Martin, VI, Prod. 5: Supplikation der Appolonia Wetzl vom 21. Februar 1551. This case is also mentioned in Kinzelbach, 'Böse Blatter', p. 32.

Elder), to the brink of financial ruin.[75] As the latter lamented in his petition of October 1564, physicians and barber-surgeons had come and gone in and out of his house on a daily basis for three years. The expensive medications for his son, whose body, in the medical practitioners' view, was afflicted, 'unfortunately, with the most severe and evil kind of Morbo Gallici', had not just swallowed up his own revenues, but also almost all of his son's maternal inheritance. With financial resources exhausted, the father wrote in despair, friends and relations were no longer able or willing to help. The last hope for his boy was a cure in the *Blatterhaus*. If Onophorius's experiences were bad, the most severe trials of all were visited upon the family of the weaver Lienhart Dörr, who applied for re-admission to the *Blatterhaus* in 1583.[76] In his petition he described how his entire family had contracted the pox in the course of the 1570s. He himself had undergone four previous *Blatterhaus* treatments, 'the first time for 5 weeks, the second and third time 10, and the fourth time 36 weeks', while his wife and three of his children aged one, five and twelve had each been admitted for three separate periods of treatment. Initially, only his five-year-old daughter had given the medical practitioners grounds for optimism. The rest of the family had been discharged with the comment that 'the pox house was not a spital' for the chronically sick. In the medical practitioners' view the Dörrs were not suffering from the pox, but from some kind of 'nasty rash', which would eventually disappear of its own accord. In discharging them, the doctor provided special skin lotion, which was to prove ineffective. Lienhart's five-year-old daughter remained six months longer in the *Blatterhaus* than the rest of the family, during which time the lesions on one of her feet had been cauterised by the barber-surgeon. But in her case, too, wrote Lienhart, the doctors had finally given up hope and 'thrown her out with open sores'. Fortunately, the Alm Lords, who administered the Pilgrims' House, had taken pity on the girl and allowed her to be treated in their institution for nearly a year, during which time her condition gradually improved. Lienhart's twelve-year-old son was less fortunate. After a brief stay in the *Blatterhaus* he, too, had been transferred to the Pilgrims' House for attention to his 'festering wounds'. The medication administered had produced no improvement, and the Pilgrim's House-appointed medical practitioners had 'sent the boy home again with four gaping sores, saying he was beyond help'. Within ten weeks this gloomy prognosis proved accurate; the boy had 'gone to his grave, which is for the best, may the Lord God grant his soul a joyful resurrection', his grieved father reported. Lienhart himself, whose condition continued to deteriorate, was denied further treatment at the *Blatterhaus*. Only the Alms Lords took pity on him, paying for him to undergo three private treatments with the Augsburg weaver and healer Samuel Zimmermann. 'With the help and grace of God', as one of his advertisement flyers

75 For the following see StAA, St Martin, VI, Prod. 37: Supplikation des Onophorius Pfefferlin vom 9. Oktober 1564.

76 For the following see ibid., Prod. 43: Supplikation des Webers Lienhart Dörr vom 26. Januar 1583.

proudly announced, he, Zimmermann, specialised in treating 'sick persons with serious diseases such as pox, paralysis, old concealed discharges, ulcers, fig warts and other similar ailments'. And his business was going well, much to the dismay of the barber, bath master and barber-surgeon craft which tried to persuade the council to ban Zimmermann and his kind from pursuing these activities.[77] But they had no success, partly because the council had an interest in allowing him to continue to practise, not least as a place of last resort to which Alms Lords could refer hopeless cases such as that of Lienhart Dörr, who had already 'been hospitalised a second, third and fourth time in the lazarett or *Blatterhaus*, where every treatment has been administered to him'.[78] In Dörr's case, unfortunately, Zimmermann's mercury vapour cure and miracle potions proved no more effective than anything he had tried before. Not only, wrote Lienhart, had they failed to 'bear fruit', in fact the treatment had made his condition even worse. '[C]onstant unceasing headaches, and a tightness around the chest as if I would die of suffocation' had now been added to his existing ailments. But Lienhart, who was as firmly convinced as ever that he was suffering from the pox, refused to give up hope. His petition of 26 January 1583 was his final attempt to return to the *Blatterhaus*. He still expected to regain his health, he wrote, hoping to be able 'to support my wife and four uneducated children by practising my trade'. The sources do not reveal if the council was magnanimous one more time; of the fate of the family nothing more is known.

Most petitioners who wrote for their families pinned the hopes on admission to the *Blatterhaus*. And rightly so, as it freed the family from the fear of infection and allowed them to hope for their loved one's speedy recovery. Moreover, it was a huge financial relief. Occasionally, however, acceptance to the *Blatterhaus* could put additional strain on family life, as confirmed by several petitions asking for re-admission to the *Blatterhaus*. The case of Anna Fick, who applied in 1596, is a telling example.[79] She had been in the pox hospital for a few weeks when she discovered that her husband had also fallen ill and was lying at home unattended. As the couple were childless and apparently could not call on the help of friends and neighbours, Anna felt obliged, despite her own fragile state of health, to nurse her husband. She repeatedly applied to the *Blatterhaus* medical practitioners for temporary leave. Owing to the seriousness of her condition, her request was rejected

77 The Augsburg sources offer little information on these private pox healers. The following case of Samuel Zimmermann is a rare exception. See StAA, Reichsstadt, Handwerkerakten, Karton 5: Bader und Barbiere 1581–1600, Fasc. 2: Streitigkeiten Samuel Zimmermanns mit den geschworenen Wundärzten vom September 1581; for itinerant healers selling their nostrums on Augsburg's marketplaces see also Stein, 'Quack', pp. 192–200.

78 This interest of city authorities in supporting itinerant healers was widespread in early modern Europe. For Italy see Pomata, *Contracting a Cure*, pp. 145–149.

79 For the following see StAA, St Martins, VI, Prod. 26: Supplikation der Anna Fick vom 11. September 1596.

each time. Finally, in total despair, Anna discharged herself without permission and secretly went home to her husband. Soon her condition deteriorated to the extent that she was unable to rise from her bed, and felt compelled to reapply for a place in the *Blatterhaus*. What the panel decided, we do not know.

Like Anna Fick, the weaver Peter Sigmayr and his wife Emerenza realised that admission to the *Blatterhaus* was not necessarily a blessing for family life.[80] The couple had been accepted by the examination panel along with two of their children. Their third child, however, who was according to the medicine team in 'good health', was refused admission. The longer their own cure lasted, the more fearful and anxious the parents became for this child, who was being looked after by acquaintances. Having failed to persuade the learned doctor to allow them to leave temporarily, they broke off their treatment prematurely and discharged themselves in defiance of the doctor's orders. However, like Anna Fick, at home their conditions deteriorated rapidly so that, after a week, they became unable to care either for the child or for themselves. They both reapplied for admission, 'so that we will not be completely ruined and will be soon able again to raise our children without too many burdens'.

Anna Fick, just like the Sigermayrs, probably knew that trying to hide the real circumstances that made them leave the pox hospital would not have gained them re-admission. Fortifying information about earlier stays in the house was immediately punished with rejection. This threat, however, did not deter some petitioners from 'dramatising' their situation in their application letters, in the hope, no doubt, of arousing the officials' sympathies and thus increasing their chances of admission. As mentioned earlier, the council was well aware of these tactics and often requested additional information from the panel members if a candidate's story appeared suspicious to them. Wolf Rottinger, in applying for his wife Katharina Blomenhauer to be re-admitted to the *Blatterhaus*, was exposed in this manner.[81] In his application letter from April 1560 Wolf had claimed that he was unable to care for his wife who was suffering from oozing pox lesions all over her body. Being 'wretchedly poor', he pretended not to be able to afford privately the medical treatment his wife so desperately needed. However, the council's discreet enquiries elicited a contrary opinion from the pox father.[82] His view was that the couple's financial circumstances were not nearly as wretched as Rottinger claimed. First of all, the couple had no children to care for and, secondly, the petitioner was a healthy, robust young man whose job as a city watchman provided at least a regular income. According to the pox father, Rottinger was perfectly able 'with God's help, to care for his wife as required'; her admission was therefore hardly a matter of urgency. The council followed his advice and supported the panel's decision that Katharina Blomenhauer should not be readmitted.

80 Ibid., Prod. 27: Supplikation des Weberehepaares Peter und Emerenza Sigmayr vom 8. Februar 1558.

81 Ibid., Prod. 30: Supplikation des Wolf Rottinger vom April 1560.

82 Ibid. Prod. 30: Bericht des Blattervaters 5. Juni 1560.

Honesty was crucial in all dealings with the authorities of the *Blatterhaus*. Any misrepresentation of one's living conditions, as in the case of Rottinger, could trigger the immediate rejection of the petition. If the panel, however, considered a petitioner's description of his or her financial distress genuine they were happy to step in and help out particularly in regard to the examination fees. As mentioned earlier, citizens paid 1 fl., while non-citizens, as long as they had worked for two years or more in the service of Augsburg citizens, paid 2 fl. until the mid-1580s, and thereafter 3 fl. Foreigners were admitted only exceptionally and if so, they had to pay the extremely high sum of 10 fl.[83] Some applicants, particularly menial staff and apprentices who were unable to pay the full amount, were often supported by their masters, such as the above-mentioned brickmaker Veit Schuster, who offered to pay for his orphaned maid in December 1584.[84] For those cases like the one of Felicitas Schneid, the widow of a municipal tower watchman, who could not call on the good will of an employer, the council stood in.[85] Her son Thomas, who had served abroad as a soldier for years and forsaken his rights of citizenship through his marriage to a foreigner, had returned with his wife Barbara to his hometown in November 1600, both of them impoverished and stricken with the pox.[86] Schneid stated in her petition that she could not afford the full inspection fee for foreigners for both, amounting as it did to 20 fl. She was more than willing, however, to pay a portion of the fee upfront and the rest in later instalments. The chief guardians of the *Blatterhaus*, who acted on behalf of the council in her case, declared themselves willing, 'in consideration of her poverty', to advance the necessary fee 'as an act of mercy, against sufficient deposit and security'. Whether she ever settled the debt is unknown. The chief guardians may have written it off as they did in the case of Jörg Sumer in July 1557.[87] Though Sumer still owed the examination fee for his first admission to the *Blatterhaus* the previous year, the chief guardians decided to forgive the debt as an act of mercy, in view of the fact that Sumer truly had 'nothing left to live off'.

The panel was sensitive not only in regard to the information about the financial situation of the candidate but also to any rumour of moral and social misconduct. The case of the carpenter's daughter, Anna Gessler, is a telling example. She found her petition of October 1562 undermined by negative reports of her personal conduct.[88] Admitting that she had been treated in the *Blatterhaus* on five previous

83 StAA, Blatterhaus, Ordnung 1581, p. 37–8.

84 StAA, St Martin, VI, Prod. 48: Supplikation des Zieglerknechtes Veyt Schuster vom 22. Dezember 1584.

85 Ibid., Prod. 78: Supplikation der Witwe Felicitas Schneid vom 7. November 1600.

86 For how to lose one's citizenship in Augsburg see Roeck, *Krieg and Frieden*, vol. 1, pp. 210–15.

87 StAA, St Martin, VI, Prod. 32: Supplikation des Hansen Mair und Hansen Hilleprands, Pfleger des Jörgen Sumer.

88 Ibid. Prod. 33: Supplikation der Anna Geßlerin.

occasions, she expressed the hope of being admitted once again due to sharp pains in her thighs, which she ascribed to the pox. When the council made discreet enquiries about Gessler's previous behaviour in the house to the pox father, the latter responded by refusing to take her back. In the women's ward, he reported, she had regularly started arguments and 'been heard uttering obscenities on many occasions'.[89] To keep peace in the house he had to segregate her from the other female inmates for almost a week and lock her in a room all by herself. Furthermore, she had refused on numerous occasions to take the medicines prescribed by the in-house physician Gereon Sailer. And most annoyingly, instead of awaiting patiently her recovery and cure, Anna had finally prematurely and wilfully run away into town to meet friends and relatives. This information was sufficient for the council to deny the woman another hospital stay.

The indecent behaviour of the above mentioned Jörg Sumer during one of his four previous stays in the *Blatterhaus* was similarly detrimental to his re-application in July 1562.[90] The deputy guardians and physician had no good word to say about him: Sumer had flouted the regulations several times, 'presuming to leave his allocated ward and visit the women and young girls, provoking them with his cunning addresses to all kinds of wanton behaviour … and perhaps even desiring to indulge in venery, had he been able to'.[91] Moreover, he had persuaded staff members to loan him several gulden which he had never returned. When finally punished for his behaviour, Sumer had even become violent. Last, but not least, during his last stay he had simply 'escaped from the *Blatterhaus* without permission'. Although Sumer promised to curb his behaviour, advancing his 'youth and lack of understanding' as an excuse for his chronic insolence, the council ruled that he should not be readmitted.

Affra Winter from Nördlingen was another candidate whose moral conduct was a matter of intense debate among the members of the examination panel and the council. Petitioning the council in July 1548, she gave her occupation as 'maid, in service in Augsburg', preferring to omit her secondary earnings as an occasional prostitute.[92] She beseeched the council 'for the Lord God's sake, to accept me into the *Blatterhaus* for treatment that I may again serve as an honest citizen'. The council had no hesitation in turning her down once the panel had reported that her alleged 'honest' services to its citizens was known to involve patrolling the streets.[93] The historian Lyndal Roper has shown in her study of sixteenth-century Augsburg that public attitudes to sex before and outside marriage gradually became more harsh over the course of the century due to the increasing success

89 Ibid., Bericht Blattervater vom 12. Oktober 1562.

90 Ibid., Prod. 32: Supplikation Hans Mair und Hans Hilleprand, Pfleger des Jörgen Sumer.

91 For the following see ibid., Prod. 32: Bericht des Unterpflegers, Doktors und Wundarztes 28. Juli 1562.

92 StAA, St Martin, VI, Prod. 1: Supplikation Affra Winterin Juli 1548.

93 StAA, Reichsstadt, Ratsprotokolle 22 (1548), 10. Juli 1548.

of Protestant moral campaigns. An early victory of the Reformers was the closing of the municipally-run brothel in 1532.[94] The council's negative verdict in regard to Affra Winter's application fits Roper's description of an increasing moralistic atmosphere in the city.

However, the *Blatterhaus* records also clearly show that prostitutes not only continued to apply for treatment but were also admitted. The 'discovery' of their secret trade by the authorities did not automatically trigger the rejection of the candidates. There is no doubt that the women's activities were considered as despicable and sinful, but the hospital records also reveal that the authorities never excluded the possibility that, at any moment, such sinning women might atone and begin to lead a godly life after all. In fact, in many cases the council explicitly wished to offer these women a chance of redemption and admitted them, sometimes even against the wishes of the *Blatterhaus* panel, as the case of Abraham Welling from February 1619 shows. Welling was the keeper of the local prison and applied for three of his female inmates – Barbara Kugler, Barbara Schwertfeger and Anna Eiseler – to be transferred to the *Blatterhaus*.[95] The chief guardians of the institution tried to block this transfer by hook or crook. Confirming in their report of 21 February that the three women had been diagnosed by the *Blatterhaus* medical practitioners as having all contracted the pox, the chief guardians acknowledged that, theoretically, the trio would be entitled to be admitted to the institution after payment of the inspection fee. Regrettably, however, their experiences with other 'profligate women' in the hospital had convinced them that the three would be unlikely to renounce their 'sinful life' once they had been cured. They had observed all too often with great sadness, they wrote, how such wretched women, after 'everything had been done to their benefit, to enable them to be cured ... wasted no time in re-treading their old footsteps'. For too long they had 'drifted through their sinful lives, many of them wantonly destroying themselves'. At bottom, wrote the chief guardians, such women were taking advantage of the council's benevolence and mercy to 'seek refuge here in the pox hospital, knowing they will be nowhere else so well cared for and cured'. If these ungrateful women were admitted for treatment, others who had 'been honest and pious from youth, and been stricken with such troubles [the pox] through no fault of their own' would have to be denied. The council, however, did not share the chief guardians' dim view of the women's future prospects and ruled, in a spirit of 'Christian forgiveness', that the three 'sinful and profligate' prison inmates be given another chance. The chief guardians were instructed on 21 February 1619 to 'do their best for the three female sinners' and to admit them immediately to the *Blatterhaus*.

---

94 Roper, *Household*, pp. 89–97, has shown that the closure of the Augsburg civic brothel was *not* related to the outbreak of the pox. Karant-Nunn, 'Continuity', pp. 23–4 supports Roper's results.

95 For the following see StAA, St Martin, VI, Prod. 88: Bericht der Oberpfleger des Blatterhauses vom 21. Februar 1619.

Whether 'fallen women' were accepted out of mercy and Christian forgiveness in the private Fugger *Holzhäuser* is unknown, as records revealing the sufferer's side of the diagnostic encounter did not survive. However, it is at least possible to reconstruct the precondition that had to be met by the applicant before his or her examination could take place. In contrast to the municipal *Blatterhaus*, the official examination, which took place in the barber-surgeon's room of each *Holzhaus*, was free of charge. However, as mentioned above, only those people who were of Catholic faith had a chance of being examined. The decision whether to admit a candidate to the examination was in the hands of a panel presided over by the in-house physician and barber-surgeon, with the wood father and the Fuggerei administrator – as the Fuggers' official representative – also in attendance. In contrast to the civic *Blatterhaus*, there was no fixed monthly public examination, and, in theory, pox victims could apply in writing to the senior heads of the two branches of the Fugger family to be admitted at any time. It was only the first examination at the very beginning of each cure year that had a fixed date (ensuring maximum use of the bed capacity from the outset). To inform potential petitioners of the date of this 'opening examination' (*Eröffnungschau*), the administrator of the Fuggerei sent invitations on behalf of the Fuggers to the bailiffs of the widely dispersed family estates.[96] These printed mandates reminded the family's subjects and those residing on the Fugger's estates of the aims of the *Holzhaus* foundations, namely to 'treat and heal through the wood cure a number of poor, sick, ailing people who have been crippled or otherwise impaired by the evil pox'.[97] Pox-infected men and women were bidden to travel from their homes to Augsburg and present themselves for examination in the Fuggerei *Holzhaus* at 7 am on the appointed day. To avoid delaying the inspection through late arrival, candidates were advised to spend the previous night in accommodation near the city walls. Those in the Fuggers' service were expressly advised not to enter the city until the actual day of examination. Perhaps the founding families were concerned they might otherwise have to pay for their bed and board. It is also quite possible that pox sufferers were prevented from entering the city any earlier by watchmen at the city's gates. To prevent an influx of paupers from the outlying countryside, the watchmen had strict instructions from the authorities to 'keep an eye out for itinerant beggars and otherwise suspicious persons' and prevent such 'vagabonds' from entering the city without permission.[98]

On the examination day candidates had to present all the necessary official documentation.[99] The most important was the 'certificate and reference' from a local priest attesting that the applicant had been to confession and received the last

96 For a reprint of one of these invitation letters of which many survived in the Fugger archive see Weidenbacher, *Fuggerei*, pp. 118–19.

97 For the following see ibid.

98 StAA, Ratserlasse 1600–1668; Ordnungen der Torleut, 10. Februar 1600, Art. 3.; see also Ordnungen und Statuten, Karton 20, Nr. 431.

99 For the following see Weidenbacher, *Fuggerei*, p. 118.

rites. This was intended to ensure that only Catholic pox sufferers were admitted, and that before beginning treatment, the patient was reconciled with the Almighty and asked for God's grace 'so that the treatment may proceed more felicitously'. In addition to the confessor's testimony, every candidate required a certificate from the bailiff of the relevant Fugger estate confirming that they were 'in service' there. Such documents were also to include information about the petitioner's general conduct. Documentation for Casper Gall from Aichbach, for example, dated 3 November 1626, indicates that the bailiff vouched that 'he, Gall, to the best of my knowledge and within my sphere of influence, has always conducted himself decently and honestly, possessing only what he has earned with the daily labour of his hands, in the course of which duties he has succumbed to this disease'.[100] The last requirement was a certificate from a medical pre-examination. To ensure that applicants did not journey to Augsburg in vain, they were to be examined by an 'experienced barber-surgeon' in their place of residence and obtain confirmation from him that they were, indeed, suffering from the pox and therefore 'would benefit from the wood cure'. Regulations drawn up by Anton Fugger and his nephews in 1548 stipulated that anyone failing to present any of these official documents at the inspection would be sent away.[101]

Only with papers in order would the panel in all three Augsburg pox hospitals proceed to the actual examination to ascertain whether the petitioner's bodily symptoms were related to the pox.

The Physical Examination

For the medical examination candidates had to strip off all clothes and present themselves to the critical eyes and experienced hands of the barber-surgeon and the learned doctor. The Augsburg barber-surgeon Joseph Schmid, who had worked many years at the *Blatterhaus*, claimed that the pox diagnosis presented one of the greatest challenges for any medical practitioner. As explained in Chapter 1 in more detail, within the explanatory framework of Hippocratic-Galenic medicine each person suffered from an individual 'version' of the pox due to his or her unique humoral mixture and his or her interaction with the environment. Thus the manifestations of the pox, Schmid rightly pointed out (echoing the pox authors), were almost innumerable. To master the pox the medical practitioner had to possess exceptional diagnostic skills otherwise the sly disease would easily deceive him.[102] Particular attention, Schmid advised, should always be paid to alterations in the throat, nose and mouth, as well as the candidate's genitals.[103]

100 F.A. 5.3.2 d, fol. 45v; fol. 75r. Gall was admitted on 24 March 1627.

101 Weidenbacher, *Fuggerei*, p. 116.

102 Schmid, *Kurtzer Bericht*, p. 146.

103 His advice is also applicable to the examination of lepers. For this see Demaitre, 'Diagnosis'; Bremen, 'Lepra–Untersuchungen', pp. 65–77; Beriou/Touati, *Leprosus*;

In close cooperation with the applicant the medical teams in all three pox hospitals had to provide answers to the following questions: First, did the signs on the sufferer's body actually belong to the pox? If they decided positively on that matter, the next challenge was to assess the severity of the pox. In a final assessment, they had to come to a decision on whether the candidate's overall physical state at the moment of the examination was stable and strong enough to allow him or her to survive the often strenuous treatment. No one should be admitted whose physical condition the medical practitioners judged as hopeless. The house rules of all pox institutions strictly instructed them to turn away all candidates 'whose wounds are such that there is no hope of cure or recovery of health … the concern being that every treatment and medicine, all care and labour would be wasted'.[104]

The individual medical criteria of the pox hospital's practitioners have not survived but is its worth examining the categories listed by Joseph Schmid in one of his treatises, as they may well have been similar. In his attempt to describe the various stages of the disease, Schmid claimed that the loss of all body hair indicated the 'mildest' form of the pox.[105] It signified that the morbid disease matter was still very weak and 'mingled with a subtle vapour or humours … which spreads through the whole body and attacks the roots of the hairs so that they all have to fall out'.[106] This early stage of the pox was little worrisome and treatable with bloodlettings and purges. A more serious stage of the disease was reached when the victim's skin became covered with red spots, yellow boils and small oozing ulcers. In such cases the French poison had already successfully disrupted the individual's humoral balance to such a degree that it could only be brought back into its healthy balance by the right choice of medication. Worse, according to Schmid, were the appearances 'here and there on the body of dry red boils or pustules'.[107] These 'flesh-devouring ulcers or abscesses' appeared first on the head, particularly the forehead and ears of the sick. They were especially dangerous because they often tended to attack and destroy the soft sensitive flesh of the mouth and nasal cavities. The appearance of such symptoms strongly suggested to a medical practitioner that the disease had already 'corrupted the liver', which, according to Hippocratic-Galenic medicine, was the very production centre of the four humours. By far the most ominous kind of the pox (categorised by Schmid as the most severe) was that which was longstanding, 'old and deeply rooted' in the

Keussen, 'Lepra-Untersuchungen', pp. 80–112; Risse, *Mending Bodies*, pp. 167–73.

104 StAA, Blatterhaus, Ordnung von 1522; StAA, Blatterhaus, Ordnung von 1535, 'They are only allowed to admit those who are suffering from the French pox'; these instructions are repeated in the house rules of 1581; see StAA, Blatterhaus, Ordnung von 1581, p. 36.

105 Schmid, *Kurtzer Bericht*, pp. 151–2.

106 Ibid., p. 144.

107 For the following see ibid., p. 145.

body.[108] This stage was recognisable by the damage to 'the thick flesh, the limbs, ligaments, membranes and nerves, causing unbearable pains, which are multiplied at night'.[109] The sufferer's body was covered all over with bulbous ulcers and boils with the regrettable result that at length 'the limbs start to rot, and begin to fall off in pieces'. In such cases, prognosticated Schmid, the sufferer was not long for this world; and it is certain that such a hopeless case would not have been admitted to the wards of the any of the three hospitals.

Having judged the state and severity of the pox, the two healers discussed whether the applicant had sufficient physical strength left to survive an exhausting course of treatment that could last several weeks. Barber-surgeon Schmid took the view that treatment was most likely to be effective with those pox victims in whom 'the disease is still new and there are not yet many symptoms; where the sick is still young and physically robust'.[110] There was little hope for those sufferers in 'whom the disease … has prevailed upon for so long and who were afflicted with such malign accidents as stubborn headaches, boils and rotting limbs, incurable ulcers; also those who are physically frail and who had been previously treated by many different healers'. Medical treatment in those cases would be of little use, according to Schmid. And any healer who claimed to be able to help such hopeless cases with expensive cures, he warned, was thinking more about his purse than the wellbeing of the sick.

However, to answer all these diagnostic and prognostic questions confidently and to assess the condition of the candidates correctly, the medical practitioners required information from the examinee. How did *they* explain their illness? What information did *they* considered necessary to provide?

Every applicant, whether Catholic or Protestant, took it for granted that his or her illness derived ultimately from the will of God. This underlying conviction is evident in all the petitions examined in this study, though it is frequently expressed in formulaic terms. Few, however, suffered more from the wrath of the Almighty than the already mentioned weaver Lienhart Dörr and his family. Dörr wrote in his petition of 26 January 1583 that he, his wife and four children had lived together honestly and faithfully for twenty-one years during which time he had 'practised [his] weaver's trade without complaint'.[111] In 1579, without warning, his entire family had been 'stricken most terribly by the Almighty Merciful God with the … dreadful malady of the French pox, perhaps in punishment of our sins'. Although he could not name the exact sin he or one of his family members had committed, Dörr was certain that it must have been a major one. Why otherwise would the Almighty have punished the family with the death of his twelve-year-old son? Most of the petitions reflect the belief that God punishes individuals, either

108 Ibid., p. 146.

109 Ibid.

110 For the following see Schmid, *Kurtzer Bericht* (1702), p. 146.

111 StAA, St Martin, VI, Prod. 43: Supplikation des Webers Leinhart Dörr vom 26. Januar 1583.

for sins they had committed personally, or as representatives for the general sins of mankind. They also indicate that the pox was held to be sent to test a victim's faith. However, the belief in God's punishment did not trigger a fatalistic attitude anymore than it did among the pox authors discussed in Chapter 1. Certainly, the belief in divine punishment did not hinder the stricken from urgently and persistently seeking treatment in the *Blatterhaus*.

The elderly supplicant Jakob Koler, while attributing his suffering to divine intervention, also connected his contraction of the pox to a particular event. A year before submitting his petition, around Candlemas 1582, Koler had visited one of the Augsburg's public baths, and was convinced he had 'emerged with Morbum Gallicum'.[112] Public baths, it was well known in Augsburg, were dangerous sources of pox infection on account of the direct physical contact with other perspiring bathers, not to mention the barber-surgeon's frequent use on several different bathers of the same instruments for cupping and bleeding.[113] The council was aware of these potential dangers to visitors' health and tried to regulate entry to these popular institutions. The edict of 1549 explicitly forbade bath-masters, barbers and barber-surgeons from admitting bathers 'who are marked with signs of disease, malady or distemper that may infect or harm others'.[114] Visitors who were suffering from the 'hideous malady of the French pox' were to be denied admission altogether. The council's ban was considered unfair by the bath owners, as their letter to the council from 1550 reveals. They complained that it was impossible to implement the edict from the previous year without suffering serious financial losses. Many of their customers refused to be closely checked by them and had left their premises in fury, never to return. Moreover, the poor quality of light in the baths in winter made it almost impossible to detect infected bathers. And if, as was so often the case with the pox, the tell-tale signs were 'on the head or the private parts', where they were easy to conceal under bathing caps or aprons, infected visitors might mingle with the healthy bathers without the bathing attendants' knowledge. Although the bath owners stressed the financial losses they had to endure due to the council's bans to stop the spread of the pox, these were not the reason for the closing down of many of the city's bathhouses at the end of the sixteenth century. Instead, the archival records clearly show that it was predominantly the dramatic increase in the price of firewood which made the running of these institutions unprofitable and was responsible for their disappearance.[115]

---

112 Ibid., Prod. 44: Supplikation des Jakoben Koler aus Lützelburg vom März 1583.

113 This is particularly evident in StAA, Reichsstadt, Handwerkerakten, Karton 5: Bader und Barbiere 1581–1600, Fasc. 2: Bericht der Bader auf die Supplikation des Lohmüllers Sebastian Ertlin vom 2. Januar 1592.

114 For the following account see StAA, Reichsstadt, Handwerkerakten, Karton 4: Bader und Barbiere 1535–1580, Fasc.1: Supplikation der geschworenen Wundärzte Georg Scholler, Moritz Stromair, Matheis Konpfler, Georg Mair, Michael Härl von 1549.

115 The archival records contain a great number of supplications from bath owners complaining about the high price of firewood and asking for civic support. See StAA,

Just as Jakob Koler blamed his contraction of the pox on a visit to the municipal baths, the day-labourer Ursula Wagner in November 1600 also attributed her illness to a critical event in her life.[116] To supplement the meagre income of her family of four, this mother of two small children had worked as a wet-nurse in the city orphanage and suckled three infants.[117] After doing this for some time, 'I became aware', she wrote in her petition, that one of the children, 'I humbly submit, was infected with the disease of the evil pox'. By the time the child died, Ursula had suffered damage to her own health. Alas, the disease had now attacked not just her, but her own two small children.

Another direct cause of the pox often cited by petitioners was exposure to unaccustomed weather conditions, particularly during travels. It is hardly surprising that such explanations are found most frequently in the petitions of soldiers. The already-mentioned impoverished widow Felicitas Schneid, for example, when petitioning for her soldier son Thomas and his wife Barbara, enclosed her son's passport as proof that he had served in the wars against Turkey, the 'arch-enemy' of Christendom, in Hungary and other countries between 1586 and 1590.[118] As the desperate mother explained, the prolonged physical exertion and travelling in unhealthy wet and cold climatic conditions had resulted in both contracting the French pox. Her son was now, 'God have mercy, so wretched and diseased in his whole body, and crippled in his hands and feet … that even with a stick, and certainly not without, he can barely cross the room unaided'. The soldier Hans Mayr was another who blamed his illness on the vagaries of military life, particularly the continuous changes of location.[119] He had first noticed signs of the pox during his last leave, having spent much of the journey back home on board a ship. His body had been subjected for too long to 'overwhelming and unbearable frost and cold upon tempestuous seas', so that the pox was an almost unavoidable result, he explained. He was not at all surprised, therefore, when, soon after 'stepping off water and on to dry land', he found the mere act of walking extremely painful. The agony had now become so excruciating that he 'could not find peace or rest by day or night'.

Divine wrath at the sins of mankind, a momentous visit to the public baths, suckling infected infants, and the climate are typical explanations that emerge from

---

Reichsstadt, Handwerkerakten, Karton 5: Bader und Barbiere 1581–1600, Fasc. 2.

116 For the following see StAA, St Martin, VI, Prod. 23: Supplikation der Tagwerkerin Ursula Wagner (mid-sixteenth century).

117 The civic orphanage was founded in 1572. See for more information Roeck, *Krieg und Frieden* I, p. 47; Roper, *Household*, pp. 7–55; Safley, *Charity and Economy*.

118 For the following see StAA, St Martin, VI, Prod. 78: Supplikation der Witwe Felicitas Schneid vom 7. November 1600. The file also contains the diagnostic verdict signed by Doktor Rumler from 16 November 1600.

119 For the following see StAA, St Martin, VI, Prod. 67: Supplikation des Simon Wöbely vom 3. November 1594.

the petitions of pox victims. It is clear that many of them saw the pox as deriving simultaneously from natural and supernatural causes (e.g. divine punishment), and that no one saw this as in any way contradictory.[120]

During the diagnostic act in the pox hospitals the medical practitioners linked these individual disease narratives to the physical signs of each candidate. The hospital records show that the two healers usually worked alongside each other for several years, sometimes even decades. Together they examined hundreds of bodies, and restored to health the great majority of their French-diseased patients. Through their long-standing close cooperation the two healers had reached a shared understanding of which physical signs of each candidate pointed to the pox's underlying invisible essence and what element of his or her disease narrative supported their own considerations. Through mutually-gained experience they were able to distinguish signs of the pox from those physical manifestations that were only accidental or fortuitous, dependent on a candidate's individual nature, natural complexion, dwelling place, nutrition, profession, age, astrological inclination and so on.

Diagnostic Results

There were three different diagnostic verdicts the medical practitioners could possibly reach. First of all, if in their opinion a petitioner's physical signs were not attributable to the pox, the petitioner was deemed 'unsuitable' (*untauglich*) for the *Blatterhaus*. Such was the verdict in the case of the elderly supplicant Elias Schmid in 1615.[121] Schmid had been to the *Blatterhaus* once already, when he complained of various 'body pains'. On that occasion, he informed the authorities, 'the disease … had raged only in my limbs'. Now, however, it had developed into an open wound, which he hoped a second stay in the *Blatterhaus* would cure. This hope was not fulfilled: at his inspection on 14 March 1615 the *Blatterhaus* medical practitioners reached the same conclusion as at his first examination, and diagnosed a 'fistulated ulcer' on his right side, affecting some of his ribs.[122] A treatment with guaiacum would be of little benefit to him, they concluded, 'for which reason they find him unsuitable for the *Blatterhaus*'. As an alternative treatment they suggested an intensive bathing cure in one of city's nearby spas.

The soldier Hans Mayr, from Nördlingen, was luckier than Elias. He attended the public examination at the *Blatterhaus* in November 1594 complaining of 'severe excruciating and ceaseless pains in the limbs especially … in the thighs',

120 This is also stressed by Jütte, *Ärzte*, p. 42, and Kinzelbach, *Gesundbleiben*, p. 284; p. 394.

121 StAA, St Martin VI, Prod. 83: Supplikation des Elias Schmid vom 10. März 1615; it also contains the decision of the physicians from 14 March 1516.

122 For the case see StAA, St Martin, VI, Nr. 47, Prod. 67: Supplikation des Simon Wöbely vom 3. November 1594. The examination result from 5 November 1594 is signed by Doctor Johann Ulrich Rumler.

and particularly intense when urinating. In his case the medical practitioners were of one mind that he was 'in need of treatment on account of his great pains and ulcers'. He was therefore judged a 'suitable' (*tauglich*) candidate who could be admitted without hesitation.

However, in a considerable number of cases the two examining medical practitioners failed to agree and stopped short of a definitive 'suitable' or 'unsuitable' verdict. Instead they judged the candidate's physical state as fluid and somewhere in between these two conditions. They could even come to the conclusion that a body was harbouring two different diseases simultaneously at the time of the examination. One of these cases has already been presented in Chapter 2. Katharina Moltenrock was admitted to the *Blatterhaus* for preliminary observation in August 1566 as her symptoms suggested to the medical practitioners both leprosy *and* the pox. Despite treatment in the pox hospital, her condition did not improve. When, in a second examination on 3 September, Moltenrock's signs were all unequivocally identified as related to leprosy, she was immediately discharged from the *Blatterhaus*.[123]

The already-mentioned Philipp Eß is another telling example of an individual whose physical signs could not be definitively judged. Eß had presented himself at the *Blatterhaus* in December 1618, and turned out to be a somewhat controversial case for the appointed medical experts.[124] After examining his naked body in detail, they agreed on the following diagnosis: his physical signs, they claimed, were ambiguous. They simultaneously pointed to the French pox and to an ailment that they identified as 'elephantiasis'. (The latter was classified as one of the four possible forms of leprosy in the popular sixteenth-century vernacular medical treatise written by the Augsburg pharmacist Christoph Wirsung.)[125] Because Eß's physical signs indicating the French disease outnumbered those pointing to elephantiasis, the two practitioners concluded that a cure at their institution would probably be beneficial. Since he fulfilled all the other requirements for admission – citizenship, poverty, and evidence of an irreproachable family and community life – the hospital's civic administrators followed the practitioners' recommendation and admitted him to the male ward. But only a few weeks later Eß's wretched body reappeared in the hospital records. His bodily signs had re-attracted the attention of the hospital's medical practitioners on one of their daily rounds. After keeping him under close supervision for a few days, the physician and the barber-surgeon came to the conclusion that his physical signs had morphed to unambiguous signs of leprosy. This new diagnosis triggered instant and dire consequences for Eß's institutional fate: he was now considered a serious health

123 For the following see StAA, Collegium Medicum. Wundärzte, Bader u. Barbire, in specie betr. von 1570–1804; c) Siechen von 1555–1649: Supplikation von Leopold Drenkel, Marcus Wind und Jeremias Martius vom 3. September 1566.

124 StAA, St Martin, VI, Prod. 7a; Prod. 86; for a more detailed analysis of this particular case see Stein, 'Meaning of Signs'.

125 See Christoph Wirsung, *Artzney Buch* (Heidelberg, 1586), pp. 510–12.

threat to his fellow convalescent inmates and was immediately expelled from the *Blatterhaus*. The sources unfortunately do not tell us whether he applied for admission at one of the city's three leprosy hospitals. From similar cases, however, we know that this would have been a likely option.

The changing diagnosis of Katharina Moltenrock's and Philip Eß's physical signs is a common phenomena in the *Blatterhaus* records and underlines the flexibility and fluidity of disease definition and classification in the early modern period, which I have explored in more detail in Chapter 1. The metamorphosis of diseases, as exemplified in the cases of Moltenrock and Eß (and others), was rooted in a particular conception of a physical sign and how its relationship to disease was understood. No physical sign (investigated by the medial practitioners together with the candidate) was automatically assigned to the pox. The decisive moment, which turned a physical sign into a sign *of* the pox was the encounter between the medical practitioner and the applicant in the examination room of one of the Augsburg pox hospitals. The meaning of any signs, the diagnostic result, was a merger between the medical practitioners' understanding of the applicant's condition and the latter's previous and/or simultaneous engagement in the same matter. The diagnostic verdict reached in the examination presented a picture of disease that seemed to all the parties involved a meaningful and explanatory reflection of the candidate's condition. However, it was also understood by all parties involved in this act that the agreement which was reached over the meaning of particular signs was not fixed, but could be altered at any moment in time due to changing diagnostic circumstances.

This is what Walburga Reuchart experienced when she brought her sick three-year-old daughter for examination to the *Blatterhaus* in May 1564.[126] The girl was a serious and heartbreaking case: she was in terrible pain, her small body covered with open lesions and ulcers. However, Doctor Zeller and barber-surgeon Hans Gablinger came to the conclusion that the girl's signs were not related to the French disease but rather to some kind of poisonous and infectious rash, which was not treated in the pox hospital. They therefore refused her admission and advised her to try the Hospital of the Ghost – an odd suggestion in view of the fact that this institution refused to accept children (or any sufferers) from open lesions identified as infectious. Walburga Reuchart was not satisfied with the practitioners' verdict. She identified her daughter's lesions as signs of the French disease. Although she had been widowed and was without any substantial financial means, she managed to obtain the opinion of several healers in town, all of whom confirmed her initial suspicion and, aware of her precarious financial situation, had advised her to apply for free treatment at the municipal pox hospital. While she was not convinced of Zeller's and Gablinger's diagnosis, and was perhaps unaware of the various health-care institutions' admissions practices, she initially followed their suggestion and took her daughter to the Holy Ghost Hospital. In the official examination certificate, the Hospital's three appointed physicians – Leopold Trenklin, Marcus Wind,

126 StAA, St Martin, VI, Prod. 35.

and Bernhard Schludi – backed Walburga's interpretation.[127] According to their medical experience they judged the girl's signs as unambiguously related to the French pox. The official diagnosis certificate, signed by three important members of Augsburg's medical elite, empowered Reuchart to return to the French-disease hospital and officially question Zeller's and Gablinger's diagnosis. Both reacted furiously, not so much because of her reappearance (many sufferers showed up several times), but because of her audacity in openly defying their diagnosis with an official certificate issued by their own colleagues. They felt that their professional honour and expertise was being attacked publicly. In a letter written to the town council, both bemoaned the three physicians' unsporting conduct. They also sought to control the smoldering reproach, sparked by Walburga and the physicians' certificate, that they had deliberately 'misread' the girl's physical signs in order to avoid burdening themselves with the admission of a complicated and labour-intensive case of the pox. Zeller and Gablinger re-emphasised their original verdict: in their professional opinion, based on their long experience with the pox, the little girl was not suffering from the French pox. Moreover, they added, even if they made a generous exception and admitted the girl, it was her overall physical state that stood against her admission: her body had been so badly ravished that little or no improvement could be expected. It was to be feared that she would become a 'permanent sick' in the institution – and it was well known, as they cleverly reminded the money-conscious hospital administrators (quoting the house rules), that they were not allowed to admit anyone whose recovery they had judged impossible.

The fate of Walburga Reuchart's daughter is unknown. Her case, however, not only stresses again the fluidity of medical diagnosis and suggests, like that of Philipp Eß, that it was understood as temporary. Moreover, the diagnostic act was strongly shaped by the immediate context in which it took place: while *Blatterhaus* practitioners Gablinger and Zeller judged the signs as not related to the pox, their peers at the Holy Ghost Hospital (according to their expertise in these matters) did.

One might be tempted to interpret the changing verdicts in the Reuchart case as an example of personal and professional rivalry over institutional funds and workloads. While such motives cannot be excluded, this interpretation assumes that all medical practitioners involved in the diagnosis intentionally 'misread' the little girl's physical signs in order to get their way. Moreover, by presuming that there is a 'right' way of reading the signs (which is withheld from the mother by the medical practitioners), this interpretation of the case does not give Reuchart any agency in the act of diagnosis. But was she really a victim of a medical world in which power is with the medical practitioners?

A less functional explanation is probably preferable. These struggles over the interpretation of physical signs (of which we can find many in the archive) may well have been a necessary consequence of a completely different understanding of the meaning of physical signs and their relation to the human body. It was widely

127 For the physicians see Martz, *Gesundbleiben*, pp. 27; 30; 36.

understood in sixteenth-century Augsburg that proper knowledge and diagnosis of the pox could not be gained by the mere act of sensing the physical sign, but only by decoding its invisible meaning. Earlier in this chapter it has been demonstrated in detail how this belief in the interpretation of the invisible in order to define the pox shaped the way its diagnosis was conducted in the three pox hospitals. In the absence of our modern distinction between a subjective and an objective gaze, as well as of standardised procedures to measure bodily functions, the identity of the French pox almost certainly could be forged only in a process of discursive mediations between the various parties involved in the very act of the diagnosis. The power of disease definition was equally shared among all participants. The opinion of academic physicians or barber-surgeons never carried absolute authority: it could, and often would, be contested by the sufferers themselves, and/or by their relatives, or even by their professional peers (as shown by the Reuchart case). The diagnosis of the pox required the subtle art of evaluation and negotiation that, in the final judgement, all parties involved accepted the 'medical portrait' of the pox drawn for that particular case.[128]

What happened to those candidates who had the good fortune (unlike Walburga's little daughter) to be univocally diagnosed with the pox? They had to first surrender their clothes to the pox/wood mother who kept them until treatment was complete and handed them back on the day of their discharge. In exchange they were given the standard hospital attire: linen nightshirt, nightcap, bathing robe and felt slippers. Their names, domicile, and date of referral were recorded by the pox/wood father in a book. Before being assigned to a bed in one of the two wards, they were given a bath by the maids, and any open sores were cleaned and bandaged by the barber-surgeon. It was then time to begin their cure.

128 For the comparison of medical diagnosis with painting see Nance, *Mayerne*, p. 78: 'Just as a good portrait conveys a sense of a person's unique being, so a good medical portrait produces a sketch of the patient's particular collection of conditions, morbid and non-morbid, recent and longstanding, the gifts of nature and the effects of nurture.'

Chapter 4
Treating the Pox

The Guaiacum Cure

From the early 1520s, guaiacum wood was considered the most efficient pox treatment in all three Augsburg hospitals. Every new inmate was prophylactically 'laid into the wood'.[1] According to medical opinion, guaiacum's primary and secondary qualities made it particularly suited to expelling the acid, cold-wet morbid matter from the poxed body, regardless of its individual complexion.[2] Guaiacum warmed and dried the elemental bodily fluids and made them thin and liquid, the barber-surgeon Joseph Schmid proclaimed. Administered as a hot potion it stimulated perspiration, thus allowing the morbid pox matter to be conveyed naturally out of the body.[3]

The wood was initially purchased in substantial quantities from pharmacists and wood dealers in or outside the city.[4] In 1563, for example, the Fuggerei administrator, Moritz Kronegger bought the stockpile of 3,555½ lb of guaiacum, purchased at 5½ fl. a cord. Kronegger had the wood sawn into small pieces, packed in linen sacks, and then stored in a dark and dry cellar. By the early 1580s, however, the quantity of guaiacum purchased at any one time was substantially reduced. Kronegger's successors bought only as much wood as might be needed for one year's treatment. This new purchasing strategy was initiated by the academic physicians who had become convinced that long periods of storage reduced the wood's healing properties. Old or even rotten wood was thought not only to be ineffective but occasionally harmful. According to Joseph Schmid, the most successful treatments were to be achieved with fresh guaiacum that was still moist at its core. It was easily recognisable, he explained, by its oily, almost black colouring.[5]

Between 1583 and 1631 the average consumption of guaiacum during the nine-month treatment period in the Fuggerei *Holzhaus* amounted to roughly 166 lb.[6] But not all the wood bought by the administrators was for the institution's own

1 F.A. 5.3.2 (a), Holzordnungen, Ordnungen Holzhaus auf dem Gänsbühl von 1568.

2 For a detailed description how the drug was thought to act in the human body see Chapter 1.

3 Schmid, *Kurtzer Bericht*, p. 173.

4 F.A. 66.1, fol. 1r. For Augsburg pharmacies see Gensthaler, *Medizinalwesen*.

5 Schmid, *Kurtzer Bericht*, p. 173.

6 For the exact amount of guaiacum consumption between 1583 and 1631 see Stein, *Franzosenkrankheit*, p. 204.

needs. Small amounts of the wood were made available to private individuals, such as the apothecary Johann Schober, who, in 1563, purchased 29¼ lb of guaiacum bark for his shop in the Steingasse.[7] However, not everyone had to pay for it. Local healers who treated pox victims outside the *Holzhaus* at the behest – and expense – of members of the Fugger families received the wood free of charge from the Fuggerei administrator.[8] Other recipients of 'free' guaiacum included Fugger servants and employees: Philipp Fugger's groom, Ulrich Zichen, received ½ lb of the wood in 1577 for his cure at a private local pox clinic of his choice.[9] Occasionally quantities of the stored guaiacum were also sent abroad: on 7 May 1546 a delivery of 10 lb of guaiacum was made to Georg Hörman, the Fuggers' agent in the Tyrolean mining town of Schwaz.[10]

While members of Augsburg's medical trade and Fugger employees received the wood gratis, members of the founding families always paid for it. In 1556 Kronegger sold 165 lb of guaiacum wood to Raymund Fugger for 11 fl.[11] Two years later Kronegger delivered a further 46½ lb to him and 13½ lb. to Marx Fugger, at a total cost of 4 fl.[12] These occasional purchases of guaiacum by Fugger family members do not necessarily indicate that they were suffering from the pox. According to Joseph Schmid, guaiacum's warm-wet qualities were also valuable in the treatment of other diseases such as 'chronic pains in the limbs, gout, winds, persistent headaches, ailments of the liver and the spleen [and] for external wounds'.[13]

The Fuggerei administrator's accounts reveal that (depending on the patient's individual physical condition) between 2 lb and 10 lb of guaiacum were required for a treatment lasting between three to six weeks.[14] At an average price of 1 fl. for 8 lb, guaiacum cure was not particularly expensive, as the anonymous Augsburg author of *A Clear Account* recorded already in 1525.[15] By the end of the sixteenth century, as Joseph Schmid reports, the wood was even considered a poor man's remedy.[16] At the beginning of the century, however, when the wood was still a novelty, local timber dealers, pharmacists and itinerant healers may well have sold

7 F.A.66.1.1, fol. 10v. Schober, who had purchased the pharmacy from Christoph Wirsung in 1557, was the Fuggerei *Holzhaus* pharmacist at the time.

8 For more examples see F.A.66.2.7, fol. 14r.

9 For more examples of Fugger family members offering guaiacum to sick employees see F.A. 66.2.4 (c), fol. 34r; F.A. 66.2.2, fol. 14r; see F.A. 66.2.3(b), fol. 98v.

10 F.A. 66.2.3 (b), fol. 98v; and F.A. 66.2.2, fol. 10r.

11 F.A. 66.1.1, fol. 47a.

12 F.A. 66.1.1, fol. 48a.

13 Schmid, *Kurtzer Bericht*, pp. 173–4.

14 For similar observations see *Ein bevert recept*, fol. Aiiia, which suggests 6 to 10 lb for a cure. The author of *Ain clarer bericht*, fol. Aiiiia, calculated 4 to 10 lb per cure.

15 Anonymus, *Ain clarer bericht*, fol. Aiiiia.

16 Schmid, *Kurtzer Bericht*, p. 174. The wood's inexpensiveness convinced Johannes Wittich to include guaiacum in his vernacular medical book for poor people. See Wittich, *Arme vnd dürfftige Leute*, pp. 116–19.

it at greatly inflated prices, as the other Augsburg anonymous author of *A Tried and Tested Prescription* complained retrospectively in 1518.[17]

How was the wonder drug from the New World prepared? To be suitable for treatment, the wood had first to be planed into small shavings, for 'only when boiled in small strips can the wood's powers be properly released' (see Figure 4.1).[18] By the mid-sixteenth century not only the wood itself, but also its shavings had to be fresh, or at least not more then two months old, to be considered therapeutically effective.[19] In each hospital the employee responsible for preparing the decoction – a female 'wood boiler' in the *Blatterhaus*, and the wood mother in the two *Holzhäusern* – was instructed to prepare the potion for each patient in strict accordance with the physician's orders. None of these instructions have survived, but some information as to how the guaiacum potion was prepared can be gleaned from *A Tried and Tested Prescription*:[20] 2 lb of fresh shavings were to be placed in a glazed clay pot and covered with six measures (i.e. 7.2 l) of fresh water. The mixture should first be allowed to draw for twenty-four hours. The next day it was covered and had to simmer on a moderate heat until a third of the liquid had evaporated.[21] The froth thus produced (being especially beneficial in treating the festering sores of the pox) was then to be skimmed off and poured into a glass. If daubed twice a day with the foam the sores would soon disappear, promised the author of *A Tried and Tested Prescription*. After removal of the froth the decoction had to simmer for another eight hours, until only half the original volume remained. The pot was never to be left unattended during the boiling period, to ensure that the mixture did not boil over or burn. Finally the pot was to be removed from the fire and the contents left to cool for twenty-four hours. It was then to be strained through a linen cloth into a glass, 'at which point the potion is ready for use'. Readers were advised that 2 lb of wood to 6 measures (7.2 l) was the right concentration for persons of average complexion or temperament. For sufferers of a more delicate complexion, the concentration should be modified accordingly, the author advised.

17 He warned his readers never to pay more than 30 fl. for a pound of guaiacum. See Anonymus, *Ain bevert recept*.

18 Schmid, *Kurtzer Bericht*, p. 175.

19 See the letter of Fuggerei Holzhaus physician Christoph Heuberger from 7 March 1577 in F.A.5.2.13, Holzhaus in der Fuggerei 1577–1662, Prod. 2, fol. 4a.

20 The instructions are similar to other guaiacum recipes. In fact, the instructions from *Ain bevert recept* can be found word for word in Wittich, *Arme vnd bedürfftige Leute*, pp. 116–19.

21 According to the house rules of all three hospitals the maid responsible for the boiling of the potion was not allowed to leave the room during this period. See StAA, Blatterhaus, Ordnung von 1581, pag. 2; and F.A. 5.3.2 (a) Holzordnungen Ordnung Holzhaus auf dem Gänsbühl von 1568.

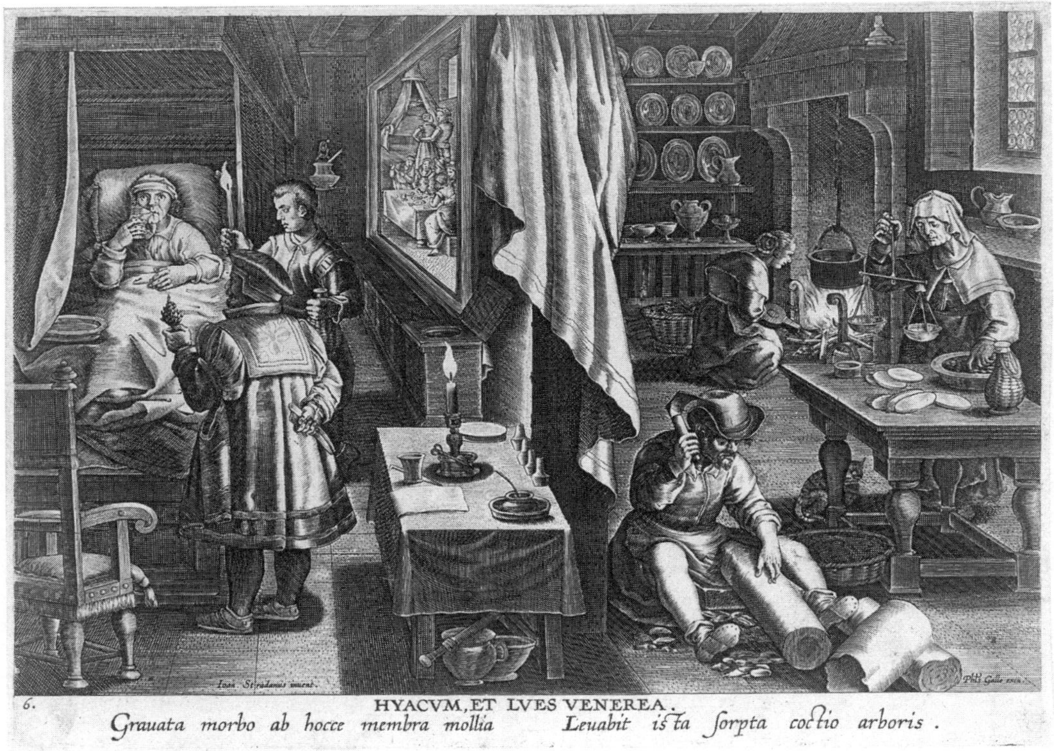

Figure 4.1 A domestic scene showing the different steps of the preparation of guaiacum and the following cure. Reproduced by courtesy of the Wellcome Library, London. Source: Engraving by Jan van der Straet after Philipp Galle

In determining the exact amount of wood to be used, the seasonal conditions had to be taken into account: on hot summer days it was advisable to use a pound of guaiacum shavings at most, 'so that it retains its taste and effectiveness', wrote the author of *A Tried and Tested Prescription*. The house rules of the *Holzhaus* on the Goosehill for 1568 indicate how seriously such instructions were taken: 'The wood potion should be adjusted ... because neither all sick are of one kind or complexion, nor of the same age. Some of them are more poisoned and damaged than others. Therefore the wood water should be boiled according to the instructions of the doctors and without their orders nothing should be changed.'[22] The maid boiling the guaiacum potion in the municipal *Blatterhaus* had to adhere to similarly strict regulations: 'she should boil the water according to the orders of the doctor who adapts [the water's or potion's] intensity to summer or winter time, cold or hot weather, the weakness or strength, youth or old age of the sick. And she should change its composition according to their [the doctors'] orders and follow them'.[23]

The potion was given to patients twice a day. In the *Holzhaus* on the Goosehill it was administered every morning two hours before the visit of the barber-surgeon, around 5 am and again at 4 pm in the afternoon.[24] Inmates of average age and complexion were given ¼ measure (300 ml), very young or elderly patients correspondingly less, approximately ⅛ measure (150 ml). To drink more of the potions than prescribed by the doctors was strictly forbidden. The Fuggerei physician Christoph Heuberger explained why:[25] it was a widespread misconception, he wrote in 1577 to the two trustees of the Fugger family, that drinking more guaiacum speeded up the healing process. Each patient could only tolerate and digest a certain amount of the sweat potion depending on his or her age and individual complexion. By consuming more than this quantity, patients could easily 'overstrain' their stomachs. Unable to 'boil it [the potion] down' quickly enough, the guaiacum then remained undigested in the patient's stomach, which could potentially worsen his or her condition, Heuberger warned.[26]

The drinking of the potion was followed by an hour of intense sweating during which great precaution was undertaken that the inmates were not exposed to cold, since, as the author of *A Tried and Tested Prescription* warned, 'a person then

22 F.A. 5.3.2 (a) Holzordnungen, Ordnung Holzhaus auf dem Gänsbühl von 1568.

23 StAA, Blatterhaus, Ordnung von 1581, pag. 22.

24 F.A. 5.3.2 (a), Holzkordnungen, Ordnung Holzhaus auf dem Gänsbühl von 1568. In the *Blatterhaus* the inmates received the potion at 4 am and at 1 pm. StAA, Blatterhaus, Ordnung von 1581, p. 18.

25 For the Catholic physician Christoph Heuberger see Martz, *Gesundheitswesen*, p. 35.

26 In this interesting letter Heuberger reported on the existing guaiacum cure and suggested some therapeutic improvements. See F.A. 5.2.13, Prod. 2, fol. 3–4, Bericht des Fuggerei Holzhausdoktors Christoph Heuberger from 7. März 1577.

exposed may be putting his life in danger'.[27] The Nuremberg barber-surgeon Franz Renner explained to his readers the medical reasoning behind this warning: guaiacum 'opens the body and skin through the heat and effects of the remedy so that impure vapours are released through the pores and expelled'. However, if patients were exposed to cold air, Renner warned, 'the pores of the skin become sensitive and close, trapping the contaminated vapours'. To prevent the pores from doing so, the patients in all three hospitals were swathed in thick eiderdown quilts and furs, and staff had strict instructions to ensure that no one heedlessly exposed and uncovered him- or herself. When they had finished sweating, patients were dried with linen towels, put into fresh nightgowns and had to rest in bed for a couple of hours.

Not everybody, however, responded positively to the guaiacum potion and the following sweating process. In those cases the medical practitioners resorted to more drastic measures.

The Mercury Cure

An inmate's physical condition had to be judged extremely serious before the medical practitioners would suggest mercury, a remedy that was widely regarded as potentially harmful to the patient. The house rules of all hospitals stated explicitly that the practitioners must 'use it with moderation, and try everything else first, before resorting to such a dangerous and sharp cure'.[28]

The toxic metal was administered in three different ways, the least dangerous of which was the so-called 'mercury water', a mercuric chloride. It was prepared by heating mercury with sulphuric acid and salt, and then applied with a brush onto the skin of the sufferer. The records reveal that the mercury water was preferably applied to those inmates whose general physical conditions were judged delicate and not robust enough to sustain a treatment with mercury ointment. The latter was specially prepared by the barber-surgeon and consisted of mercurium principatum[29] mixed with wax, various oils, animal and/or human fat, turpentine and various dried flowers and herbs to reduce (so it was believed) the metal's toxicity.[30] The appropriate quantity to be administered to each patient was determined by the learned physician, who also advised the barber-surgeon

27 Anonymus, *Ain bevert recept*, fol. Aiib.

28 See, for example, the rules for the *Holzhaus* on the Gänsbühl, F.A. 5.3.2. (a), Holzordnungen, Ordnung Holzhaus auf dem Gänsbühl 1568.

29 Mercurium Principatum was a mixture of mercury and aqua fortis. A contemporary preparation can be found in Renner, *Handbüchlein*, fol. 148–50.

30 Many of the barber-surgeon's shopping lists survive in the archives. Unfortunately they do not tell us anything about the dosage of the mercury used. For examples see F.A. 66.1.1, fol. 49v: (1563); F.A. 66.2.4 (b), fol. 29v (1576); F.A. 66.2.4 (g), fol. 30r–31r (1580); F.A. 66.2.4 (h), fol. 25v–26v (1581); F.A. 66.2.4 (r), fol. 14v–16r (1585); and for

where exactly to apply the ointment on the patient's skin.[31] For his own protection the barber-surgeon should always wear gloves when doing so, advised Joseph Schmid.[32] His Nuremberg colleague Franz Renner nurtured a mercury-phobia and maintained that during all his years of practice he had never once applied a mercury salve himself, 'for, though beneficial to the patient, it is dangerous for the practitioner'.[33] After applying the ointment (the hospital records suggest that this was done by the patients themselves) they were left to sweat, 'as the nature and quality of mercury is such that it very subtly filters through, dissolves and distributes the moist vapours, which then depart with the sweat through the pores. [It] also stimulates the uprising of moist vapours so that they come out through the mouth and in anal excretions'.[34] The continuous dripping of saliva or other fluids from the patients' mouths and other bodily openings during this treatment, or even the appearance of blood in their stools, was generally interpreted, 'not as ominous, but rather as a sign of hope of recovery', visible proof that the pox's morbid matter was finally leaving the body.[35] But to the experienced medical practitioner in charge of the treatment, such symptoms also indicated that it was high time to stop the treatment. Mercury ointments, wrote Schmid, should 'continue to be applied until the patient begins to complain of pains in his teeth and everything in his mouth is sore, and his whole mouth begins to slaver, the saliva runs out of his mouth. These signs would generally appear on the third, fourth, fifth and sixth day', he explained.[36] At that stage, he advised, the treatment should cease forthwith. Where the mercury had caused inflammation of the mucous membrane in the mouth, patients should be given a cup of soothing gargle water of sweet almonds, rose honey and liquorice.

Only in 'hopeless cases', in which neither the mercuric chloride nor the more aggressive ointment had achieved lasting results, was fumigation called for. This was considered by far the most dangerous of the three forms of mercury treatment. Schmid counselled its use only in extreme cases because 'the symptoms that follow the use of mercury vapour treatment are much more severe, painful and dangerous than in the ointment cure'.[37] As the mercury fumes, a mix of cinnabar, herbs, incenses and spices, could be potentially dangerous for other inmates 'because they are forced to inhale such poisonous vapours' those patients

the *Holzhaus* on the Gänsbühl F.A. 88.2., fol. 33r/v (1574); F.A. 88.2, fol. 3r (1584); F.A. 88.3, fol. 3a (1600).

31 For instructions on how to prepare mercury ointments see Renner, *Handbüchlein*, fol. 146–8; for the instructions of the barber-surgeon in the house rules StAA, Blatterhaus, Ordnung von 1581, p. 43

32 Schmid, *Kurtzer Bericht*, p. 202.

33 Renner, *Handbüchlein*, fol. LXXr.

34 Ibid., fol. IIIIr.

35 Ibid.

36 Schmid, *Kurtzer Bericht*, p. 204.

37 Ibid., pp. 207–8.

who had been selected for fumigation were confined to the two small extra rooms on the ground floor of the *Holzhäuser*.[38] They had to take off all clothing and might be given a heart-strengthening remedy before treatment, as recommended by Schmid, to 'drive the poison inhaled with the vapour away from the heart and thus defend it'.[39] Then the door to their rooms was locked, and the patients themselves poured the mercury mixture into a red-hot pan. They would then inhale the vapours for a period of time, either standing over the pan or, if too weak, lying on the bed as Figure 4.2 shows. Alternatively, they exposed only certain parts of the body to the vapours. Depending on the severity of each patient's condition, the fumigation could be repeated several times. Only when the patient 'complains of a sore mouth and his saliva begins to run should one cease the treatment and make good use of warm gargle water', the hospital sources report.[40] As with the other forms of mercury treatment, the inhalation of mercury vapours was followed by at least an hour's rest, when the patients, under supervision, were to lie in bed on their respective wards and sweat.

All three mercury treatments ended with a final purging of the patient, 'so that what is still existing of the sharp and slimy disease matter will be driven from the body entirely and all the inner organs and bowels will be cleansed from such dirtiness and impurity'.[41]

Surgery

The barber-surgeon not only prepared all the mercury-containing treatments, but also all the other, less dangerous salves and plasters. Accompanied by the learned physician, he and his apprentice visited the wards twice a day, cleaning and dressing wounds. If necessary, he also performed surgical operations, including the cauterisation of ulcers, the removal of gangrenous flesh and, occasionally, amputations.[42] The latter became necessary when a limb had been completely ravaged by the pox and both medical practitioners feared that the poisonous pox matter accumulated in the rotten limb would possibly spread to other areas of the body. Such was the fate of Peter Gansmair from Oberndorf, admitted to the Fuggerei for a salve treatment on 4 July 1544 on Anton Fugger's recommendation.[43]

---

38 For the quotation see StAA, Blatterhaus, Ordnung von 1581. For more information on mercury fumigation see Lesky, *Quecksilber und Quecksilberverbindungen*, p. 3202. For the ingredients used in the Fuggerei *Holzhaus* see F.A.66.1.3, fol. 25a (1585).

39 Schmid, *Kurtzer Bericht*, p. 212. However, according to Schmid's experience, this was only the case after five to nine fumigations.

40 For the following see F.A. 66.1.3, fol. 16r (1585).

41 Schmid, *Kurtzer Bericht*, p. 204.

42 Renner, *Handbüchlein*, fol. CVr–v offers a vivid description of such an amputation.

43 For the following see F.A. 66.2.1, fol. 167v.

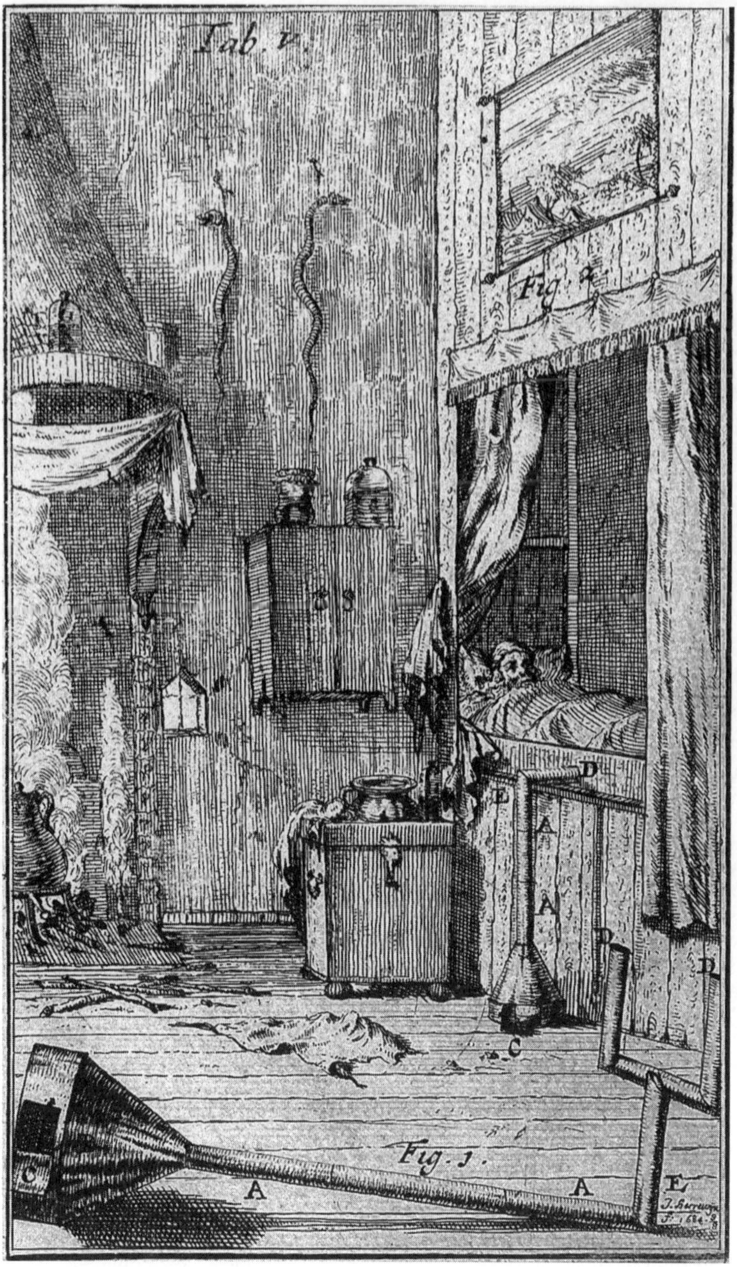

Figure 4.2 The sweating cure showing a patient lying in bed over a hot tube. Reproduced by courtesy of the Wellcome Library, London. Source: Engraving by J. Harrewijns, in Stephen Blaankart, *Venus belegert en ontset* (Amsterdam, 1685)

But his condition did not improve. On the contrary, Gansmair developed gangrene in his right foot. By 23 July, finding the pain unbearable, he begged the presiding physician Adolph Occo I to instruct his colleague, the barber-surgeon master Joseph, to put an end to his torment and to amputate the diseased limb. After prolonged consultation between the two medical practitioners, Gansmair's morbid wish was finally granted and the foot was cut off. His determination seems to have paid off: his condition noticeably improved, so that on 24 September he was discharged as 'cured'.

Whether Gansmair replaced his lost foot with an artificial one we do not know, but Augsburg's barber-surgeons certainly would have offered him a variety of different prostheses to choose from.[44] In fact, for many of them the manufacture of artificial limbs was a lucrative extra source of income. A real 'moneyspinner' in Joseph Schmid's assortment was a little metal plate for pox victims whose palates had been so badly eaten away by the disease that 'they will never again be able to speak clearly'.[45] Schmid produced these small removable palate replacements from white tin or gold and silver, depending on the size of the sufferer's purse. 'The plate', he explained, 'has to be a bit wider than the hole in the bone of the palate and thick as a groat, and curved in the shape of the palate so that it fits better. On top of the plate pointing toward the brain fix a little sponge that will catch the humidity dropping from the brain. The sponge will swell with the humidity and keep the plate in position so that it cannot fall out and the person can speak properly again.' Schmid not only fabricated plates for the palate, but also provided new noses for those who had lost theirs to the ravages of the pox.[46] The customers could choose from a selection of wooden, ebony or metal noses, which were tied with a ribbon behind the wearer's head. For male customers Schmid fitted his noses with a moustache in various colours and shapes.

Also for male patients who had lost their private parts to the pox, Schmid manufactured wooden or metal urination tubes, which the patient attached before urinating. The production of these tubes, it appears, was something of a tradition in the Schmid family. He reported that his father Balthasar Schmid had already made them for the pox patients he treated at the family home. His son Joseph remembered very vividly the case of a tailor's apprentice from the city of Kaufbeueren.[47] His father had treated the young man over a couple of weeks

44 For reconstructive surgery in the early modern period see Mariacarla Gadebusch Bondio, *Medizinische Ästetik. Kosmetische und plastische Chirurgie zwischen Antike und früher Neuzeit* (München, 2005).

45 For the following see Schmid, *Kurtzer Bericht*, pp. 259–61. His Nuremberg colleague Franz Renner, however, considered these metal plates rather unpractical because they were, in his view, difficult and painful for the patient to remove. Sometimes they got loose, fell out and into the throat, causing suffocation. He himself preferred small leather pieces on which he had fixed pieces of sponge. See Renner, *Handbüchlein*, fol. LXXXVIr.

46 For nose prosthetics see Gadebusch Bondio, *Plastische Chirurgie.*

47 For the following see Schmid, *Kurtzer Bericht*, p. 223.

during which his phallus was completely eaten by the pox and 'peeled at the front, like an onion'. It was only thanks to his father's tubes that he was able to urinate and thus to survive. Joseph Schmid continued this family tradition with similar success. He prided himself that during the occupation of the city in the Thirty Years' War, one of his products saved the life of a Swedish officer in 1633, 'whose whole organ was infected with gangrene right up to his stomach'. To Schmid's greatest astonishment, the rotting member of the Swedish soldier, having fallen off at some point, was 'given [a] proper burial' to which he had been invited.

Regiment of Life: The Six Non-Naturals

The guaiacum and/or mercury treatments as well as all surgical procedures were accompanied by a strict regiment aimed at controlling each patient's interaction with the six 'non-naturals': air, evacuation and retention, food and drink, motion and rest, sleeping and waking, and the passions of the soul.[48] It was the medical practitioner's responsibility to influence these in such a way that the patient's individual nature would be strengthened in its struggle against the pox.

Air

In all three hospitals the greatest attention was paid to the quality and quantity of air since it was believed that it penetrated the body at will through the pores of the skin and other bodily orifices. The belief in air's potentially harmful effects influenced the course of the pox cure in several ways. First of all, certain months of the year were regarded as more propitious than others for commencing treatment. According to medical opinion, the cold-moist quality that characterised the pox matter made the spring, summer and early autumn months, with their warm temperatures, especially suitable. According to Schmid, 'this sort of air is suitable for all cold diseases … In late autumn almost all diseases tend to last longer, and they produce worst results. Because the expulsion [of diseased matter] through sweat, urine, defecation and sputum are hampered by the general dampness of that season, they have to be artificially brought about by laxative measures and sweating'.[49] It was for this reason (besides the economic considerations mentioned earlier) that the Fugger *Holzhäuser* houses were only open for cures from mid-March to early November. The municipal *Blatterhaus*, in contrast, accepted patients all year round, although its archival records do not reveal whether it actually carried out treatments during the cold season or merely offered pox sufferers a warm place to stay with the promise of treatment the following spring.

---

48 For the detailed discussion of the 'six non-naturals' see Niebyl, *Non-naturals*, pp. 486–92; Rather, *Non-Natural*, pp. 337–47; Mikkeli, *Hygiene*, pp. 14–92.

49 Schmid, *Kurtzer Bericht*, p. 158.

As much as the body was believed to be constantly under attack from the surrounding air, so were all hospital medications. Great pains were taken to ensure that medicines were not exposed to corrupted air. The guaiacum decoction was regarded as particularly susceptible. The maid responsible for boiling the wood in the *Blatterhaus* was instructed to allow the potion to cool down after boiling, before storing it in the cool cellar, 'so that the cellar is not made steamy and the potion ruined'.[50]

Maintaining a consistent temperature in all rooms, but especially in the sick wards, was a daily challenge for the hospital staff trying to follow medical orders. The physician ruled that 'the sick shall be kept in the same moderate temperature all day, except that at four o'clock in the morning (an hour before the sweat potion [guaiacum] is administered at five) the rooms may be heated a bit more'.[51] Abrupt changes in temperature through the sudden opening of windows or doors were to be avoided at all costs. Thick woollen curtains over the glass windows protected patients in the two *Holzhäusern* from harmful draughts. In the *Holzhaus* on the Goosehill, the first bed by the door in each ward was shielded by a black woollen curtain suspended from iron rods to ensure that the patient was not exposed to unnecessary health risks whenever the door was opened.[52]

Although the doctors laid great stress on the constancy of room temperatures, they were equally concerned with the importance of fresh air. The Fuggerei physician Christoph Heuberger warned that patients deprived of fresh air were at risk from their own fetid exhalations.[53] The maids were instructed to open the ward windows for a few minutes several times a day, so that 'the air may be purged and purified'. During these airings they were to ensure that all patients remain in their beds, securely covered by eiderdowns and furs. Since air could penetrate the body not just through natural orifices such as mouth, nose, anus and pores, but also through open wounds and oozing ulcers, these were to be covered and protected at all costs by bandages and plasters. When, twice a day, in the early morning and in the late afternoon, the barber-surgeon in the *Blatterhaus* changed the bandages, he was urged to work as fast as possible so as not to leave the lesions long uncovered, 'for waiting with uncovered wounds is both painful and harmful'.[54]

50 StAA, Blatterhaus, Ordnung von 1581, p. 22; see also the instructions in later house rules StAA, Blatterhaus, Ordnung von 1535; a similar instruction can be found for the *Holzhaus* on the Goosehill F.A. 5.3.2 (a) Holzkurordnung vom 1. September 1568.

51 F.A. 5.2.13, Prod. 2, fol. 3–4: Bericht des Fuggereiholzhausdoktors Christoph Heuberger vom 7. März 1577.

52 F.A. 5.3.2 (c), Holz- und Schneidhaus Inventare 1572–1669: Inventar vom März 1584.

53 For the following see F.A. 5.2.13, Prod. 2, fol. 3–4: Bericht des Fuggereiholzhausdoktors Christoph Heuberger vom 7. März 1577.

54 StAA, Blatterhaus, Ordnung von 1581, p. 43. This instruction can already be found in the house rules of 1535, see StAA, Blatterhaus, Ordnung von 1535.

The fear of random 'air assaults' on the unprotected inner body through natural orifices and uncovered lesions was also one of the reasons why patients were strictly forbidden to leave the hospital during treatment. Even after recovery they were detained on the doctor's orders for another week or two to make sure that their recovery was permanent, although they no longer slept in their ward beds to avoid being infected again by the exhalations of the sick. During their recuperation they were encouraged by the staff to perform small tasks in and outside the hospital to build up their physical strength, and, more importantly, to accustom their body to the qualities and temperature of the outside air.[55]

Evacuation and Retention

The secretion of bodily fluids including the expulsion of morbid disease matter, as well as the intake of liquids were processes much easier for the hospitals' medical practitioners to control than the patient's atmospheric environment. Three distinct methods enabled them to influence the processes of secretion: bloodletting, purging and bathing.

Immediately after admission the inmate was bled and purged by the barber-surgeon under the physician's supervision. Both measures were designed to counter the 'fullness and malignity of the disease matter'.[56] At the same time they were supposed to thin the bodily fluids and dissolve any obstructions in the patient's body so that the 'channels and ducts by which excretion may be achieved are opened so that the wood [guaiacum] and other adopted cures can be more effective'.[57]

For purging (even more than for bloodletting) the taking into account of the patient's individual complexion and the way the seasons influenced this individual mixture of humours was vital. According to the tenets of Galenic-Hippocratic medicine, a body of an innately dry complexion, for instance, had to be purged less than one with a more moist temperament. The amount that had to be purged depended on the doctor's calculations as to how much morbid pox matter he suspected in the individual's body. The spring and early summer were generally believed to be the most favourable seasons for cleaning the body of morbid fluids

55 F.A. 5.3.2 (a) Holzkurordnung vom 1. September 1568; for similar instructions in the civic pox hospital see StAA, Blatterhaus, Ordnung von 1535 and StAA, Blatterhaus, Ordnung von 1581, p. 28.

56 Schmid, *Kurtzer Bericht*, pp. 166–7.

57 Ibid., p. 168. For Schmid's interesting discussion on bloodletting see ibid., p. 166. For the instructions in the pox hospitals see F.A. 5.3.2 (a), Holzhausordnung auf dem Gänsbühl 1568. F.A. 5.2.13, p. 1, Holzordnung in der Fuggerei von ca. 1525, reprinted in Weidenbacher, *Fuggerei*, p. 112; StAA, Blatterhaus, Ordnung von 1581, p. 41.

because its mild temperatures were thought to make all bodily humours thin and fluid and thus easier to expel.

In the pox hospitals the purgatives, adapted in substance and dosage to each individual patient, were administered as a soluble powder or in pill form. In order not to get confused over who had what and when, the in-house physician in the *Holzhaus* on the Goosehill noted all prescribed purgatives and other remedies in a book. During his ward rounds patients were encouraged to give full account of all bodily changes having occurred since they first took the purgatives so that the physician could record the results. The pox father in the *Blatterhaus* and the wood fathers in the Fugger *Holzhäusern* were responsible for administering the medication, and together with their staff had to ensure that the inmates 'diligently [took] the prescribed purgatives or other potions, electuaries or pills'.[58] The maid who fetched the purgatives and other medicines for the doctor from one of the city apothecaries had to guarantee that each patient received the medicine actually prescribed for him or her. They were instructed 'to take great care not to spill the potions, to administer the right medicine to each patient and not let anything fall in'.[59] To moderate a medicine's often unpleasant taste or help a patient whose throat was affected by the disease swallow the pills and potions, the maids would offer them a slice of soft white bread or spoonful of honey or juice with the remedy.[60]

Besides bloodletting and purging, the third corrective measure designed to influence the patient's humoral composition and quantity of the morbid matter was bathing.[61] This processes was enhanced by bath additives made of herbs and plants whose qualities (according to the 'contraria principle' of Hippocratic-Galenic medicine) were thought to counter those of the diseased matter.[62] In all three hospitals the daily hot water or steam bath (sometimes lasting over one hour) was an essential part of the treatment. In the *Blatterhaus* the bath maid heated the bath every morning at 5 am, so that 'the men may enter at 6, and the women soon after'.[63] Patients in the *Holzhaus* on the Goosehill were given a 'sweating potion of theriac' (a then very popular antidote believed to be effective against almost any disease).[64]

58 StAA, Blatterhaus, Ordnung Holzhaus auf dem Gänsbühl von 1568, p. 3.

59 F.A. 5.3.2 (a), Ordnung Holzhaus auf dem Gänsbühl von 1568. See also StAA, Fuggerei, Ordnung von 1555; StAA, Blatterhaus, Ordnung von 1535.

60 F.A. 5.3.2 (a), Ordnung Holzhaus auf dem Gänsbühl vom 1568; StAA, Blatterhaus, Ordnung von 1581, p. 20.

61 For the value of baths see StAA, Blatterhaus, Ordnung von 1576, p. 8.

62 F.A. 66.2.6 (e), fol. 7b. For the preparation of baths see Wirsung, *Arztney Buch*, pp. 503–4.

63 StAA, Blatterhaus, Ordnung von 1576, p. 8.

64 StAA, Fuggerei, Ordnung Holzhaus auf dem Gänsbühl von 1568. See also Schmid, *Kurtzer Bericht*, p. 169, who also advised to administer theriac in order to intensify the sweating process. On early modern theriac see Jütte, *Ärzte*, p. 79. See also Michael McVaugh, 'Theriac at Montpellier', *Sudhoffs Archiv* 56 (1972), pp. 113–43; Gilbert Watson, *Theriac and Mithridatium: A Study in Therapeutics* (London, 1966).

When and how often a patient should bathe or sweat during treatment was a matter of dispute among the doctors in the three hospitals. The *Blatterhaus* physicians, whose views have survived in more detail, were of the opinion that every patient should sweat intensely only for the first two weeks of treatment.[65] After that, they argued, such measures had no longer an impact on the quantity of morbid matter in the body. To submit patients to more hot baths after that period would be dangerous because excessive heat, they warned, would tire them and ultimately weaken their individual nature in its struggle to prevent 'further poisoning of the blood'. Excessive bathing could lead to the blood 'becoming inflamed and the sick [becoming] less inclined to sweating'. The maids and orderlies in all three hospitals were under strict instruction never to leave the patients in the bath unsupervised to ensure that no one 'drinks in the bath'.[66] To imbibe liquids while sweating was regarded as both counterproductive and dangerous, since the very point of the baths was to excrete harmful humours. It was foolish, the doctors argued, to give the moist-cold matter of the pox fresh nourishment by taking in fluids at the same time. Another reason why staff were to stay in the room with the sweating patients was 'to come to the aid of any [of them] who are suddenly overcome with exhaustion'. An hour of sweating in the heat without taking in fluids drove many patients to the limits of their physical strength. Fainting fits and sudden bouts of weakness often occurred.

Food and drink

The patients' daily food intake was as closely monitored and regulated by the learned physicians as the surrounding atmospheric condition and bodily evacuations and retentions. Dishes that were not specifically prescribed by the physician were strictly forbidden.[67] Hence, in the *Holzhaus* on the Goosehill the wood mother and their maids were instructed to monitor all gifts that were brought in to ensure that 'the sick do not eat and drink foodstuff secretly brought in by friends or strangers which was not prescribed by the doctors and would thus potentially harm them'.[68] Food given as alms by Augsburg citizens (a widespread practice during the sixteenth century) could not be used by the pox mother until the doctor 'had examined beforehand whether it was stale or fresh, fit or unfit for the sick, and to whom it might be given, since what is right for one sick person is not right for another'.[69]

---

65 For the following see StAA, Blatterhaus, Ordnung von 1576, p. 9.

66 For the following see StAA, Blatterhaus, Ordnung von 1581, p. 23, F.A. 5.3.2 (a), Ordnung Holzhaus auf dem Gänsbühl von 1568.

67 StAA, Fuggerei, Ordnung Holzhaus Fuggerei von 1555; StAA, Fuggerei, Ordnung Holzhaus auf dem Gänsbühl von 1568; StAA, Blatterhaus, Ordnung von 1581.

68 F.A. 5.3.2. (a), Ordnung Holzhaus auf dem Gänsbühl von 1568.

69 StAA, Blatterhaus, Ordnung von 1535.

The reason for such strict regulation was the importance assigned by Galenic-Hippocratic medicine to food and its specific qualities in preserving humoral balance explained in more detail in Chapter 1. All foodstuff was believed to influence the individual mixture of the humours in the blood and the slightest changes in one's daily eating habits could lead to dangerous imbalances and provoke various illnesses – including the French pox. However, due to the intimate links between the quality and quantity of foodstuff and the human complexion, food and drink could also be ascribed healing properties.[70] Properly used, their specific qualities could restore the body to its natural state of balance. Following the ancient 'contraria principle', the qualities of foodstuff should be diametrically opposed to the qualities attributed to the disease. Accordingly, in the case of the cold and wet pox, ailments of warm-dry quality were especially suitable.[71]

In the *Holzhaus* on the Goosehill the patients, some of whom spent several weeks in treatment, were not offered much variety. Apart from the week of fasting before Easter, during which they were given a fine milk purée containing sliced apple and sweet almonds, they were fed twice a day – in summer at 9 am, and in winter at 10, and between 5 and 6 in the evening – a meal of boiled chicken, veal or mutton.[72] With their ascribed warm and dry qualities these meats were thought to be light and easily digestible, especially when boiled rather than roasted, and 'so constituted that they create but little excrement and faeces'.[73] To be avoided at all costs were meats such as beef, pork and fish, which were believed to produce black bile and phlegm and thus threatened to increase the pox matter. Great importance was attached both to the quality of the meat at the point of purchase, and to observance of the physician's instructions during preparation. The wood mother went to the butcher in person to select the meat and had it cut into portions as specified by the physician.[74] For 1582, weekly and annual meat consumption in the *Holzhaus* on the Goosehill can be gleaned from the surviving shopping lists of the wood mother, Katharina Hochenauer. For an average of eleven patients during a thirty-three week treatment from 17 March to 22 October, she bought a total of 1,500 lb of veal and mutton. Average weekly consumption was therefore

70 Thomas Ehlert, 'Wissensvermittlung in deutschsprachiger Fachliteratur des Mittelalters, oder: Wie kam die Diätetik in die Kochbücher?', *Würzburger medizinhistorische Mitteillungen* 8 (1990), pp. 137–59.

71 See the lists of appropriate foodstuff in Alexander Seitz in Ukena, *Seitz*, pp. 21–4.

72 StAA, Fuggerei, Ordnung Holzhaus aus dem Gänsbühl von 1568; see also the weekly shopping lists for the Fuggerei Holzhaus F.A. 88.2 – 88.6.

73 Schmid, *Kurtzer Bericht*, p. 159.

74 Unfortunately the individual size of these portions is unknown. For similar instructions for the wood mother of the Fuggerei hospital see StAA, Blatterhaus, Ordnung Holzhaus in der Fuggerei von 1555.

approximately 45 lb per week.[75] With the boiled meat the patients were served unsalted white bread, which was also thought to be easy to digest.[76] The bread was not to be fresh, however, because that would only make the patients thirsty, and any additional liquid intake was to be avoided. Although patients were not served generous portions, the daily consumptions of veal, mutton and bread baked from wheaten flour must have presented a novelty for many of them. In sixteenth-century Augsburg these were 'luxury foods' which would only rarely have found their way on to the plates of the patient in the pox hospitals, all of whom came from the less affluent parts of the city's population.[77] When at home their daily meals would have consisted mainly of pork and beef, sausages and innards that poor butchers or butchers' widows sold at the entrance to the city's meat market. Also, the pauper of Augsburg rarely could have afforded wheat bread. Their cereal was rye from which more bread could be made than from wheat, and which could be stored longer.[78]

The daily meals in the *Holzhaus* on the Goosehill were supplemented by dishes that were considered to dilute the blood and benefit the digestion, like prunes, raisons or rice. Spices were used only sparingly in the kitchen and if, only those that were believed to help purify the blood, such as nutmeg, cloves or coriander.[79] In all three hospitals the consumption of salt was carefully monitored since the doctors believed that its specific qualities favoured the production of the morbid moist and cold matter of the pox and hampered the therapeutic effects of the guaiacum wood. Most meals were therefore salt-free.[80]

In constructing a bill of fare for the pox hospitals, it was not only the primary and secondary qualities of foodstuff that had to be considered. Equally important were the size of the portions deemed healthy for each inmate which were decided by the physician taking into consideration the patient's age, the state of his or her illness, and overall physical condition.[81] During treatment, the body was supposed to concentrate its efforts on excreting morbid matter, and not waste its strength on

75 F.A. 5.3.2 (d), fol. 7r–39v. In the Fuggerei *Holzhaus* the meat consumption in 1582 during the 37-week cure (12 March – 12 November) amounted to 2,544 lb, 68 lb weekly. In total there were 54 patients admitted during that time. See F.A. 66.1.2, fol.48b; F.A. 66.1.2, fol. 48b; 66.2.4 (k), fol. 10r–11v; fol. 17r.

76 The average consumption of bread is unknown in all hospitals.

77 For the following see Roeck, 'Brot', pp. 47–55; 150; 92; see also Anton Werner, 'Der ungarische Ochsenhandel und das Augsburger Metzgergewerbe', *Der Sammler* 74 (1911), pp. 3–5.

78 For the consumption of cereal in the early modern period see also Uwe Dirlmeier, *Untersuchungen zu Einkommensverhältnissen und Lebenshaltungskosten in oberdeutschen Städten des Spätmittelalters* (Mitte 14. bis Anfang 16. Jahrhundert) (Heidelberg, 1987).

79 F.A. 5.3.2 (d), fol. 7–39.

80 StAA, Fuggerei, Ordnung Holzhaus auf dem Gänsbühl von 1568. For the use of salt during pox treatment see also Chapter 1.

81 Ibid.

the various decoctions of food in the liver.[82] For this reason, fasting during pox treatment was seen in a positive light. Ancient medical theory taught that during the fast, when the body's substance was not fully replenished, all the body's passages opened, obstructions were removed and excretions facilitated. Raw material was properly boiled and its qualities improved; thin and useless fluids were evaporated; thick viscous fluids were set in motion and prepared to be expelled.[83] Though light fasting was seen as beneficial, the general rule was that patients were not to be debilitated by being undernourished. In the *Blatterhaus* pregnant women and small children 'who lack strength' were therefore given an additional morning broth on the physician's instructions.[84] Alternative foodstuff, such as porridge made of milk and flour, were also given to those patients whose pox lesions in the throat made it impossible for them to swallow the 'common fare'.[85] If an inmate had no appetite at the appointed mealtime, the portion was kept in the kitchen and served to him or her later in bed by the maids. Such measures were supposed to stop those with no appetite giving their portion to hungry fellow-patients or – even worse in the eyes of the hospital's authorities – selling it to the highest bidder. For the same reason leftovers, especially uneaten bread, were collected by the maids immediately after the meal and taken back to the bread cellar.[86]

It has already been shown that the taking of any form of liquids was strictly regulated by the doctors to avoid 'nourishing' the wet-cold morbid pox matter. What this strict denial of liquid entailed for patients undergoing lengthy sweat cures and repeated purges is hard to imagine today. The inmates in the *Holzhaus* on the Goosehill, for example, had to wait until 2 pm to quench their thirst with the first cold drink of boiled guaiacum – in a lesser concentration than the morning and evening 'sweat potions'.[87] All other beverages were only allowed if the doctor had prescribed them as a tonic in individual cases, such as a glass of wine after bloodletting.[88]

The huge importance attached to daily food intake in relation to health and disease is epitomised in the instructions to patients upon discharge. Once back in their homes, the doctors instructed them, to make every effort to consolidate their recovery by maintaining as good a regimen as when they were in hospital so that their cure remained permanent. It often happened, however,

82 See here also the explanations of Alexander Seitz in Ukena, *Seitz*, p. 23.

83 Müller, *Humoralmedizin*, p. 85. For a sixteenth-century explanation of the effects of fasting during pox treatment see Renner, *Handbüchlein*, fol. XXXIIIIr.

84 StAA, Blatterhaus, Ordnung von 1581, p. 26.

85 F.A. 66.2.4 (ss) fol. 11r.

86 StAA, Fuggerei, Ordnung Holzhaus auf dem Gänsbühl vom 1568; see the identical instructions for the *Blatterhaus* StAA, Blatterhaus, Ordnung von 1581, pp. 12; 27.

87 StAA, Fuggerei, Ordnung Holzhaus auf dem Gänsbühl von 1568.

88 In the Goosehill hospital weak and middle-aged patients received an extra ¼ l of wine; children were served milk. StAA, Fuggerei, Ordnung Holzhaus auf dem Gänsbühl von 1568. See also Schmid, *Kurtzer Bericht*, p. 16.

the doctors lamented, that after their release people would devour hungrily whatever they desired and could put their hands on. Such uncontrolled eating habits could result, they warned, in many of them returning to the pox hospital soon afterwards.[89]

Motion and Rest

After air, secretion and nutrition, the next factor to be considered in the treatment of the pox was the interplay between physical activity and rest. Physical movement was believed to augment the body's internal heat, which would consequently activate the humours, with beneficial results for both food concoctions in the liver and secretions.[90] However, while movement in moderation was healthy and necessary, excessive physical activity was considered harmful, since it consumed too much of the body's substance and cooled and weakened it. A further risk was that the pox poison, often hiding or stuck within the body, would be suddenly released, causing all kinds of skin ulcers, abscesses, and putrefactive fevers. Thus, patients in the pox hospitals were discouraged from engaging in too much physical activity. As long as they drank guaiacum water, bathed, sweated or underwent various mercury treatments, they were to enjoy complete rest, to allow all treatments to have maximum effect. During these periods of rest the patients were closely supervised by a maid or male servant who were exempt from other domestic duties at such times so that they could devote themselves entirely to supervising and – in emergencies – hurrying to the aid of fainting inmates.[91] On doctors' orders, those patients whose constitutions were judged sufficiently robust were to rise from their beds after breakfast and walk around their wards in dressing gown and slippers for at least an hour, 'for such moderate exercise cleans up all rubbish [in the body] and supports a good digestion'.[92] In the *Blatterhaus* such patients were even encouraged, with the doctors' approval, to perform minor domestic tasks such as carrying firewood and helping out in the kitchen.[93]

89 StAA, Blatterhaus, Ordnung Holzhaus auf dem Gänsbühl von 1568.

90 Johannes Wittich's, *Praeservator Sanitatis*, p. 26, contains an interesting section on the benefits and dangers of bodily movement.

91 StAA, Blatterhaus, Ordnung von 1581, pp. 19–20. For the Gänsbühl *Holzhaus* see StAA, Fuggerei, Ordnung Holzhaus auf dem Gänsbühl von 1568.

92 Schmid, *Kurtzer Bericht*, p. 160. See also the various instructions F.A.5.3.2 (a) Ordnung für das Holzhaus auf dem Gänsbühl von 1568; according to the instructions of the *Blatterhaus* patients had to stay awake for at least two hours. See StAA, Blatterhaus, Ordnung von 1535.

93 StAA, Blatterhaus, Ordnung von 1581, p. 30.

Sleeping and Waking

Closely connected to the interplay between physical movement and rest was the relationship between sleeping and waking. Sleep meant respite from movement, with the senses dormant. Physical powers that had been dissipated and depleted by work and wakefulness were refreshed and renewed.[94] But necessary though sleep was for the health of the human body, it was important to avoid it in excess. Too much sleep, the physicians believed, could dull the senses and make them lethargic; it also produced mucous fluids that cooled and moistened the body. Wakefulness, by contrast, aroused the senses and enhanced bodily strength, accelerated the concoction process and stimulated secretion. But again, excessive wakefulness had also to be avoided because it potentially consumed too much bodily strength, slowed down the concoction process, confused mind and senses, and inflamed the gall bladder.

Consequently, patients in the pox hospitals were urged to sleep only at night. During the day, especially immediately after a meal, sleep was to be avoided if possible, unless 'a person is so weak that he cannot stay up, or was unable to sleep the previous night'.[95] Sleeping during the day was considered particularly dangerous for pox sufferers. While nocturnal slumber would 'settle and strengthen spent powers', sleeping by day, warned Joseph Schmid, 'might give rise to all kinds of corrupt humidity'.[96] To assure patients' adequate sleep during the healthy nocturnal hours, the wards in the *Holzhaus* on the Goosehill, for instance, were locked by key at 8 pm so that the inmates could 'give themselves to rest'.[97] Nothing and no one was to disturb this nocturnal peace, unless a patient's condition required a night-time visit by one of the medical practitioners. The night ended in all pox hospitals around 5 am when the maids distributed the first hot guaiacum potion.

The Passions

The passions of the soul were the last of the six non-naturals to be carefully monitored during pox treatment. As discussed in Chapter 1, the passions were believed to have a direct impact on the humours, altering their balance and leading

94 For a sixteenth-century description of the benefits and dangers of sleep see Johannes Wittich, *Praeservator Sanitatis*, p. 25; for the following see also Müller, *Humoralmedizin*, p. 87.

95 F.A. 5.3.2 (a), Holzordnungen, Ordnung auf dem Gänsbühl von 1568.

96 Schmid, *Kurtzer Bericht*, p. 160.

97 For the following see F.A. 5.3.2 (a) Ordnung für das Holzhaus auf dem Gänsbühl von 1568; for similar instructions in the civic pox house see StAA, Blatterhaus, Ordnung von 1576, p. 11.

in unfortunate cases to illness or even death. Regarded as possible direct causes of disease, they were therefore treated accordingly.[98]

In the pox hospitals, the staff was instructed to 'protect' patients from abrupt 'movements' of their passions. The barber-surgeon Schmid advised his readers in no uncertain terms, 'anger and all other emotions are to be avoided as potentially harmful; a peaceful and friendly atmosphere should be created'.[99] If the authorities of each of the pox hospitals insisted rigorously on peace and harmony, it was predominantly out of concern that unrest among the patients could obstruct the healing process. Anything 'by which the patients may be moved to argue with each other' was to be avoided.[100] In the wards of the *Blatterhaus* and the two Fugger *Holzhäusern*, inmates were forbidden, on pain of punishment, to do anything that might distress others and disturb their rest and sleep, such as 'using lewd, obscene language, singing worldly songs, chattering needlessly or playing games'.[101]

But the authorities had other reasons for insisting on a 'friendly atmosphere' in the pox hospitals. Disrespectful behaviour among the inmates was also believed to insult the glory of God, on whose grace and mercy each patient's recovery ultimately depended. If a patient's conduct under therapy gave the Almighty cause for annoyance or anger, He might use His divine powers to delay or even prevent recovery: 'For how can God, who is a God of peace, allow such abhorrent persons to prosper and be well,' the *Blatterhaus* regulations reminded its inmates.[102] In all hospitals patients were required before cure began to 'make peace with God and begin a new life', because 'no one knows what awaits him in the cure'.[103] Inmates were encouraged to pray together several times a day. Before and after meals one patient in each ward of the Catholic *Holzhaus* on the Goosehill led his fellow patients in saying 'the Lord's Prayer, followed by the Ave Maria and the Credo, which the others shall repeat'.[104] In the *Blatterhaus*, which catered for both confessions, prayers for the success of the treatment were also uttered before and after meals. Some of the younger patients seem not to have taken this prayer obligation seriously enough, since the pox father was obliged to remind them repeatedly of the virtues of 'godliness, prayer and gratitude, both in and out of the wood cure'.[105] For dying patients, the pox father might summon a minister 'either of the old Catholic religion, or of the Augsburg confession', so that 'none

98 For a contemporary description of the harmful effects of uncontrolled emotions see Johannes Wittich, *Praeservator Sanitatis*, p. 25.

99 Schmid, *Kurtzer Bericht*, p. 161.

100 StAA, Blatterhaus, Ordning von 1576, p. 6.

101 Ibid. See also the identical instructions for the Fugger *Holzhaus* StAA, Fuggerei, Ordnung Holzhaus auf dem Gänsbühl von 1568; StAA, Fuggerei, Ordnung Holzhaus in der Fuggerei von 1555.

102 StAA, Blatterhaus, Ordnung von 1576, p. 6.

103 Ibid., pp. 3–4.

104 F.A. 5.3.2 (a), Holzordnungen, Ordnung auf dem Gänsbühl von 1568.

105 StAA, Blatterhaus, Ordnung von 1581, p. 24.

shall be troubled against his conscience' on their deathbeds.[106] Similarly, in the Catholic *Holzhäusern* great value was attached to a 'good death'.[107] If an inmate lay dying, a priest was immediately called in 'to give the Holy Sacraments and last rites in accordance with Catholic custom, so that he may die and be buried in the faith'.[108]

Besides disturbing a patient's humoral balance and invoking the wrath of God, unseemly behaviour in the hospitals was also thought to offend the dignity and honour of 'the authority invested by God'.[109] Inmates in the *Blatterhaus* were regularly reminded in the readings of the house rules on Sundays that their stay in the hospital 'is not a matter of justice or necessity, but a great act of mercy, organised by the honourable Council, for the Glory of God and for the best for its poor subjects'.[110] In return, the council expected patients to be both grateful and obedient. In their prayers they were to pray not just for their own recovery, but also for the councillors and pious citizens who had given alms to the hospital. The Catholic Fuggers could take it for granted that patients in their *Holzhäuser* would pray several times a day for members of the founding family, for the souls of those dead and the welfare of those still living: 'they should diligently consider why they are there, namely for the attainment of health, and that such accommodation is not justice or necessity but an act of mercy born of Christian sympathy, wherefore they should every day call earnestly upon the Almighty and beseech Him to graciously grant them the strength to be cured. They should also pray for the well being of those who donated these alms, whether they be dead or alive.'[111]

In sum, from the authorities' point of view, disruptive behaviour by inmates had a threefold dimension. First of all, spontaneous emotions exploding into outbursts of anger or violent arguments were believed to directly affect the patient's own and possibly also his or her fellow-patients' humoral balance and thus might delay or obstruct the healing process. Quarrels and brawls also compromised the spiritual relationship with God. If roused to anger, the Almighty might withdraw His goodwill both from the individual patient and the institution as a whole. Catholics and Protestants alike believed that, in the absence of divine goodwill, no lasting cure could be achieved. Finally, disruptive behaviour in the hospitals put a strain on the inmates' relationship with the divinely appointed secular authority to which they owed gratitude and obedience and for whose preservation they were expected

106 Ibid., p. 30.

107 There is much literature on the topic of a 'good death' in the Middle Ages and the early modern period. Useful is Marcus Wenninger (ed.), 'du guoter tot'. *Sterben im Mittelalter – Ideal und Realität* (Klagenfurt, 1998).

108 StAA, Fuggerei, Ordnung Holzhaus auf dem Gänsbühl von 1568.

109 For this quote and more details on the understanding of the council as God's deputy and the guardian of the Christian civic community see StAA, Blatterhaus, Ordnung von 1581, p. 17.

110 StAA, Blatterhaus, Ordnung von 1576, p. 1.

111 StAA, Fuggerei, Ordnung Holzhaus auf dem Gänsbühl von 1568.

to pray every day. For ensuring peace and order in the hospital the caretakers and staff were responsible.[112] However, they did not have the authority to punish patients' misdemeanours themselves; they were required to report any occurrences first to the learned doctor', who was the only one officially authorised 'to punish such persons according to the nature of their offence'.[113] Since the hospital staff could not be ever-present in the wards, an inmate was chosen from each ward to remind his fellow roommates of their obligations and report any infringements to the pox or wood father.[114]

While the inmates' conduct was monitored by the staff, that of the staff was monitored by the inmates. If, for example, patients in the *Holzhaus* on the Goosehill had grounds for complaint about the behaviour of personnel, they were entitled to bring it up with the medical practitioners during the morning visits.[115] And as the records show, the inmates were as much concerned about the impact of disruptions as were the practitioners and hospital authorities. In 1590, for example, patient complaints even brought about the dismissal of the *Blatterhaus*'s learned physician Johann Scheurlin.[116] Scheurlin suffered from an alcohol problem so serious that he repeatedly 'forgot' to show up for his joint morning rounds with the barber-surgeon Diel. With Scheurlin often failing to appear, Master Michel Diel had treated the patients on several occasions 'in the absence of the doctor' with, however, tragic results, according to patients' complaints. Diel's treatment of two of their fellow inmates had resulted in 'such injury to private parts, and general damage to other areas', they reported, 'that both it is feared will forfeit their lives'. Worried about their own lives and also God's anger at Scheurlin's behaviour (which might in turn affect their recovery too), the patients shared their anxieties with the chief guardian and demanded the doctor's dismissal. After a thorough examination of this sensitive issue, it was granted by the council and a new doctor was hired who took his job more seriously.

Although in the Scheurlin case the patients had reported correctly what had happened, there were obviously some who did try to exploit the system; hence the forceful admonition in the house rules to tell the truth in such matters and not

112 StAA, Fuggerei, Ordnung Holzhaus in der Fuggerei von 1555; StAA, Blatterhaus, Ordnung von 1581, p. 20.

113 F.A. 5.3.2 (a), Ordnung für das Holzhaus auf dem Gänsbühl von 1568. Für das Holzhaus auf dem Gänsbühl siehe F.A. 5.3.2 (a), Ordnung für das Holzhaus auf dem Gänsbühl von 1568.

114 F.A. 5.3.2 (a), Ordnung für das Holzhaus auf dem Gänsbühl von 1568; StAA, Blatterhaus, Ordnung von 1581, p. 15.

115 StAA, Fuggerei, Ordnung Holzhaus auf dem Gänsbühl von 1568; StAA, Fuggerei, Ordnung Holzhaus in der Fuggerei 1555; StAA, Blatterhaus, Ordnung von 1576, p. 9.

116 For the following see StAA, St. Martin, VI, Prod. 3: Supplikation der Oberpfleger über das Blatterhaus vom Juni 1590.

'discredit with lies' either doctors or staff out of personal animosity or 'lust for revenge'.[117]

Any inmate who, despite frequent warnings, continued to cause disruption in the hospital was 'despatched from the house without mercy' as a warning and deterrent to others and told that he or she could never return.[118] We have already seen that disruptive behaviour was one of the reasons why Katharina Blomenhauer, Wolf Rottinger's wife, was refused re-admission to the *Blatterhaus*. The complaints against Blomenhauer were summarised by the in-house physician Gereon Sailer. During the whole of her stay, he complained, she 'caused disquiet in the ward with screaming, singing, scolding, squabbling and other disturbances', unsettling the hospital as a whole.[119] Furthermore, she had 'ignored and refused to take her medicine, so that I was obliged to throw away the pills specifically prescribed for her'. Frequent warnings and minor punishments failed to have an effect; indeed, she had caused such a riot in the women's ward that all thirteen patients had been repeatedly disturbed in their sleep. Sailer had been compelled to segregate her from the other patients and confine her to a separate room. He refused to go through it again and urged the council to reject her application, advising that she was 'an impudent, wicked person' who had obstructed the healing process for other patients. The council acted on his recommendation.

Leaving the Pox Hospital

In all three Augsburg pox hospitals the doctors were adamant that patients should not put their health at risk by leaving the hospital prematurely. But neither, for obvious reasons of cost, should anybody stay longer than necessary. If the practitioners on their daily rounds established that a patient's condition had clearly improved and the defining moment of crisis had passed, the person was officially 'declared healthy' in a final examination. The criteria used by practitioners to make these judgements are unknown, but probably resembled those of the Augsburg barber-surgeon Joseph Schmid, who discharged patients from his private pox clinic only 'when all headaches and limb pains have ceased, pustules, ulcers, tumours and boils have healed and disappeared', in sum 'when all symptoms have abated, which may happen sooner with some than with others'.[120]

Health in the sixteenth century, as we have seen was a relative concept and assessed in terms of an individual's ability to function socially. To the medical

117 F.A. 5.3.2 (a) Holzkurordnungen, Ordnung Holzhaus auf dem Gänsbühl von 1568; StAA, Blatterhaus, Ordnung von 1576, p. 7.

118 StAA, Blatterhaus, Ordnung von 1576, p. 7; F.A. 5.3.2 (a) Holzkurordnungen, Ordnung Holzhaus auf dem Gänsbühl 1568.

119 For the following see StAA, St Martins, VI, Prod. 30: Bericht des Doktor Gereon Seiler vom April 1560.

120 Schmid, *Kurtzer Bericht*, p. 179.

practitioners, patients were healthy when they were able to resume daily tasks to earn a livelihood without too many difficulties. To be released it was not considered necessary that the patient was completely free of all pain or all physical symptoms. Hence the discharge in September 1544 of Peter Gansmair after the amputation of his right foot with the comment that he was 'completely healthy and cured'.[121]

As soon as patients in one of the pox hospitals had been declared officially cured, they stopped taking the guaiacum remedy and were given a slightly richer diet. They were also encouraged over the next week or fortnight to spend more time outdoors and to undertake small household duties in order gradually to become re-accustomed to the climatic conditions outside the hospital. As we have seen, the length of treatment depended on a number of factors, including the patient's humoral complexion, age, general physical condition and, last but not least, the degree of severity of the pox. No medical practitioner in the hospitals was able or willing to predict how long a patient's cure might take. Again, Joseph Schmid was probably typical among the Augsburg's medical community. 'While some may be cured within three or four weeks, others might not after three or four months,' he declared.[122] Particularly with 'old pox', it was wise not to make any prognostic predictions, he warned, but instead prepare for further deterioration in the patient's health, since such advanced conditions had been known with time to turn into other diseases. 'Most distressing', he continued, 'are those pox conditions that are old and long-established in which the inner organs are ravaged and the lungs rotted, giving rise to consumption, in which they [the patients] produce a ceaseless flow of semen from the kidneys, a continuous rupturing of the intestines, corruption of the uterus in women and a simultaneous paralysis or palsy leading to leprosy or dropsy which, at last, will suffocate the patient most wretchedly.'[123]

That treatment could be of different duration for different patients is clear from the records of the *Holzhaus* at the Fuggerei, which in many cases record the length of an inmate's stay.[124] While some patients remained only a few days, others stayed for weeks or even months. Not infrequently it is recorded that the pox mutated into another condition altogether, as happened in the case of Catharina Pastenecker.[125] Catharina had worked as a maid at an inn near Augsburg when she fell seriously ill with the pox 'in her throat and private parts'. The village pastor had asked Hans Jakob Fugger to allow her to undergo guaiacum treatment at the Fuggerei *Holzhaus*. But as there was no bed free, so between 29 April and 17 June 1547 she was treated at the private home of the Fuggerei resident, Elspeth Sunthaimer. Initially her condition improved. It was not long, however, before the *Holzhaus*'s two medical practitioners who visited her on a daily basis realised that this apparent improvement had merely been the prelude to more dramatic

121 F.A. 66.2.1, fol. 145r.

122 Schmid, *Kurtzer Bericht*, p. 180.

123 Ibid., p. 182.

124 See for example the list of the year 1586, F.A. 66.2.4 (ss), fol. 16r–20r.

125 For the following see F.A. 66.2.3 (b), fol. 144v.

developments. Concluding that 'the dropsy has broken out in her', the doctor and the barber-surgeon ruled that Catharina Pastenecker was highly unlikely to recover. She was sent home with some well-intentioned medical advice.[126]

Once patients had been declared cured by the doctors and re-acclimatised to conditions outside the hospital, the clothing in which they arrived was returned to them. We know from the *Holzhaus* records that some patients 'arrived here quite naked', or at least with torn clothing.[127] Upon discharge such patients received new clothing.[128] The hospital's caretaker recorded the patient's name, date of discharge and the length of time they spent in hospital. Almost all those discharged by the Fugger hospitals received a small allowance from the Fuggerei administrator to arm them for what might be a long journey home and to try to ensure that they 'do not collapse again' en route. Patients whose health was considered still fragile were sent, at the Fuggers' expense, to one of the nearby spas to further consolidate their recovery.

From the available source material is it is impossible to guess the number of patient cases per year in which treatment was ineffective, or the number of patients who were left 'uncured' or even died in hospital. However, the few references that survive suggest that these were relatively small. In 1582, for example, a total of thirty-three patients were treated in the *Holzhaus* on the Goosehill, seventeen women and sixteen men.[129] While twenty-seven of those recovered their health, in six cases the guaiacum and even the aggressive mercury treatments were unsuccessful. In the Fuggerei *Holzhaus*, in 1592, a total of seventy-seven patients were treated of whom only one died.[130] In 1621 the patient list of the Goosehill *Holzhaus* does include a record of those who died: out of a total of forty-two patients treated in the course of that year's opening period, only two women died.[131] The others were discharged as entirely 'fit and healthy'.

The following table of patient numbers (Table 4.1), taken from the surviving records of the *Holzhaus* in the Fuggerei, indicate that over the course of sixty-two years a total of 3,420 pox patients were treated in the Fuggerei *Holzhaus* and discharged as 'cured and healthy'.

126 For another Fuggerei *Holzhaus* case see e.g. Anna Schweiger from March 1544, who developed dropsy and was then transferred into private care. F.A.66.2.1, fol. 114r.

127 F.A. 66.1.1, fol. 52b.

128 For example, see F.A. 66.1.1, fol. 52b; F.A. 66.1.1, fol. 48b.

129 F.A. 66.1.2, fol. 48v.

130 F.A. 66.1.2, fol. 17r

131 F.A. 66.1.2, fol. 43v.

Table 4.1 Total number of patients treated per annum in Fuggerei *Holzhaus*, 1544–1632

Year	*Total*	*Year*	**Total**	*Year*	*Total*	*Year*	**Total**	*Year*	*Total*
1544	84[132]	-	-	**1593**	77	**1607**	47	**1621**	49
-	-	**1580**	60[133]	**1594**	67	**1608**	48	**1622**	46
1546	35[134]	**1581**	60[135]	**1595**	76	**1609**	44	-	-
1556	77	**1582**	54[136]	**1596**	69	**1610**	48	**1624**	26[137]
1557	80	**1583**	68[138]	**1597**	75	**1611**	46	**1625**	25
1558	79	**1584**	72	**1598**	62	**1612**	48[139]	**1626**	27
-	-	**1585**	76	**1599**	58	**1613**	54	**1627**	29
1563	67	**1586**	76	**1600**	66	**1614**	54[140]	**1628**	15
-	-	**1587**	81	**1601**	58[141]	**1615**	58	**1629**	25
1571	57	**1588**	69	**1602**	57[142]	**1616**	35	**1630**	47[143]
-	-	**1589**	76	**1603**	56[144]	**1617**	43	**1631**	31[145]
1576	57[146]	**1590**	95	**1604**	49[147]	**1618**	36	**1632**	11[148]
1577	56[149]	**1591**	62	**1605**	54[150]	**1619**	39	-	-
1578	58[151]	**1592**	77[152]	**1606**	47[153]	**1620**	42	-	-

Source: Weidenbacher, *Fuggerei*, Table 7, with additions and corrections from author.

Given that deaths were relatively rare, the cure of the pox in the three Augsburg hospitals can be deemed enormously successful.

132 F.A. 66.2.1, fol. 35r–47r.
133 F.A. 66.1.2, fol. 47b.
134 F.A. 66.2.3 (a), fol. 55r.
135 F.A. 66.2.4 (h), fol. 18v.
136 F.A. 66.2.4 (t), fol. 18v.
137 F.A. 66.2.8 (p), p. 50.
138 F.A. 66.2.4 (n), fol. 9r.
139 F.A. 66.1.5, fol. 60.
140 F.A. 66.2.7 (b), fol. 4a.
141 F.A. 66.2.6 (c), fol. 8b.
142 F.A. 66.1.4, fol. 141a.
143 F.A. 66.2.8 (gg), fol. 26r.
144 F.A. 66.1.4, fol. 148a.
145 F.A. 66.2.8 (hh), fol. 22v.
146 F.A. 66.2.4 (b), fol. 48r.
147 F.A. 66.1.4, fol. 161a.
148 The cure ended on 21 May 1632 due to the Swedish occupation of the city. The eleven inmates had to leave prematurely. The *Holzhaus* closed and was used by the Swedish troops as a stable. Even after the end of the Thirty Year War the *Holzhaus* remained closed and was eventually converted into dwellings. See F.A. 66.2.8 (mm), fol. 22v.
149 F.A. 66.2.4 (c), fol. 47r.
150 F.A. 66.2.6 (k), fol. 34a.
151 F.A. 66.1.2, fol. 16v.
152 F.A. 66.2.5 (i), fol. 17r.
153 F.A. 66.1.5, fol. 9a.

Conclusions

This study has been concerned with the socio-cultural construction of the French pox in the imperial city of Augsburg in the sixteenth century. To employ the concept of constructionism in this area of history is of course hardly novel. That our view of the natural world, including diseases, and the way we investigate it is influenced and shaped by society's values and norms at a particular moment in time is a view that has been in fashion for the past three decades at least. Yet, even if the term has lost much of its earlier potential for academic and public controversy (as in the 'science wars' of the 1980s), it remains a popular notion in the humanitities. Indeed, the number of social studies bearing 'construction' in their title is so extensive that the philosopher of science Ian Hacking has come to wonder if there is any heuristic value left to it.[1] Every aspect of human biology and culture, he observes, is now potentially 'socially constructed': nature, nationalism, human bodies, quarks, technology, emotions, illness and health, gender, homosexuality, religion, childhood, reality, serial homicide, authorship and so on. However, this popularity, supported by the emergence of postmodern thinking since the 1980s, has not contributed to the clarification of the concept. Instead, it has become something of a code, overused and increasingly obscure.[2] What's the point of further using it, Hacking asked?

I agree with Hacking's spirited critique, and regret that I read his study only after I had reached my conceptual framework for this study. Nevertheless, I believe that in the field of the history of disease there is still some point in pursuing constructionism. One reason is that, where the concept of constructionism has been applied in the history of medicine, it has been done unimaginatively. This is particularly apparent in the history of pre-nineteenth-century diseases. Most studies that claim to investigate the socio-cultural construction of a particular early modern disease content themselves with reconstructing only social and cultural *responses*. How contemporaries actually constructed the physical reality of disease is not addressed. Further, the nosological picture of early modern disease remains sketchy, its relationship to the human body hardly explored. How early modern understandings of this physicality shaped or were shaped by wider socio-cultural practices in particular locations, and at particular moments in time, remains largely uncharted. This study, attentive to time and space, has devoted itself precisely to these conceptual and socio-cultural interactions with disease.

Fundamental has been the claim that the sixteenth-century French pox was not our modern disease of venereal syphilis, the conceptualisation of which is

1 Ian Hacking, *The Social Construction of What?* (Cambridge, MA, 1999), p. VII.

2 Ibid.

intrinsically linked to the emergence of laboratory medicine at the end of the nineteenth century. My analysis of vernacular German treatises on the pox aimed at demonstrating that, unlike ourselves, no early modern person perceiving the pox understood it as etiologically, morphologically and symptomatically separate from other disease entities. Their perception, couched within the reasoning of Hippocratic-Galenic medicine and Aristotelian natural philosophy, did not allow the pox to manifest itself physically in the same way in different individuals. Thus, to the consternation of medical practitioners and sufferers, there were hundreds of different species of the pox which were believed to originate from subtle and innumerable differences in the mixture of the four vital humours.

By refusing to identify the pox with venereal syphilis, and thus putting its identity into question, my object has not been to deny the 'reality' of the pox. Of course the pox, a new disease that appeared suddenly all over Europe at the end of the fifteenth century, was 'real' for those who suffered and died from it. And its sudden unexpected appearance also prompted 'real' socio-cultural reactions, such as the publication of medical advice books and the opening of new hospitals for pox victims.

This study has sought to represent the sixteenth-century pox as both 'real' and 'constructed' on the grounds that 'reality' itself is an ongoing negotiation. This understanding follows those who argue that reality refers not to a single overarching thing existing independent from human society, but rather something endlessly re-processed along with language and life itself.[3] The aim of this study was thus to reconstruct the negotiated 'reality' of the pox. To achieve this, it investigated the socio-cultural responses of sixteenth-century society to the new ailment, *at the same time as* the ways in which contemporaries perceived and explained its causes, courses, symptoms and signs. In so doing, I sought to bring together two areas that in the history of medicine are usually kept separate: the world of medical semiotics and the daily practice of diagnosing and treating disease within a particular local context. In short, what I wanted to capture was the 'pox concept in action'.

My textual analysis has confirmed the work of scholars claiming that disease definition in the early modern period was fluid, flexible, and always temporary. This flexibility was based on a fundamentally different understanding than ours of how the meaning of physical signs was to be established. What early modern diagnosis aimed at was the identification of the invisible essence or nature of diseases hidden in the body by means of reading outer sensible physical signs. Diagnosing the pox was a complicated and subtle business that relied as much on the opinions and interpretations of the sufferer as on the professional expertise of the medical practitioner. A diagnosis had to establish multiple links between the microcosm of the human body and the God-created macrocosm. The result was a picture of the pox to which all parties involved in the act of diagnosis could agree. No one, however, considered the verdict written in stone. It was agreed that the

3 Hilary Putman, 'Sense, Nonsense and the Senses: an Inquiry into the Powers of the Human Mind', *The Journal of Philosophy* 91 (1994), p. 452.

pox could alter its ways, change its appearance rapidly, even mutate into different diseases, such as dropsy or leprosy.

The exploration conducted here into the surviving archival records of Augsburg's three pox hospitals has gone a step further to suggest that the identity of the pox was not only fluid and temporary, but also ultimately locally defined. As much as the pox 'acted upon' sixteenth-century Augsburg society, its reality was shaped by the existing socio-cultural landscape in which it was perceived and understood. Hence the impact of the pox was often far *less* dramatic than historians have supposed. Its arrival did not seriously challenge medical practice and theory, despite what might be surmised from the prompt opening of the new *Blatterhaus* for its victims, an event hailed by historians as 'revolutionary' in the history of hospitals. As we have seen, while academically trained healers in the city were initially unsure how to integrate the new ailment into their learned framework, their artisanal colleagues treated the pox confidently from the start. Moreover, the establishment of the *Blatterhaus* itself was not merely a preventive act fuelled by panic and confusion about an unknown disease; rather, it was driven by the city council's ambition publicly to challenge the authority of the Catholic Church over matters of charity. The process of the communalisation of civic charity, which had already begun in the mid-thirteenth century, reached its peak around the time the pox struck the city. The spread of new reformed ideas, which led to the official introduction of the Reformation in the city in 1537, culminated in *all* health institutions coming under the control of the city council. The opening of the two pox hospitals by the Fugger families in 1523/24 and 1572 were exceptional and reflect more this particular Catholic family's exalted social and political status in the city. Their hospitals were intended to demonstrate and celebrate the Catholic faith in a predominantly Protestant environment; they were not intended as a means to cash in on the family's monopoly on guaiacum, as some historians have suggested. In fact, as my reading of the archives indicates, a Fugger monopoly on the wood from the New World never existed.

Augsburg's pox hospitals were not the only institutions specialised in treating a particular disease phenomenon. They were not the precursors of the eighteenth-century clinic, as historians of hospitals have claimed. They were a part of an elaborate network of institutions that, for financial and administrative reasons, divided up the care of specific physical conditions. How those conditions were defined and differentiated involved constant negotiations between the inmates, the appointed medical practitioners and staff, and the civic authorities that oversaw the particular institution.

In the case of the pox the process of defining and fixing clinical responsibilities took over twenty years of intense debates between medical practitioners and administrators in the *Blatterhaus*. Only at the end of those protracted struggles did the pox diagnosis and its cure come to rest authoritatively with the academic physicians. Thus, this 'success' story cannot be understood simply as rooted in academic credentials. The physicians' triumph over other healers was in any case intimately linked to their close social ties with the city's ruling elite. The physicians' close proximity to political power also made it relatively easy for them to influence major decisions in the area of public health. But even though Augsburg's academic healers gained official control over the treatment of the pox, their authority was never total. Their colleagues, the barber-surgeons, whose professional duties were increasingly restricted in the course of the sixteenth century, constantly challenged learned medical expertise. Moreover, as the example of Walburga Reuchart and her daughter suggests, pox suffers and their families considered themselves competent judges of their physical condition, and were always ready to fight against professional verdicts.

As the early modern understanding of the meaning of physical signs was responsible for the flexible and changing identity of the pox, so the concept of signs was also responsible for the changing authority of those who interpreted physical signs. Verdicts were always temporary and closely linked to the particular space in which the diagnostic act took place. As we saw, medical practitioners at the Holy Ghost Hospital often identified a patient's physical signs differently from their colleagues in the *Blatterhaus*. Diagnostic results were thus ever open to question, along with the authority of those who had reached them.

If, as the study has suggested, diagnosis and disease definition in the early modern period were fluid, temporal, and local, it would be instructive to pursue the 'pox concept in action' in other early modern German communities. For Cologne, a city comparable in size to Augsburg, it is known that the academic medical practitioners held no power over the treatment of this disease. It was entirely in the hands of the barber-surgeons' guild who – in contrast to Augsburg – dominated and controlled the city's medical services. Further studies will have to determine what such different distributions of professional power over the human body mean for the diagnosis and treatment of early modern diseases.

This study has contributed to an approach to early modern disease that goes beyond simply the investigation of social responses. It has sought to take the historicity of the human body and its functioning as a part of the problem facing historians in the study of disease. To explore the identity of past diseases such as the pox requires us to look at both – that is, to look at the specific socio-cultural environment in which the disease occurred and was dealt with, *and* the world of early modern medical and philosophical reasoning that explained the functioning of the human body. It is surely the combination of both approaches that will yield insight into the reality and the contructedness of the past and the study of the body in disease.

Bibliography

1. Primary Sources: Archival

Stadtarchiv Augsburg: Bestand Reichsstadt

Baumeisteramt:

Baumeisterbücher: 1496–1632 (Nr. 90–217)

Blatterhaus:

Blatterhausordnungen 1495; 1522; 1535; 1576; 1581; 1789
Inventar des Blatterhauses (after 1671)
Urkunde betreffend die Aufsicht über die Klöster St Martin, St Margarethen und St Nikolaus vom 22. März 1581

Collegium Medicum:

1. Verzeichnis der öffentlichen Anschläge und Verordnungen die Sanität betreffend, 1563–1793
2. a. Wundärzte, Bader u. Barbiere, in specie betr. von 1570–1804; b. Rettungsanstalten bei Ertrunkenen, Erstickten, Erhängten von 1751–1805; c. Siechen von 1555–1649; d. Lohbad betr. von 1592
3. Acta, die Stadt-und Pestphysicos betr. von 1548–1789, Fasc. 5; Bericht über Vorgänge in den Brechhäusern 1563/64
4. Doctores Medicinae in genere betr. von 1548–1795
5. Apotheker von 1564 bis 1804, Tom I
6. Apotheker von 1557–1641, Tom I
7. Acta materiam contagionis von 1708–1780 und Kontagionsanstalten von 1563–1724
8. a. Lazareth in der Stadt in genere von 1693–1795; b. Lazareth außer der Stadt von 1632–1794, Fasc. 16
9. Pfuscher, hiesige und Fremde betr. von 1562–1793, Fasc. 8
10. Hiesige Ärzte als Zahn-, Hüneraugen-, Schnittärzte, Occultisten, Brüchschneider, Operateurs, Waldmänner betr. von 1548–1761
11. Ärzte, Ordnungen und Decreta von 1525–1804

Ratsprotokolle 22 (1548), 10. Juli 1548
Ratserlasse 1600–1668

Evangelisches Wesensarchiv:

Nr. 325: Die Herren Administratoren und andern Bediensteten bei St. Servatii Siechenhaus betr. 1552–1730
Nr. 326: Acta Siechenordnung betr. 1595–1739

Fuggerei:

Ordnung Holzhaus in der Fuggerei 1555
Ordnung Holzhaus auf dem Gänsbühl 1568

Heilig-Geist-Spital:

Tit. I, Tom 48
Tit. III, Tom 1; 2; 111; 225; 226; 227; 252–254; 256; 258–262
Camera Kasten, Hospitalordnungen, Ordnungen des Spitals zum Heiligen Geist 1521

Historischer Verein Schwaben:

Nr. 34/1: Collegium Medicum Protokollbände 1490–1638

Literalien Sammlung:

Kiste 1551
Ordnungen und Statuten, Karton 20, Nr. 430; 431

St Martinsstiftung:

C. Blatterhaus
I. Blatterhaus-Aufnahme und Wirtschaft (Kt. VI., Nr.47/48)
Nr. 47: Suppliken an die Stadtpfleger; Bürgermeister und den Rat um Aufnahme in das Blatterhaus und zur Erteilung von Almosen
Nr. 48: Blatterhaus – Ökonomie

II. Blatterhaus – Personal (Kt. VI. Nr. 50/51 und Kt. VII. Nr. 52–54)
Nr. 50: Aufnahme und Besoldung der Medici, 1562–1643. 1780: Prod. 1–10
Nr. 51: Blatterhaus – Wundärzte oder Barbiere, 1562–1593.1793.1796: Prod. 1–9.
Nr. 52: Aufnahme und Besoldung der Unterpfleger, 1581–1630.1763: Prod.1–10.
Nr. 53: Aufnahme und Besoldung der Blatterhausväter und Versorgung ihrer Witwen, 1558–1804: Prod. 1–12
Nr. 54: Blatterhaus-Dienstboten 1757–1783: Prod. 1–5

III. Blatterhaus – Rechnungen und Bausachen (Kt. VII. Nr. 55–62)
Nr. 55: Blatterhaus-Rechnungen, 1549–1589; Prod. 1–8
Nr. 59: Blatterhaus und Bleicherzettel, 1510–1528, Blatterhaus und Bleicherzettel aus den Jahren 1510, 1515,
Nr. 61: Blatterhaus – Bausachen, 1513; 1567, Prod. 1–2
Nr. 62: Miscellanea, 1573–1626

D. Lazarette, Sanität und St. Sebastiankapelle (Kt. VIII, Nr. 63–71)
Nr. 63: Ordnung über das Brechhaus, 1585–1638, Prod. 1–7
Nr. 64: Aufnahme der Pestilentiarii u.a.
Nr. 66: Aufnahme der Wundärzte und Barbiere des Lazaretts 1564–1633. 1713: Prod. 1–11
Nr. 67: Aufnahme der Lazarettväter u. Unterpfleger u.a. 1568, 1613. 1703
Nr. 68: Die Trostknechte im Lazarett, 1610–1626

Zünfte, Handwerkerakten, Bader und Barbiere
Kt. 4: Fasc. 1
Kt. 5: Fasc. 2; Fasc. 3
Kt. 16: Fasc. 15

Fürstliches und Gräfliches Fuggersches Familien- und Stiftungsarchiv Dillingen

F.A. 66.1.1; F.A. 66.1.2; F.A. 66.1.3; F.A. 66.1.5; F.A. 66.1.7; F.A. 66.1.8; F.A. 66.1.9; F.A. 66.1.10; F.A. 66.2.1; F.A. 66.2.1; F.A. 66.2.3; F.A. 66.2.4; F.A. 66.2.5; F.A. 66.2.6; F.A. 66.2.7; F.A. 66.2.8; F.A. 66.2.9.
F.A. 88.1; F.A. 81.3; F.A. 81.6; F.A. 82.3;F.A. 86.1; F.A. 86.2; F.A. 86.3; F.A. 86.4; F.A. 88.2; F.A. 88.3; F.A. 88.4; F.A. 88.5; F.A. 88.6.
F.A. 5.1.8(b); F.A. 5.1.10; F.A. 5.2.9; F.A. 5.2.11; F.A. 5.2.13; F.A. 5.2.15(a); F.A. 5.3.2; FA. 5.3.3; F.A. 19.2.

2. Primary Sources: Printed

Ahorner von Ahornrain, Joseph, *Catalogus Medicorum Augustanorum* (Augsburg 1800).
Anonymus, Ein clarer bericht wie man alte schaden, löcher und bülen heylen soll mit dem holtz Guaiaco ... (Strasbourg, 1525).
Anonymus, *Hienach volgt ain bevert recept von ainem holtz genannt Guaiacanum wechst in Antilles in ainer Insel gehaissen la isola spagola: fast hailsam für all alt schäden vnd die kranckhait der Frantzosen* (Augsburg, 1519).
Aristoteles, *Werke*. Alexander von Frantzius (ed.) [1833] (reprint, Aalen, 1978).
Casas, Bartolomé des las, *Historia de las Indias* (5 vols, Madrid, 1876).

Fries, Lorenz, *Spiegel der artzney* (Strasbourg, 1532).

Fuchs, Conrad Heinrich, *Die ältesten deutschen Schriftsteller über die Lustseuche in Deutschland von 1495 bis 1510, nebst mehreren Anecdotis späterer Zeit, gesammelt und mit literaturhistorischen Notizen und einer kurzen Darstellung der epidemischen Syphilis in Deutschland* (Göttingen, 1843).

Galen, *Opera Omnia*. C. G. Kühn (ed.) [1833] (reprint, Hildesheim, 1964).

Girtanner, Christoph, *Abhandlungen über die venerische Krankheit* (3 vols, Göttingen 1788/89).

Grünpeck, Joseph, *Ein hübscher Tractat von dem vrsprung der Bösen Franzo, das man nennet die Wylden wartzen. Auch ein Regiment wie man sich regiren soll in diser zeyt* (Augsburg, 1496), in: Karl Sudhoff (ed.), *Zehn Syphilisdrucke aus den Jahren 1495–1498* (Milan, 1924), pp. 71–115.

Hensler, Philipp-Gabriel, *Geschichte der Lustseuche, die zu Ende des fünfzehnten Jahrhunderts in Europa ausbrach* (Altona, 1789).

Hundt, Magnus, *Eyn kurtzes vnd sehr nutzbarlichs Regiment wider dye schwynde vnd erschreckliche kranckheit der Pestilentz auß bewerten vn[d] geübten Ertzten tzu samen getragen, sampt einem kurtzen bericht der schweysskrankheyt. Meher eyn nutzlichs Regiment wider die weltleuftige un[d] und vnsauber kranckheit der Frantzosen. Dortzu eyn bericht der gebranthen wasser zu gebrauchen durch Magistram magnum Hund von Magdeburgk des Fürste[n] Collegiums tzu Leiptzigk Collegaten aussgangen* (Magdeburg, 1529).

—, in ibid. (ed.), 'Das Regiment wider die Frantzosen von Magnus Hundt II. Ein Beitrag zu den Sammelwerken der ältesten Schriften über Syphilis', *Medicinisch-Chirurgisches Central-Blatt* 15 (1880) 74, pp. 37–8; 5, pp. 49–50; 7: p. 73; 8, p. 85.

Hutten, Ulrich von, *Ulrich vo[n] Hutten eins teutschen Ritters von der wunderbarliche[n] artzney des holtz Guaiacum genant, und wie man die frantzosen oder blattere[n] heilen sol. Durch den hochgelerte[n] herre[n] Thoma[n] Murner der heilige[n] geschrifft vo[n]beider rechten Doctor geteutschet und verdolmetschet* (Augsburg, 1519), in Eduard Böcking (ed.), *Ulrich von Hutten. Schriften* (5 vols, Leipzig, 1861), vol. 5, pp. 399–497.

Jöcher, Christian Gottlieb, *Allgemeines Gelehrten-Lexikon* (Leipzig, 1750–51).

Knobloch, Tobias, *De Lue Venerea. Von Frantzosen kurtzer Bericht. Was für ein Kranckheit, von deroselben Anfang, Ursachen vnd Zeichen, Auch wie Gesunde zu präserviren, Kranke aber oder Inficierte zu curiren, vnd in währender Chur in einem vnd anderem sich verhalten sollen. Gestellet Dem gemeinen Mann zum besten, Durch Tobiam Knoblochium* (Giessen, 1620).

Luther, Martin, D. *Martin Luthers Werke. Kritische Gesamtausgabe* (Weimar 1912–).

Montaigne, Michel de, *The Journal of Montaigne's Travels in Italy by Way of Switzerland and Germany*, W. G. Waters (ed.) (3 vols, London, 1903), vol. 1, pp. 129–44.

Mülich, Hector, *Chronik des Hector Mülich. Mit Zusätzen von Demer, Walther und Rem*, in *Die Chroniken der deutschen Städte* (Leipzig, 1894), vol. 23.

Oviedo y Valdés, Gonzalo Fernández de, *Historia general y natural de las Indias*, José Amador de los Rios (ed.) (Madrid, 1851), vol. 1.

Reischlin, Michael, *Wie man es währen des Sterbens in den Brechhäusern gehalten*, in Friedrich Roth (ed.), *Deutsche Städte Chroniken* vol. 32 ([1917] (reprint Göttingen, 1966), pp. 485–95.

Renner, Franz, *Ein new wol gegründet nützlichs vnnd haylsams handtbüchlein, gemeiner Practick, aller innerlicher vnd eusserlicher Erztney, so wider die erschröckliche, abscheuliche Kranckheit der Frantzosen vnd Lemung, auch für all ander seuchten, so auß disen Kranckheyten erfolgen, vnnd wider die erkent, vnd zu gründlicher Cur mögen gebracht werden* (Nuremberg, 1559).

—, *Ein köstlich vnd bewärtes Artzney büchlein aller inner= vnnd eusserlichen Arztney, wider die abschewliche kranckheit der Frantzosen Vnd Lähmung. Auch vor alle andere Seuchten, so auß dieser kranckheit erfolgen, wie die recht erkent, vnd zu gründlicher Cur gebracht werden mögen* (Amberg, 1609).

Rosenbaum, Julius, *Geschichte der Lustseuche im Alterthume, nebst ausführlichen Untersuchungen über den Venus- und Phallus cultus, Bordelle, Nousos thelēia der Skythen, Paederastie und andere geschlechtlichen Ausschweifungen der Alten. Als Beiträge zur richtigen Erklärung ihrer Schriften für Aerzte, Philologen und Alterthumsforscher* (Halle, 1845).

Ryff, Walter, *New erfundne heylsame, und bewärte artzney, gewusse hülff unnd raht, nit alein die Frantzosen oder bösen blatern, sonder auch andere gebrechen, menschlichs leybs, so sich eüsserlichen oder innerlichen ergeben, aber bißher für vnheylbar geacht worden, gründtlichen vnd gäntzlichen zu vertreiben, heylen vnd Curieren* (Strasbourg, 1559).

Schmid, Joseph, *Examen chirurgicum: Das ist, Wie alle junge angehende Feldscherer, Barbier un[d] Wundärzt sollen befragt warden, wie sie sich in allen begebende Verwundungen in deß Menschen Leib vom Haupt bis auff die Fußsohlen verhalten sollen, In gleichen wie alle Chirurgische Instrumenten zugericht, vnd gebraucht warden, in kupffer vor Augen gestellt* (Augsburg, 1649).

—, *Kurtzer iedoch Gewisser bericht, dreyer Erblicher kranckheiten, alß da sein, die Pest, Frantzosen, vnd Scharbock, wie sie mögen curirt warden ...* (Augsburg, 1667).

—, *Kurtzer iedoch Gewisser bericht, dreyer Erblicher kranckheiten, alß da sein, die Pest, Frantzosen, vnd Scharbock, wie sie mögen curirt werden* (Augsburg, 1702).

Seitz, Alexander, *Ein nutzlich regiment wider die bösen frantzosen mit etliche[n] clugen fragstucken durch Alexander Sytzen zu Marbach beschriben (Pforzheim, 1509)* in Peter Ukena (ed.), *Alexander Seitz sämtliche Schriften* (Göttingen, 1970) vol. 1, pp. 7–29.

Stetten, Paul von (the younger), *Beschreibungen der Reichs-Stadt Augsburg, nach ihrer Lage, jetzigen Verfassung, Handlung und den zu solcher gehörenden Künsten und Gewerben, auch ihren andern Merkwürdigkeiten* (Augsburg, 1788).

Stetten, Paul von (the older), *Geschichte der Heil. Röm. Reichs Freyen Stadt Augsburg, aus Bewährten Jahr=Büchern und Tüchtigen Urkungen gezogen und an das Licht gegeben* (2 vols, Frankfurt and Leipzig, 1743/1758).
Wirsung, Christoph, *Artzney Buch.* (Heidelberg, 1586).
Wittich, Johannes, *Artzneybuch für alle Menschen sonderlich aber Für arme vnd dürfftige Leute, denen bißweilen die Sonne ehe im Hauß kommt, dann das liebe Brodt* (Leipzig, 1596).
—, *Von dem Ligno Guyaco, Wunderbawm, res nova genandt, von der China Ex Occidentali India, von der Sarsaparilla, von dem Fenchelholtz Sassafras, und von dem Grießholtz, so man Lignum Nephriticum nennet, Welche alle zum theil wieder die flechten der Indianische Seuche* ... (Arnstadt, 1603).
—, *Praeservator Sanitatis: Ein Nützlicher Bericht, von den Sechß unvermeidlichen dingen zur Gesundheit gantz ersprießlichen* ... (Arnstadt, 1607).

3. Secondary Sources

Abramowitz, William, 'Historical Points of Interest in the Mode of Action and Ill Effects of Mercury', *Bulletin of the New York Academy of Medicine*, 56 (1978), pp. 695–705.
Achelis, Johann Daniel, 'Über die Syphilisschriften des Theophrastus von Hohenheim. I. Die Pathologie der Syphilis', *Sitzungsberichte der Heidelberger Akademie der Wissenschaften, Mathematisch-Naturwissenschaftliche Klasse* 9 (1938), pp. 3–42.
Aderbauer, Herbert, *Das Tübinger Hospital. Vom Pfründnerheim zur Armen- und Arbeitsanstalt und der Wandel der sozialen Funktion in der frühen Neuzeit* (Tübingen, 1997).
Aikema, B. and Meijers, D., *Nel regno dei poveri. Arte e storia dei grandi ospedali veneziani in età moderna, 1474–1797* (Venice, 1989).
Allgemeine Deutsche Biographie (56 vols, Munich 1875–1912).
Alvarez-Pélaez, Raquel, *La Conquista de la Naturaleza Americana* (Madrid, 1993).
Amelang, James S. (ed.), *A Journal of the Plague Year: The Diary of the Barcelona Tanner Miquel Parets, 1651* (New York and Oxford, 1991).
Amundsen, Darrel W., 'Caring and Curing in Medieval Catholic Tradition', in ibid., *Medicine, Society, and Faith in the Ancient and Medieval Worlds* (Baltimore and London, 1996).
— and Ferngren, Gary, 'Evolution of the Patient-Physician Relationship: Antiquity through the Renaissance', in Earl E. Shelp (ed.), *The Clinical Encounter: The Moral Fabric of the Patient-Physician Relationship* (Dordrecht and Boston, 1983), pp. 3–46.
Andreski, S., 'The Syphilitic Shock: A New Explanation of the "Great Witch Craze" of the 16th and 17th Centuries in the Light of Medicine and Psychiatry', *Encounter* 58 (1982), pp. 7–26.

Anschütz, Felix, *Ärztliches Handeln. Grundlagen, Möglichkeiten, Grenzen, Widersprüche* (Darmstadt, 1987).

Appelboom, E. A., 'Can a Diagnosis be Made in Retrospect? The Case of Desiderius Erasmus', *The Journal of Rheumatology* 13 (1986), pp. 1181–4.

Arends, Dietrich, Hickel, Erika and Schneider, Wolfgang, *Das Warenlager einer mittelalterlichen Apotheke* (Braunschweig, 1960).

Arksey, Hilary, 'Expert Knowledge and Lay Participation in the Construction of Medical Knowledge', *Sociology of Health and Illness* 16 (1994), pp. 449–67.

Arnold, Werner, *Die Flugschriften der frühen Neuzeit. Die Erforschung der Buch- und Bibliotheksgeschichte Deutschlands* (Wiesbaden, 1987).

Arrizabalaga, Jon, 'Medicina universitaria y Morbus Gallicus en la Italia de finales del siglo XV: El arquitra pontificio Gaspar Torella (c. 1452–c. 1520)', *Asclepio* 40 (1988), pp. 3–38.

—, 'Medical Responses to the 'French Disease' in Europe at the Turn of the Sixteenth Century', in Kevin Siena (ed.), *Sins of the Flesh: Responding to Sexual Disease in Early Modern Europe* (Toronto, 2006), pp. 33–55.

—, 'Sebastiano d'ell Aquila (c. 1440–c. 1510), el "mal francés" y la "dispita de Ferrara" (1487), *Dynamis* 14 (1994), pp. 227–247.

—, 'Syphilis', in Kenneth F. Kiple (ed.), *The Cambridge World History of Human Disease* (Cambridge, 1993), pp. 1025–33.

—, and French, Roger, 'Coping with the French Disease: University Practitioners' Strategies and Tactics in the Transition from the Fifteenth to the Sixteenth Century', in Roger French et al., *Medicine from the Black Death to the French Disease* (Aldershot, 1998), pp. 248–87.

—, Henderson, John and French, Roger, *The Great Pox: The French Disease in Renaissance Europe* (New Haven, 1997).

Baader, Gerhard and Keil, Gundolf, 'Mittelalterliche Diagnostik', in Christa Gork et al. (eds), *Medizinische Diagnostik in Geschichte und Gegenwart. Festschrift für Heinz Gork* (Munich, 1978), pp. 122–44.

— und Winau, Rolf (eds), 'Die Hippokratischen Epidemien. Theorie – Praxis – Tradition', *Sudhoffs Archiv* 27 (1989).

Bachoffner, Pierre, 'Notes sur la Guaiac au XVe et au début du XVIIe siècle', *Veröffentlichungen der internationalen Gesellschaft für Geschichte der Pharmazie* (1970), pp. 17–25.

Bachtin, Michail, *Rabelais und seine Welt. Volkskultur als Gegenkultur* (Frankfurt, 1995).

Bäumler, Ernst, *Amors vergifteter Pfeil. Kulturgeschichte einer verschwiegenen Krankheit* (Hamburg, 1976).

Baier, A. L. and Finlay, R. (eds), *London 1500–1700: The Making of Metropolis* (London, 1986).

Barkan, Leonard, *Nature's Work of Art: The Human Body as Image of the World* (New Haven and London, 1975).

Barrera-Osorio, Antonio 'Local Herbs, Global Medicine: Commerce, Knowledge, and Commodities in Spanish America', in Pamela Smith and Paula Findlen,

Merchants & Marvels: Commerce, Science and Art in Early Modern Europe (New York and London, 2002), pp. 163–81.

Barrera-Osorio, Antonio, *Experiencing Nature: Spanish American Empire and the Scientific Revolution* (Houston, 2006).

Barry, Jonathon and Jones, Colin, *Medicine and Charity Before the Welfare State* (London and New York, 1991).

Bartstra, J. J. J., 'Syfilis als dagelijkse host', *Geschiedenis der Geneisekunde* 2 (1995), pp. 107–9.

Barwig, Edgar and Schmitz, Ralf, 'Narren, Geisteskranke und Hofleute', in Ulrich Hergemöller, *Randgruppen der spätmittelalterlichen Gesellschaft. Ein Hand- und Studienbuch* (Warendorf, 1990), pp. 167–99.

Bátori, Ingrid, *Der Reichsstadt Augsburg im 18. Jahrhundert. Verfassung, Finanzen und Reformversuche* (Göttingen, 1969).

Bauer, Max, *Der Dirne und ihr Anhang. Ein Beitrag zur Geschichte des Geschlechterlebens* (Dresden, 1930).

—, *Das Geschlechtsleben in deutscher Vergangenheit.* (Dresden, 1930).

Benedek, Thomas G., 'The Influence of Ulrich von Hutten's Medical Descriptions and Metaphorical Use of Medicine', *Bulletin of the History of Medicine* 66 (1992), pp. 355–75.

Benthien, Claudia, *Haut. Literaturgeschichte, Körperbilder, Grenzdiskurse* (2 vols, Reinbeck, 1999).

Benzenhöfer, Udo (ed.), *Paracelsus* (Darmstadt, 1993).

Bériac, Francois, *Histoire des lépreux au Moyen Age. Une société exclus* (Paris, 1988).

Benzing, Josef, *Die Buchdrucker des 16. und 17. Jahrhunderts im deutschen Sprachgebiet* (Wiesbaden, 1926).

—, *Ulrich von Hutten und seine Drucker. Eine Bibliographie der Schriften Huttens im 16. Jahrhundert* (Wiesbaden, 1956).

—, 'Walter H. Ryff und sein Werk. Eine Bibliographie', *Philobiblion* 2 (1958), pp. 126–55; 203–25.

Bériou, Nicole and Toutati, Francois-Olivier, *Voluntate dei Leprosus. Les lépreux entre conversation et exclusion aux XIIème et XIIIème siècle* (Spoleto, 1991).

Bernsdorf, B., 'Art. Prostitution', in *Religion in Geschichte und Gegenwart* (Tübingen, 1961), vol. 5, pp. 640–45.

Berridge, Virginia and Strong, Philip, 'AIDS and the Relevance of History', *Society for the Social History of Medicine* 4 (1991), pp. 129–38.

Biernoff, Suzannah, *Sight and Embodiment in the Middle Ages* (Houndmills, 2002).

Biraben, J.-N., *Les hommes et la peste en France et dans les pays européens et méditerranées* (2 vols Paris, 1975–1976).

Bisle, Max, *Die öffentliche Armenpflege der Reichsstadt Augsburg mit Berücksichtigung der einschlägigen Verhältnisse in anderen Reichsstädten Süddeutschlands* (Paderborn, 1904).

Bitz, Matthias, *Badewesen in Südwestdeutschland 1550–1840. Zum Wandel von Gesellschaft und Architektur* (Idstein, 1989).

Blaser, Robert-Henri, 'Hutten und Paracelsus, zwei Schicksale der deutschen Renaissance', *Nova Acta Paracelsica* (1977), pp. 69–97.

Bleker, Johanna, 'Die Kunst des Harnsehens – ein vornehm und nötig Gliedmaß der schönen Artzeney', *Hippokrates* 41 (1970), pp. 385–95.

Blickle, Peter, *Deutsche Untertanen. Ein Widerspruch* (Göttingen, 1981).

Bloch, Iwan, 'Aufgaben und Ziele der Sexualwissenschaft', *Zeitschrift für Sexualwissenschaft* 1 (1914/15), pp. 2–11.

—, *Das erste Auftreten der Syphilis (Lustseuche) in der europäischen Kulturwelt: gewürdigt in seiner weltgeschichtlichen Bedeutung, dargestellt nach Anfang, Verlauf und voraussichtlichem Ende. Vortrag gehalten in der staatswissenschaftlichen Vereinigung zu Berlin am 12. November 1903* (Jena, 1904).

—, 'Die primitiven Wurzeln der Prostitution', *Zeitschrift zur Bekämpfung der Geschlechtskrankheiten* 13 (1911), pp. 143–60.

—, 'Ist die Prostitution ein notwendiges Übel?', *Die neue Generation* 5 (1909), pp. 179–90.

— and Loewenstein, Georg, *Prostitution* (2 vols, Berlin, 1912/1925).

—, *Das Sexualleben unserer Zeit in seinen Beziehungen zur modernen Kultur* (Berlin, 1907).

—, *Der Ursprung der Syphilis. Eine medizinische und kulturgeschichtliche Untersuchung, Teil I: Ursprung der Syphilis* (Jena, 1901); *Teil 2: Kritik der Lehre von der Altertumssyphilis* (Jena, 1911).

Boedecker, Dieter, 'Die Entwicklung der Hamburger Hospitäler aus ärztlicher Sicht' (dissertation, Hamburg, 1977).

Boehrer, Bruce Thomas, 'Early Modern Syphilis', in John C. Font (ed.), *Forbidden History: The State, Society and the Regulation of Sexuality in Modern Europe* (Chicago, 1992), pp. 11–28.

Bourdieu, Pierre, 'Ökonomisches Kapital, kulturelles Kapital, soziales Kapital', in Reinhard Kreckel (ed.), *Soziale Ungleichheiten* (Göttingen, 1983), pp. 183–98.

Brady, Thomas A., 'Göttliche Republiken. Die Domestizierung der Religion in der deutschen Stadtreformation', in Andreas Lindt and Alfred Schindler (eds), *Hoffnung der Kirche und Erneuerung der Welt. Beiträge zu den ökumenischen, sozialen und politischen Wirkungen des Pietismus* (Göttingen, 1985), pp. 109–36.

— et al. (eds), *Handbook of European History 1400–1600. Late Middle Ages, Renaissance and Reformation* (2 vols, Leiden, 1995).

Brandt, Allan, *No Magic Bullet: A Social History of Venereal Disease in the United States Since 1988* (New York and Oxford, 1985).

Brecht, M., *Martin Luther. Sein Weg zur Reformation 1483–1521* (Stuttgart, 1981).

Bremen, Otto von, 'Die Lepra-Untersuchungen der Kölner Medizinischen Fakultät von 1491–1664', *Westdeutsche Zeitschrift für Geschichte und Kunst* 18 (1899), pp. 65–77.

Briffault, Robert, *Sin and Sex* (London, 1931).

Broadhead, Philip, 'Popular Pressure for Reform in Augsburg 1524–1534', in Wolfgang J. Mommsen et al. (eds), *Stadtbürgertum und Adel in der Reformation* (Stuttgart, 1979), pp. 80–87.

Brockliss, Laurence and Jones, Colin, *The Medical World of Early Modern France* (Cambridge, 1997).

Brody, Saul Nathaniel, *The Disease of the Soul: Leprosy in Medieval Literature* (Ithaca, 1974).

Brown, Kevin, *The Pox: The Life and Near Death of a Very Social Disease* (Phoenix Mill, 2006).

Burckhardt, Jacob, *Die Kultur der Renaissance in Italien/Die Kunst der Renaissance in Italien* (Munich, 1997).

Brundage, James A., *Law, Sex, and Christian Society in Medieval Europe* (Chicago, 1987).

Brunner, Otto, 'Zum Begriff des Bürgertums', in Th. Meyer (ed.), *Untersuchungen zur gesellschaftlichen Struktur der mittelalterlichen Städte in Europa* (Konstanz and Stuttgart, 1966), pp. 13–24.

Bühler, Hans Viktor, 'Das Ärztegeschlecht der Occo', *Sudhoffs Archiv für Geschichte der Medizin und Naturwissenschaften* 28 (1935), pp. 14–42.

Buff, Adolf, 'Der Apotheker Claus Hofmair, die Augsburger Apotheker des 14. Jahrhunderts und Magister Ulrich Hofmair, Protonotar von Kaiser Ludwig dem Bayer', *Zeitschrift des historischen Vereins für Schwaben und Neuburg* 16 (1889), pp. 161–209.

Bullough, Vern L., 'Sex in History', in Jacqueline Murray and Konrad Eisenbichler (eds), *Desire and Discipline: Sex and Sexuality in the Premodern West* (Toronto, 1996), pp. 13–22.

—— and Bullough, Bonnie, *Sin, Sickness, and Sanity: A History of Sexual Attitudes* (New York, 1977).

Bulst, Neithard, 'Krankheit und Gesellschaft in der Vormoderne. Das Beispiel der Pest', in Neithard Bulst and Robert Delort (eds), *Maladies et société (XIIe–XVIIIe siècle). Actes du colloque de Bielefeld, novembre 1986* (Paris, 1989), pp. 17–47

——, 'Vier Jahrhunderte Pest in niedersächischen Städten. Vom Schwarzen Tod (1349–1351) bis in die erste Hälfte des 18. Jahrhunderts', in Cord Meckseper (ed.), *Stadt im Wandel* (4 vols, Stuttgart, 1985), vol. 4, pp. 251–70.

Burgun, René, 'Mésure contre la Syphilis à Strasbourg (1495–1789): Das Blatterhaus', in Georges Livet and Georges Schaff (eds), *Mèdicine et assistance en Alsace XVIe–XXe siècle* (Strasbourg, 1976), pp. 62–7.

Bylebyl, Jerome J., 'The Manifest and the Hidden in the Renaissance Clinic', in W.F. Bynum and Roy Porter (eds), *Medicine and the Five Senses* (Cambridge, 1993), pp. 40–60.

—, 'The Medical Side of Harvey's Discovery: The Normal and the Abnormal', in ibid. (ed.), *William Harvey and His Age: The Professional and Social Context of the Discovery of the Circulation* (Baltimore, 1979), pp. 28–102.

Bynum, William F., *Science and the Practice of Medicine in the Nineteenth Century* (Cambridge, 1994).

Cadden, Joan, 'Und er schuf Mann und Weib: Geschlecht und Wissenschaft im Werk der Hildegard von Bingen', in Barbara Orland and Elvira Scheich (eds), *Geschlecht der Natur. Feministische Beiträge zur Geschichte und Theorie der Naturwissenschaften* (Frankfurt a. M., 1995), pp. 224–39.

—, *Meanings of Sex Differences in the Middle Ages: Medicine, Science, and Culture* (Cambridge, 1993).

Calvi, Giulia, *Histories of a Plague Year: The Social and the Imaginary in Baroque Florence* (Berkeley, 1989).

—, 'A Metaphor for Social Exchange: The Florentine Plague of 1630', *Representations* 13 (1986), pp. 139–63.

Campbell, Mary B., 'Fracastoro's *De Syphilis* and the Discovery of the New World', in Daniel Segal (ed.), *Crossing Cultures. Essays in the Displacement of Western Civilization* (Tuscon, 1992), pp. 3–32.

Carlino, Andrea, *Books of the Body: The Anatomical Ritual and Renaissance Learning* (Chicago and London, 1999).

Carmichael, Anne G., *Plague and the Poor in Renaissance Florence* (Cambridge, 1987).

—, 'Syphilis and the Columbian Exchange: Was the New Disease Really New?', in Mario G. Marques and John Cule (eds), *The Great Maritime Discoveries and the World Health* (Lissabon, 1991), pp. 189–90.

Carter, Codell K., *The Rise of Causal Concepts of Disease* (Aldershot, 2003).

Chapman, Allan, 'Astrological Medicine', in Charles Webster (ed.), *Health, Medicine and Mortality in the Sixteenth Century* (Cambridge, 1979), pp. 175–300.

Chickering, Roger, *Karl Lamprecht: A German Academic Life (1856–1915)* (Atlantic Highlands, 1993).

Chrisman, Miriam Usher, *Lay Culture, Learned Culture: Books and Social Change in Strasbourg, 1480–1599* (New Haven and London, 1982).

Cipolla, Carlo M., *Miasmas and Disease. Public Health and the Environment in the Pre-Industrial Age* (London, 1992).

Cipriani, Marina, 'Mercurio e mercurialisti, guaiaco e guaiacofili, e "fenomeno Fugger"', *Rivista di Storia della Medica* 6 (1962), pp. 87–113.

Clasen, Claus-Peter, 'Arm und Reich in Augsburg vor dem Dreißigjährigen Krieg', in Gunther Gottlieb et al. (eds), *Geschichte der Stadt Augsburg von der Römerzeit bis zur Gegenwart* (Stuttgart, 1984), pp. 312–36.

—, 'Armenfürsorge im 16. Jahrhundert', in Gunther Gottlieb et al. (eds), *Geschichte der Stadt Augsburg von der Römerzeit bis zur Gegenwart* (Stuttgart, 1984), pp. 363–85.

——, 'Armenfürsorge in Augsburg vor dem Dreißigjährigen Krieg', *Zeitschrift des historischen Vereins für Schwaben* 78 (1984), pp. 65–115.

——, Die Augsburger Weber. *Leistungen und Krisen des Textilgewerbes um 1600* (Augsburg, 1981).

Cohen, Ester, 'Towards a History of European Physical Sensibility: Pain in the Later Middle Ages', *Science in Context* 8 (1995), pp. 47–74.

Cook, Harold J., 'Good Advice and Little Medicine: The Professional Authority of Early Modern English Physicians', *Journal of British Studies* 33 (1994), pp. 1–31.

Conrad, Lawrence I. and Wyjastyk, Dominik (eds), *Contagion: Perspectives from Pre-Modern Societies* (Aldershot, 2000).

Corbin, Alain, *The Foul and the Fragrant: Odor and the French Social Imagination* (Leamington Spa, 1986).

Coulter, Harris Livermore, *AIDS and Syphilis: The Hidden Link* (Berkeley, 1987).

Crookshank, F. C., *The Importance of a Theory of Signs and a Critique of Language in the Study of Medicine: The Meaning of Meaning* (New York, 1923).

Cross, James, *When Plague Strikes: The Black Death, Smallpox, Aids* (New York, 1995).

Cunningham, Andrew, 'Identifying Diseases in the Past: Cutting Through the Gordian Knot', *Asclepio* 54, 1 (2002), pp. 13–34.

——, 'Transforming Plague: The Laboratory and the Identity of Infectious Disease', in Cunningham and Perry Williams (eds), *The Laboratory Revolution in Medicine* (Cambridge, 1992), pp. 209–43.

Curry, Patrick, *Prophecy and Power: Astrology in Early Modern England* (Cambridge, 1989).

Czerny, Albin, 'Der Humanist und Historiograph Kaiser Maximilians I. Joseph Grünpeck', *Archiv für österreichische Geschichte* 73 (1888), pp. 315–64.

Dannenfeldt, Karl, 'Sleep: Theory and Practice in the Late Renaissance', *Journal for the History of Medicine and Allied Sciences* 41 (1986), pp. 415–41.

Daston, Lorraine, 'Die Kultur der wissenschaftlichen Objektivität', in Otto Gerhard Oexle (ed.), *Naturwissenschaft, Geisteswissenschaft, Kulturwissenschaft. Einheit – Gegensatz – Komplementarität* (Göttingen, 1998), pp. 9–39.

——, 'Wunder, Naturgesetze und die wissenschaftliche Revolution des 17. Jahrhunderts', *Jahrbuch der Akademie der Wissenschaften zu Göttingen* (1991), pp. 99–122.

——, 'The Nature of Nature in Early Modern Europe', *Configurations* 6 (1998), pp. 149–72.

——, and Park, Katharine, *Wonders and the Order of Nature, 1150–1750* (New York, 1999).

Davenport-Himes, Richard, *Sex, Death and Punishment. Attitudes to Sex and Sexuality in Britain Since the Renaissance* (London, 1990).

Davidson, Arnold I., *The Emergence of Sexuality: Historical Epistemology and the Formation of Concept* (Cambridge, MA, 2002).

Debus, Allen, G., *Chemistry, Alchemy and the New Philosophy, 1550–1700* (London, 1987).

Degenhart, Armin von, *Das Klistier* (Flensburg, 1985).

Deininger, Friedrich, 'Das Collegium Medicum Augustanum', *Deutsches Ärzteblatt* 61 (1964), pp. 1239–43.

Delkeskam-Hayes, Corinna and Gardell Cutter, Mary Ann (eds), *Science, Technology, and the Art of Medicine: European-American Dialogues* (Dordrecht and Boston, 1993).

Delumeau, Jean, *Angst im Abendland. Die Geschichte kollektiver Ängste im Europa des 14. bis 18. Jahrhunderts* (Hamburg, 1989).

Demaitre, Luke, 'The Description and Diagnosis of Leprosy by Fourteenth-Century Physicians', *Bulletin of the History of Medicine* 59 (1985), pp. 327–44.

——, *Leprosy in Premodern Medicine: A Disease of the Whole Body* (Baltimore, 2007).

Dennie, Charles Clayton, *A History of Syphilis* (Springfield, 1962).

Dinges, Martin, 'Neue Wege in der Seuchengeschichte?', in Martin Dinges and Thomas Schlich (eds), *Neue Wege in der Seuchengeschichte* (Stuttgart, 1995), pp. 7–24.

——, 'Nord-Süd-Gefälle in der Pestbekämpfung. Italien, Deutschland und England im Vergleich', in Wolfgang U. Eckhart and Robert Jütte (eds), *Das europäische Gesundheitssystem: Gemeinsamkeiten und Unterschiede in historischer Perspektive* (Stuttgart, 1994), pp. 19–51.

——, 'Social History of Medicine in Germany and France in the Late Twentieth Century: From the History of Medicine towards a History of Health', Frank Huisman and John Harley Warner (eds), *Locating Medical History: The Stories and their Meaning* (Baltimore, 2003), pp. 209–36.

——, *Stadtarmut in Bordeaux 1525–1675. Alltag, Politik, Mentalitäten* (Bonn, 1988).

Dirlmeier, Uwe, *Untersuchungen zu Einkommensverhältnissen und Lebenshaltungskosten in oberdeutschen Städten des Spätmittelalters (Mitte 14. bis Anfang 16. Jahrhundert)* (Heidelberg, 1987).

Döhner, O., *Krankheitsbegriff, Gesundheitsverhalten und Einstellungen zum Tod im 16. bis 18. Jahrhundert* (Frankfurt, Bern and New York, 1986).

Dohi, K., *Beiträge zur Geschichte der Syphilis* (Tokyo, 1923).

Dols, Michael, *The Black Death in the Middle East* (Princeton, 1977).

Duby, Gorges, 'Réflection sur la douleur physique au Moyen Age', in Geneviève Lévy (ed.), *La Douleur* (Paris, 1992).

Duden, Barbara, *The Woman Beneath the Skin: A Doctor's Patients in Eighteenth-Century Germany* (Cambridge, MA, 1991).

——, 'Medicine and the History of the Body: The Lady of the Court', in Gunnar Stollberg and Jens Lachmund (eds), *Social Construction of Illness. Historical, Sociological and Anthropological Perspectives* (Stuttgart, 1992), pp. 23–38.

Dutour, Olivier et al. (eds), *L'origine de la syphilis en Europe. Avant ou après 1493?* (Paris, 1994).

Eamon, William, 'Cannibalism and Contagion. Framing Syphilis in Counter-Reformation Italy', *Early Science and Medicine* 3, 1 (1998), pp. 1–31.

—, *Science and the Secrets of Nature: Books on Secrets in Medieval and Early Modern Culture* (Princeton, 1994).

Eatough, Geoffrey, *Fracastoro's 'Syphilis'. Introduction, Text, Translation and Notes* (Liverpool, 1984).

Ebstein, Erich, 'Zur Geschichte der venerischen Krankheiten in Göttingen', *Janus* 10 (1905), pp. 178–96.

Ecker-Offenhäußer, Ute, 'Joseph Schmid. Handwerkschirurg und Schriftsteller in Augsburg im 17. Jahrhundert', *Medizin, Gesellschaft und Geschichte* 15 (1997), pp. 117–39.

—, *'Pest, Franzosen, Scharbock' – Krankheitserfahrung und medizinischer Alltag des 17. Jahrhunderts im Spiegel der Werke des Augsburger Wundarztes Joseph Schmid* (MA dissertation, Augsburg, 1994).

Egger, Bernhard, 'Iwan Bloch und die Konstituierung der Sexualwissenschaften als eigene Disziplin' (Düsseldorf, 1988).

—, 'Ein neues Verhältnis: Sexualwissenschaften und Sozialwissenschaften bei Iwan Bloch', in Rolf Gindorf and Edwin J. Haeberle (eds), *Sexualität als sozialer Tatbestand. Theoretische und empirische Beiträge zu einer Soziologie der Sexualitäten* (Berlin, 1986).

Ehlert, Thomas, 'Wissensvermittlung in deutschsprachiger Fachliteratur des Mittelalters, oder: Wie kam die Diätetik in die Kochbücher?', *Würzburger medizinhistorische Mitteillungen* 8 (1990), pp. 137–59.

Eich, Wolfgang, *Medizinische Semiotik (1750–1850). Ein Beitrag zur Geschichte des Zeichenbegriffs in der Medizin* (Freiburg, 1986).

Eisenstein, Elizabeth L., *The Printing Press as an Agent of Change: Communication and Cultural Transformation in Early-Modern Europe* (Cambridge, 1979).

—, *The Printing Revolution in Early Modern Europe* (Cambridge, 1983).

Elkeles, Barbara, 'Aussagen zu ärztlichen Leitwerten, Pflichten und Verhaltensweisen in berufsvorbereitender Literatur' (dissertation, Hannover, 1979).

Engelhardt, Dietrich von, *Krankheit, Schmerz und Lebenskunst. Eine Kulturgeschichte der Körpererfahrung* (Munich, 1999).

Engelsing, Rolf, *Analphabetentum und Lektüre. Zur Sozialgeschichte des Lesens in Deutschland zwischen feudaler und industrieller Gesellschaft* (Stuttgart, 1973).

Epstein, Steven, *Impure Science: AIDS, Activism, and the Politics of Knowledge* (Berkeley, 1996).

Erickson, Carolly, *The Medieval Vision: Essays in History and Perception* (New York, 1976).

Essed, Wilhelm Frederik Robert, *Over den Oorsprung der Syphilis. Een kritisch-historischepidemiologische Studie tevens ontwerp eener Theorie* (Amsterdam, 1933).

Eulner, Hans-Heinz, *Die Entwicklung der medizinischen Spezialfächer an den Universitäten des deutschen Sprachgebietes* (Stuttgart, 1970).

Fabricius, Johannes, *Syphilis in Shakespeare's England* (London, 1994).

Fallet, Marius, 'Medizin, Zeitmessung und Uhrmacherkunst', *Ciba-Zeitschrift* 2 (1935), pp. 748–57.

Fanghauser, Werner, *Basels Maßnahmen gegen die Syphilis in den verflossenen Jahrhunderten* (Basel, 1931).

Fee, Elizabeth, 'The Wages of Sin? Struggles over the Social Meaning of Venereal Disease and AIDS', in *Proceedings of the 13th Symposium on the Comparative History of Medicine, 4–10 September 1988* (Brentwood, 1993).

—, and Fox, Daniel M. (eds), *AIDS: The Making of a Chronic Disease* (Berkeley, Los Angeles and London, 1992).

Feher, Michel, Naddaff, Ramona and Tazi, Nadia (eds), *Fragments for a History of the Human Body* (3 vols, New York and Cambridge, MA, 1990).

Figlio, Karl, 'The Historiography of Scientific Medicine: An Invitation to the Human Sciences', *Comparative Studies in Society and History* 19 (1977), pp. 162–286.

Finnerud, Clark W., 'Ferdinand von Hebra and the Vienna School of Dermatology', *Archives of Dermatology and Syphilology* 87 (1953), pp. 223–32.

Fisch, Max, *Nicolaus Pol Doctor 1494* (New York, 1947).

Fischer, Alfons, *Geschichte des deutschen Gesundheitswesens* [1933] (Hildesheim, 1965).

Fischer, Hermann (ed.), *Schwäbisches Wörterbuch* (Tübingen, 1904–1936).

Fischer, I., *Ärztliche Standespflichten und Standesfragen. Eine historische Studie* (Wien, 1912).

Fischer, Thomas, *Städtische Armut und Armenfürsorge im 15. und 16. Jahrhundert. Sozialgeschichtliche Untersuchungen am Beispiel der Städte Basel, Freiburg i. Br. und Straßburg* (Göttingen, 1979).

Fischer, Wilhelm, *Die Prostitution. Ihre Geschichte und ihre Beziehungen zum Verbrechen und den kriminellen Ausartungen des modernen Geschlechtslebens* 2nd edn (Leipzig, 1920).

Fischer-Homberger, Esther, *Medizin vor Gericht. Gerichtsmedizin von der Renaisance bis zur Aufklärung* (Bern, 1983).

Fissell, Mary, *Patients, Power, and the Poor in Eighteenth-Century Bristol* (Cambridge, 1991).

—, *Vernacular Bodies: The Politics of Reproduction in Early Modern England* (Oxford, 2004).

Fleck, Ludwik, *Entstehung und Entwicklung einer wissenschaftlichen Tatsache. Einführung in die Lehre vom Denkstil und Denkkollektiv [1935]* (Frankfurt, 1993).

Fleischmann, Josef, 'Die Ärztefamilie Jung', *Lebensbilder aus dem bayerischen Schwaben* 4 (1955), pp. 14–25.

Flint, J.G., 'Eine der ersten Guajakschriften', *Janus* 36 (1932), pp. 384–91; 37 (1933), pp. 320–22.

Foa, Anna, 'The New and the Old: The Spread of Syphilis (1494–1530)', in Edward Shorter, and Guido Ruggiero (eds), *Sex and Gender in Historical Perspective* (Baltimore, 1990), pp. 26–45.

Foucault, Michel, *The Birth of the Clinic: An Archeaology of Medical Perception* [1963] (London and New York, 1994).

—, *The Order of Things: An Archeaology of the Human Sciences* [1966] (London, 2003).

French, Roger, 'The Arrival of the French Disease in Leipzig', in Neithard Bulst und Robert Delort (eds), *Maladies et société XIIe–XVIIIe siècle. Actes du colloque de Bielefeld, novembre 1986* (Paris, 1979), pp. 133–41.

—, 'Sign Conceptions in Medicine from the Renaissance to the Early 19th Century', in Roland Posner, Klaus Robering and Thomas A. Sebeok (eds), *Semiotik. Ein Handbuch zu den zeichentheoretischen Grundlagen von Natur und Kultur* (3 vols, Berlin and New York, 1997–1999), vol. 2, pp. 1354–61.

—, *The Anatomical Tradition* (London, 1993).

— et al. (eds), *Medicine From the Black Death to the French Disease* (Aldershot, 1998).

Fried, Pankratz, *Die Fugger in der Herrschaftsgeschichte* (Munich, 1976).

Friedrich, Herbert, *Das Armen- und Fürsorgewesen in Zwickau bis zur Einführung der Reformation* (Würzburg, 1934).

Fries, Karl, 'Die Pest zu Augsburg im dreißigjährigen Krieg: Ein Beitrag zur Geschichte der Pest' (Augsburg, 1887).

Fröhlich, Sigrid, *Die soziale Sicherung bei Zünften und Gesellenverbänden. Darstellung, Analyse, Vergleich* (Berlin, 1976).

Fürstenwerth, Ludwig, *Die Verfassungsänderungen in den oberdeutschen Reichsstädten zu Zeit Karls V.* (Göttingen, 1892).

Fuhse, F., 'Hygiene und Heilkunde in der Stadt Braunschweig während des 16. Jahrhunderts', *Niederdeutsche Zeitschrift für Volkskunde* 4 (1926), pp. 23–44.

Gadebusch Bondio, Mariacarla, *Medizinische Ästetik. Kosmetische und plastische Chirurgie zwischen Antike und früher Neuzeit* (Munich, 2005).

Galdston, Iago, 'Diagnosis in Historical Perspective', *Bulletin of the History of Medicine* 9 (1941), pp. 367–84.

García-Ballester, Luis, 'Galen as a Medical Practitioner: Problems in Diagnosis', in Vivian Nutton (ed.), *Galen: Problems and Prospects* (London, 1981), pp. 13–46.

—, 'Medical Ethics in Transition in the Latin Medicine of the Thirteenth and Fourteenth Centuries: New Perspectives on the Physician-Patient Relationship and the Doctor's Fee', in Andrew Wear, Johanna Geyer-Kordesch and Roger French (eds), *Doctors and Ethics: The Earlier Historical Setting of Professional Ethics* (Amsterdam and Atlanta, 1993), pp. 38–70.

— et al. (eds), *Practical Medicine from Salerno to the Black Death* (Cambridge, 1994).

Gariepy, Thomas P., 'Gyaiacum et Lues Venerea', *Journal of the History of Medicine and Allied Sciences* 35 (1981), pp. 325–33.

Garin, Eugenio, *Astrology in the Renaissance: The Zodiac of Life* (London, 1983).

Geffken, Peter, 'Rehm (auch Rem)', in Wolfgang Baer et al. (eds), *Augsburger Stadtlexikon. Geschichte, Gesellschaft, Kultur, Recht, Wirtschaft* (Augsburg, 1985), pp. 301f.

Gensthaler, Gerhard, *Das Medizinalwesen der freien Reichsstadt Augsburg bis zum 16. Jahrhundert mit Berücksichtigung der ersten Pharmakopöe von 1564 und ihrer weiteren Ausgaben* (Augsburg, 1973).

Gentilcore, David, 'Contesting Illness in Early Modern Naples: Miracolati, Physicians and the Congregation of Rites', *Past and Present* 148 (1995), pp. 117–48.

—, *Healers and Healing in Early Modern Italy* (Manchester, 1998).

Gerbi, Antonello, *Nature and the New World* (Pittsburg, 1985).

Gier, Helmut et al. (eds), *Augsburger Buchdruck und Verlagswesen. Von den Anfängen bis zur Gegenwart* (Wiesbaden, 1997).

Giesecke, Michael, *Der Buchdruck in der frühen Neuzeit. Eine historische Fallstudien über die Durchsetzung neuer Informations- und Kommunikationstechnologien* (Frankfurt, 1998).

Gilman, Sander L., *Disease and Representation: Images of Illness from Madness to AIDS* (Ithaca, 1988).

Gottlieb, Gunther et al. (eds), *Geschichte der Stadt Augsburg von der Römerzeit bis zur Gegenwart* (Stuttgart, 1984).

Christoph Gradmann, *Krankheit im Labor: Robert Koch und die medizinische Bakteriologie* (Göttingen, 2005).

Grafton, Anthony, *Cardanos Kosmos: Die Welten und Werke eines Renaissance Astrologen* (Berlin, 1999).

—, Siraisi, Nancy and Shelford, April, *New Worlds, Ancient Texts: The Power of Tradition and the Shock of the New* (Cambridge, MA, 1992).

Granshaw, Lindsay and Porter, Roy (eds), *The Hospital in History* (London, 1989).

Grell, Ole Peter, 'The Protestant Imperative of Christian Care and Neighbourly Love', in ibid. and Andrew Cunningham, *Health Care and the Poor in Medieval and Renaissance Europe: Italy and England Compared* (London, 1997), pp. 43–65.

—, and Cunningham, Andrew, *The Four Horseman of the Apocalypse: Religion, War, Famine and Death in Reformation Europe* (Cambridge, 2000).

—, and Cunningham, Andrew (eds), *Medicine and the Reformation* (London, 1993).

—, and Cunningham, Andrew, *Religio Medici: Medicine and Religion in Seventeenth-Century England* (Aldershot, 1996).

Grenzmann, Lutger, *Traumbuch Artemidori: Zur Tradition der ersten Übersetzung ins Deutsche durch W. H. Ryff.* (Baden-Baden, 1980), pp. 26–37.

Grimm, Jakob and Grimm, Wilhelm, *Deutsches Wörterbuch* (11 vols, Leipzig, 1873).

Grmek, Mirko D., *History of AIDS: Emergence and Origin of a Modern Pandemic* (Princeton, 1990).

—, *Les maladies à l'aube de la civilisation occidentale. Recherche sur la réalité pathologique dans le monde grec préhistorique, archaique et classique* (Paris, 1983).

Guerra, Francisco, 'The Dispute Over Syphilis Europe Versus America', *Clio Medica* 13 (1978), pp. 39–61.

Gurlt, Ernst Julius, *Geschichte der Chirurgie und ihrer Ausübung. Volkschirurgie, Altertum, Mittelalter, Renaissance (1898)* (reprint, Hildesheim, 1964).

Habrich, Christa, Margruth, Frank and Wolf, Jörn Henning (eds), *Medizinische Diagnostic in Geschichte und Gegenwart. Festschrift für Heinz Goerke* (Munich, 1978).

Hacking, Ian, *The Emergence of Probability: A Philosophical Study of the Early Ideas about Probability, Induction and Statistical Inference* (Cambridge, 1975).

—, *Historical Ontology* (Cambridge, 2001).

—, *Representing and Intervening: Introductory Topics in the Philosophy of Natural Science* (Cambridge, 1983).

—, *The Social Construction of What?* (Cambridge, MA, 1999).

Häbler, Konrad, 'Die Stellung der Fugger im Kirchenstreit des 16. Jahrhunderts', *Historische Vierteljahrszeitschrift* 1 (1898), pp. 473–510.

Hamlin, C., 'Predisposing Causes and Public Health in Early Nineteenth-Century Medical Thought', *Social History of Medicine* 5 (1992), pp. 43–70.

Hammerstein, Notker R., 'The Battle of the Booklets: Prognostic Tradition and Proclamation of the World in Early Sixteenth-Century Germany', in P. Zambelli (ed.), *Astrologi Hallucinati: Stars and the End of the World in Luther's Time* (Berlin, 1986), pp. 129–51.

Hammond, Mitchell Love, 'The Origins of Civic Health Care in Early Modern Germany' (Dissertation, University of Virginia, 2000).

—, 'Paracelsus and the Boundaries of Medicine in Early Modern Augsburg', in Gerhild Scholz Williams and Charles Gunnoe (eds), *Paracelsian Moments* (Kirksville, 2002), pp. 19–33.

Handel – Huren – Huayacan. Ursprung und Verwendung des Heiligen Holzes seit Columbus. Ausstellungskatalog 13. Oktober – 22. Oktober 1992, I.N.K.A. (ed.) (Olching, 1992).

Hannaway, Caroline, *AIDS and the Public Debate: Historical and Contemporary Perspectives* (Amsterdam, Oxford and Tokyo, 1995).

—, 'Environment and Miasmata', in William F. Bynum und Roy Porter (eds), *Companion Encyclopedia of the History of Medicine* (London, 1993), vol. 1, pp. 292–308.

Harig, G., *Bestimmung und Intensität im medizinischen System Galens* (Berlin, 1974).

Hartmann, Fritz, 'Hausvater und Hausmutter als Hausarzt in der Frühen Neuzeit. Hausgewalt und Gesundheitsfürsorge', in Historisches Seminar der Universität Hannover (ed.), *Stadt und Gesellschaft im Mittelalter und Früher Neuzeit. Gedenkschrift für Joachim Leuscher* (1983), pp. 151–76.

—, 'Diagnose', in Eduard Seidler (ed.), *Wörterbuch medizinischer Grundbegriffe. Eine Einführung in die Heilkunde in 86 Artikeln* (Freiburg, 1979), pp. 68–75.

Hartung, Wolfgang, 'Gesellschaftliche Randgruppen im Spätmittelalter. Phänomen und Begriff', in B. Kirchgäßner and F. Reuter (eds), *Städtische Randgruppen und Minderheiten*) (Sigmaringen, 1986), pp. 49–114.

Hartwich, Carl, *Die Bedeutung der Entdeckung Amerikas für die Drogenkunde* (Berlin, 1892).

Hatje, Frank, *Leben und Sterben im Zeitalter der Pest. Basel im 15. bis 17. Jahrhundert* (Basel and Frankfurt, 1992).

Haustein, Hans, 'Die Frühgeschichte der Sphilis 1495–1498. Eine historisch-kritische Untersuchung auf Grund von Archiven und Stadtdokumenten', *Archiv für Dermatologie und Syphilis* 161 (1930), pp. 255–88.

Heckel, Martin, 'Autonomia and Pacis Compositio. Der Augsburger Religionsfrieden in der Deutung der Gegenreformation', *Zeitschrift der Savigny-Stiftung für Rechtsgeschichte, Kanonistische Abteilung* 76 (1959), pp. 141–248.

—, *Deutschland im konfessionellen Zeitalter* (Göttingen, 1983).

Heidel, G., 'Zur wahrscheinlich ältesten deutschen Übersetzung des Syphilisgedichtes von Girolamo Fracastoro', *Dermatologische Monatsschrift* 169 (1983), pp. 130–35.

Heindl-Heinz, Idamarie, 'Das Gesundheitswesen der Stadt Augsburg im 17. und 18. Jahrhundert' (dissertation, Munich, 1950).

Henderson, John, 'The Hospital of Late-Medieval and Renaissance Florence: A Preliminary Survey', in Lindsay Granshaw, and Roy Porter (eds), *The Hospital in History* (London, 1989), pp. 63–92.

—, 'The Parish and the Poor in Florence at the Time of the Black Death: The Case of S. Frediano', *Charity and the Poor in Medieval and Renaissance Europe. Continuity and Change* 3 (1988), pp. 247–72.

—, *Piety and Charity in Late Medieval Florence* (Oxford, 1994).

—, *The Renaissance Hospital: Healing the Body and Healing the Soul* (New Haven, 2006).

Hendrikson, G. L., 'The "Syphilis" of Girolamo Fracastoro', *Bulletin of the History of Medicine* 2 (1934), pp. 515–46.

Herbrand-Hochmuth, Grete, 'Systematisches Verzeichnis der Arbeiten Karl Sudhoffs', *Sudhoffs Archiv* 27 (1934), pp. 134–86.

Herberger, 'Die Seelhäuser und die Seelgeräthe in Augsburg', *Zeitschrift des historischen Vereins für Schwaben und Neuburg* 3 (1876), pp. 283–96.

Hergemöller, Bernd-Ulrich (ed.), *Randgruppen der spätmittelalterlichen Gesellschaft. Ein Hand– und Studienbuch* (Warendorf, 1990).

Herrmann, Bernd, *Mensch und Umwelt im Mittelalter* (Stuttgart, 1986).

Herzlich, Claudine, and Pierret, Janine, 'The Social Construction of the Patient: Patients and Illnesses in Other Ages', *Social Science and Medicine* 20 (1985), pp. 145–51.

——, *Kranke gestern, Kranke heute. Die Gesellschaft und das Leiden* (Munich, 1991).

Hess, Volker, *Von der semiotischen zur diagnostischen Medizin. Die Entstehung der klinischen Methode zwischen 1750 und 1850* (Husum, 1993).

Hesse, Peter G. and Hohmann, Joachim S., *Friedrich Schaudinn, 1871–1906. Sein Leben und Wirken als Mikrobiologe. Eine Biographie* (Frankfurt and New York, 1995).

Hildebrandt, Reinhard, *Die 'Georg-Fuggerischen-Erben'. Kaufmännische Tätigkeit und sozialer Status 1555–1600* (Berlin, 1966).

Hirsch, August (ed.), *Biographisches Lexikon der hervorragenden Ärzte aller Zeiten und Völker* (4 vols, Berlin and Wien, 1929–1934).

Höfler, Max, *Deutsches Krankheitsnamen-Buch* [1899] (reprint Hildesheim, 1970).

Höriger, Hermann, 'Krankheit und religiöses Tabu – die Lepra in der mittelalterlichen und frühneuzeitlichen Gesellschaft', *Gesnerus* 1 (1982), pp. 327–44.

Hörmann, Ludwig, 'Zur Geschichte des Heilig-Geist-Hospitals in Augsburg', *Zeitschrift des Historischen Vereins für Schwaben und Neuburg* 6 (1879), pp. 145–76.

Hoffmann, Robert, 'Die Augsburger Bäder und das Handwerk der Bader', *Zeitschrift des Historischen Vereins für Schwaben und Neuburg* 12 (1885), pp. 1–33.

Hofmann, Anton, 'Entwicklung der Gesundheitspflege im alten Würzburg', *Sitzungsberichte der physikalischen medizinischen Gesellschaft zu Würzburg*, 19 (1920), pp. 3–10.

Hofmann, Siegfried, 'Blatter- Brech- und Siechenhäuser in Ingolstadt', *Ingolstädter Heimatblätter* 28 (1965), pp. 85–112.

Holborn, Hajo, *Ulrich von Hutten* (Leipzig, 1929).

Holcomb, Richard, 'Ruy Diaz de Isla and the Haitian Myth of European Syphilis', *Medical Life* 43 (1936), pp. 270–315.

Horden, Peregrine (ed.), *Music as Medicine: The History of Music Therapy Since Antiquity* (Aldershot, 2000).

Huerkamp, Claudia, *Der Aufstieg der Ärzte im 19. Jahrhundert* (Göttingen, 1985).

Hunter, Kathryn Montgomery, *Doctor's Stories: The Narrative Structure of Medical Knowledge* (Princeton, 1991).

Keith Hutchison, 'Dormative Virtues, Scholastic Qualities, and the New Philosophies', *History of Science* 29 (1991), pp. 245–78.

——, 'What Happened to the Occult Qualities in the Scientific Revolution?', *Isis* 73 (1982), pp. 233–53.

Iggers, Georg G., 'Historicism: The History and Meaning of the Term', *Journal for the History of Ideas* 56 (1995), pp. 129–52

Imhoff, Arthur E. (ed.), *Biologie des Menschen in der Geschichte. Beiträge zur Soziologie der Neuzeit aus Frankreich und Skandinavien* (Stuttgart, 1978).

—, '1580–1650 als Forschungsaufgabe für die Sozialgeschichte. Deutsche und schweizerische Beispiele', in Martin Bircher et al. (eds), *Schweizerisch-deutsche Beziehungen im konfessionellen Zeitalter. Beiträge zur Kulturgeschichte 1580–1650* (Wiesbaden, 1984), pp. 1–55.

—, 'Die Funktion des Krankenhauses in der Stadt des 18. Jahrhunderts', *Zeitschrift für Stadtgeschichte, Stadtsoziologie und Denkmalpflege* 4 (1977), pp. 215–42.

— (ed.), *Leib und Leben in der Geschichte der Neuzeit. L'homme et son corps dans l'histoire moderne. Vorträge eines internationalen Colloquiums (Berlin, 1.– 3.12.1981)* (Berlin, 1983).

— and Larsen, Oivid (ed.), *Sozialgeschichte und Medizin. Probleme einer quantifizierenden Quellenbearbeitung in der Sozial- und Medizingeschichte* (Oslo and Stuttgart, 1976).

Immenkötter, Herbert, 'Kirche zwischen Reformation und Parität', in Gunther Gottlieb et al. (eds), *Geschichte der Stadt Augsburg von der Römerzeit bis in die Gegenwart* (Stuttgart, 1984), pp. 391–412.

Irsigler, Franz, and Lassotta, *Arnold, Bettler und Gaukler, Dirnen und Henker. Außenseiter in einer mittelalterlichen Stadt Köln 1300–1600* (Cologne, 1984).

Jacquart, Danielle, 'Theory, Everyday Practice, and Three Fifteenth-Century Physicians', *Osiris* 6 (1990), pp. 140–60.

—, and Thomasset, Claude, *Sexuality and Medicine in the Middle Ages* (Princeton, 1988).

Jahn, Joachim, 'Augsburgs Bevölkerungszahl im 16. Jahrhundert – ein statistischer Versuch', *Zeitschrift für bayerische Landeskunde* 39 (1976), pp. 379–96.

Jeanselme, Antoine Eduard, *Histoire de la syphilis. Son origine, son expansion: progrès realises dans l'étude de cette maladie depuis la fin du XVe siecle jusqu'à l'époque contemporaine* (Paris, 1931).

— et al., *Histoire de la syphilis, vol. 1: Traité de la syphilis* (Paris, 1931).

Jegel, August, 'Geschlechtskrankheiten vor der Entdeckung Amerikas', *Archiv für Geschichte der Medizin* 26 (1933), pp. 289–307.

—, 'Nürnberger Gesundheitsfürsorge vorallem des 16. und 17. Jahrhunderts', *Archiv für Geschichte der Medizin* 26 (1933), pp. 1–29.

Jesse, Horst, *Die Geschichte der Evangelischen Kirche in Augsburg* (Pfaffenhofen, 1983).

Jetter, Dieter, 'Gemeinschaft und Absonderung der Kranken als antagonistische Faktoren historischer Hospitäler 1500–1900', *Medizinhistorisches Journal* 5 (1969), pp. 121–38.

—, *Geschichte des Hospitals* (Wiesbaden, 1966).

Jillings, Lewis, 'The Aggression of a Cured Syphilitic: Ulrich von Hutten Projection of His Disease as a Metaphor', *The German Quarterly* 68 (1995), pp. 1–18.

Johns, Adrian, *The Nature of the Book: Print and Knowledge in the Making* (Chicago, 1998).

Jones, Colin, 'The Construction of the Hospital Patient in Early Modern France', in Norbert Finzsch, and Robert Jütte (eds), *Institutions of Confinement: Hospitals, Asylums, and Prisons in Western Europe and North America, 1500–1950* (Cambridge, 1996), pp. 55–74.

—, and Barry, Jonathan (eds), *Medicine and Charity Before the Welfare State* (London and New York, 1991).

—, and Porter, Roy (eds), *Reassessing Foucault: Power, Medicine, and the Body* (London, 1994).

—, 'Plague and Its Metaphors in Early Modern France', *Representation* 53 (1996), pp. 97–127.

Jütte, Robert, 'Aging and Body Image in the 16th Century: Hermann Weinsberg's (1518–1597) Perception of the Aging Body', *European History Quarterly* 18 (1988), pp. 259–90.

—, Ärzte, *Heiler und Patienten. Medizinischer Alltag in der frühen Neuzeit* (Munich and Zurich, 1991).

—, 'Der anstößige Körper. Anmerkungen zu einer Semiotik der Nacktheit', in Klaus Schreiner and Norbert Schnitzler (eds), *Gepeinigt, begehrt, vergessen. Symbolik und Sozialbezug des Körpers im späten Mittelalter und der frühen Neuzeit* (Munich, 1992), pp. 109–130.

—, 'Bader, Barbiere und Hebammen. Heilkundige als Randgruppe?', in Bernd-Ulrich Hergemöller (ed.), *Randgruppen der spätmittelalterlichen Gesellschaft. Ein Hand- und Studienbuch* (Warendorf, 1995).

—, '"Disziplin zu predigen ist eine Sache, sich ihr zu unterwerfen eine andere" (Cervantes). Prolegomena zu einer Sozialgeschichte der Armenfürsorge diesseits und jenseits des Fortschritts', *Geschichte und Gesellschaft* 17 (1991), pp. 91–110.

—, 'Entdeckungen des "Inneren Menschen", 1500–1800', in Richard von Dülmen (ed.), *Erfindung des Menschen. Schöpfungsträume und Körperbilder 1500–2000* (Weimar, 1998), pp. 241–58.

—, '"Es will erlitten seyn...". Pein und Weh im kulturellen Wandel', *Bild der Wissenschaft* 10 (1993), pp. 67–9.

—, 'Funktion und Zeichen. Zur Semiotik herrschaftlicher Kommunikation in der Stadtgesellschaft', *Anzeiger des Germanischen Nationalmuseums* (1993), pp. 13–21.

—, *Die Geschichte der Sinne. Von der Antike bis zum Cyberspace* (Munich, 2000).

—, 'Gesundheit, Krankheit und medikale Kultur in historischer Perspektive', *Religion und medizinische Ethik* (Ulm, 1993), pp. 72–90.

—, 'Krankheit bei Hofe: Zwischen Aderlaß und Holzkur', *DAMALS* 31 (1999), pp. 36–42.

——, '"La douleur des dents est la plus grande". Zur Geschichte des Zahnschmerzes in der Frühen Neuzeit', *Medizin, Gesellschaft und Geschichte* 15, pp. 37–54.

——, 'Lepra-Simulanten "De iis qui morbum stimulant"', in Martin Dinges and Thomas Schlich (eds), *Neue Wege in der Seuchengeschichte* (= *Medizin, Gesellschaft und Geschichte* 6), (Stuttgart, 1995), pp. 25–42.

——, 'Die medizinische Versorgung der Stadtbevölkerung im 16. und 17. Jahrhundert am Beispiel der Reichsstadt Köln', *Medizinhistorisches Journal* 22 (1987), pp. 173–84.

——, 'Norm und Praxis in der medikalen Kultur des Mittelalters und der Frühen Neuzeit am Beispiel des Aderlasses', in Gerhard Jaritz (ed.), *Norm und Praxis im Alltag des Mittelalters und der Frühen Neuzeit. Internationales Round-Table-Gespräch. Krems an der Donau 7. Oktober 1996* (Vienna, 1997), pp. 95–106.

——, *Obrigkeitliche Armenfürsorge in deutschen Reichsstädten der frühen Neuzeit. Städtisches Armenwesen in Frankfurt a. M. und Köln* (Cologne and Vienna, 1984).

——, *Patient und Heiler in der vorindustriellen Gesellschaft. Krankheit – und Gesundheitsverhalten im frühneuzeitlichen Köln* (habilitation Bielefeld, 1989).

——, 'Seuchen – Eine Strafe Gottes?', *DAMALS* 25 (1993), pp. 26–7.

——, 'Seuchen im Spiegel der Geschichte', S*pektrum der Wissenschaft*, Dossier. Seuchen 3 (1997), pp. 6–13.

——, 'A Seventeenth-Century German Barber-Surgeon and His Patients', *Medical History* 33 (1989), pp. 184–98.

——, 'The Social Construction of Illness in the Early Modern Period', in Jens Lachmund und Gunnar Stollberg (eds), *The Social Construction of Illness. Illness and Medical Knowledge in Past und Present* (Stuttgart, 1992), pp. 23–8.

——, 'Sozialgeschichte der Medizin. Inhalte – Methoden – Ziele', *Medizin, Gesellschaft und Geschichte* 9 (1990), pp. 149–63.

——, 'Zur Sozialgeschichte der Handwerkschirurgen im 16. Jahrhundert', in Heinz Dopsch und Peter F. Kramm (eds), *Paracelsus und Salzburg* (Salzburg, 1994), pp. 45–60.

——, 'Syphilis and Confinement: Early Modern German Hospitals for Syphilitics', in Norbert Finzsch and Robert Jütte (eds), *Institutions of Confinement: Hospitals, Asylums, and Prisons in Western Europe and North America, 1500–1950* (Cambridge, 1996), pp. 97–116.

——, '"Wo kein Weib ist, da seufzet der Kranke" – Familie und Krankheit im 16. Jahrhundert', *Jahrbuch des Instituts für Geschichte der Medizin der Robert Bosch Stiftung* 7 (1989), pp. 7–24.

Kaiser, Ernst, 'Paracelsus', *Selbstzeugnissen und Bilddokumenten* (Hamburg, 1969).

Kannengiesser, C., '"Job" (le livre de)', in *Dictionnaire de spiritualité ascétique et mystique: doctrine et histoire* (Paris 1974) vol. 8, pp. 1201–25.

Karant-Nunn, S. C., 'Continuity and Change: Some Effects of the Reformation of Zwickau', *Sixteenth Century Journal* 12 (1982), pp. 17–42.

Karg, Franz, 'Emersacker im 17. Jahrhundert. Zur Erwerbung durch die Fuggerschen Stiftungen', *Jahrbuch des Historischen Vereins Dillingen* 93 (1991), pp. 391–403.

—, 'Die Fugger im 16. und 17. Jahrhundert', in Renate Eikelmann (ed.), *'Lautenschlagen lernen und lieben'. Die Fugger und die Musik. Anton Fugger zum 500. Geburtstag* (Augsburg, 1994), pp. 99–110.

Keil, Gundolf, 'Aussatz', *Lexikon des Mittelalters* (Munich and Zurich, 1980) vol. 1, pp. 1249–57.

—, 'Der Aussatz im Mittelalter', in Jörn Henning Wolf (ed.), *Aussatz, Lepra, Hansen-Krankheiten: ein Menschheitsproblem im Wandel, Teil II* (Munich, 1986), pp. 85–102.

—, *Der Hausvater als Arzt* (Sigmaringen, 1991).

—, 'Paracelsus und die neuen Krankheiten', in Volker Zimmermann (ed.), *Paracelsus. Das Werk – die Rezeption* (Stuttgart, 1995), pp. 17–45.

—, 'Seuchenzüge des Mittelalters', in Bernd Herrmann (ed.), *Mensch und Umwelt im Mittelalter* (Stuttgart, 1986), pp. 109–28.

—, 'Sudhoffs Sicht vom deutschen Mittelalter', *Nachrichtenblatt der Deutschen Gesellschaft der Medizin, Naturwissenschaften und Technik e.V. 31* (1981), pp. 94–129.

—, 'Virtus occulta. Der Begriff des "empiricum" bei Nicolaus von Polen', in August Buck (ed.), *Die okkulten Wissenschaften in der Renaissance* (Wiesbaden, 1992), pp. 159–96.

—, and Daems, Willem, 'F. Paracelsus und die "Franzosen". Betrachtungen zur Venerologie Hohenheims, I: Pathologie und nosologisches Konzept', *Nova Acta Paracelsica* 9 (1977), pp. 99–151.

Kellenbenz, Hermann, *Die Fugger in Spanien und Portugal. Ein Großunternehmen des 16. Jahrhunderts* (2 vols, Augsburg, 1990).

—, *Die Fugger in Spanien und Portugal: Dokumente* (Augsburg, 1990).

—, *Die Fuggersche Maestrazgopacht (1525–1542). Zur Geschichte der spanischen Ritterorden im 16. Jahrhundert* (Tübingen, 1967).

—, *'Fuggersche Sozialpolitik', Staatliche, städtische, betriebliche und kirchliche Sozialpolitik vom Mittelalter bis zu Gegenwart* (Stuttgart, 1992), pp. 65–88.

—, 'Die sozialgeschichtliche Bedeutung der Fuggerei', *Schwäbische Blätter* 22 (1971), pp. 105–17.

—, 'Wirtschaftsleben der Blütezeit (Augsburg)', in Gunther Gottlieb et al. (eds), *Geschichte der Stadt Augsburg von der Römerzeit bis zur Gegenwart* (Stuttgart, 1984), pp. 258–301.

— and Preysing, Maria von (eds), 'Jakob Fuggers Stiftungsbrief von 1521', *Zeitschrift des historischen Vereins für Schwaben* 68 (1974), pp. 95–116.

Kellner, Martin, '"In allen Instrumenten liegt Nahrung für die Seele". Zur Bedeutung von Musik in der europäischen und arabischen Humoralmedizin', *Curare* 20 (1997), pp. 43–8.

Keussen, Hermann, 'Beiträge zur Geschichte der Kölner Lepra-Untersuchungen', *Lepra Bibliotheca Internationalis* 14 (1913), pp. 80–112.

Kießling, Rolf, *Bürgerliche Gesellschaft und Kirche in Augsburg im Spätmittelalter. Ein Beitrag zur Strukturanalyse der oberdeutschen Reichsstadt* (Augsburg, 1971).

King, Lester S., 'What is a Disease?' in Arthur Caplan et al. (eds), *Concepts of Health and Disease: Interdisciplinary Perspective* (Reading, MA, 1981), pp. 107–18.

Kinzelbach, Annemarie, '"Böse Blatter" oder "Franzosenkrankheit": Syphiliskonzept, Kranke und die Genese des Krankenhauses in oberdeutschen Reichsstädten in der frühen Neuzeit', in Martin Dinges and Thomas Schlich (eds), *Neue Wege in der Seuchengeschichte* (Stuttgart, 1995), pp. 43–69.

—, *Gesundbleiben, Krankwerden, Armsein in der frühneuzeitlichen Gesellschaft. Gesunde und Kranke in den Reichsstädten Überlingen und Ulm, 1500–1700* (Stuttgart, 1995).

—, 'Heilkundige und Gesellschaft in der frühneuzeitlichen Reichsstadt Überlingen', *Medizin, Gesellschaft und Geschichte* 8 (1989), pp. 119–49.

Kirchgässner, Bernhard and Reuter, Fritz (eds), *Städtische Randgruppen und Minderheiten* (Sigmaringen, 1986).

Klibansky, Raymond, Panofsky, Erwin and Saxl, Fritz, *Saturn and Melancholy: Studies in the History of Natural Philosophy, Religion and Art* (London, 1964).

Knefelkamp, Ulrich, *Das Gesundheits- und Fürsorgewesen der Stadt Freiburg im Breisgau im Mittelalter* (Freiburg, 1981).

—, *Das Heilig-Geist-Spital in Nürnberg vom 14.–17. Jahrhundert. Geschichte, Struktur, Alltag* (Nuremburg, 1989).

Koutná-Karg, Dana, 'Die Ehre der Fugger', in Johannes Burckhard (ed.), *Augsburger Handelshäuser im Wandel des historischen Urteils* (Berlin, 1996), pp. 87–106.

Kraus, Jürgen, *Das Militärwesen der Reichsstadt Augsburg 1548–1806. Vergleichende Untersuchungen über städtische Militäreinrichtungen in Deutschland vom 16.–18. Jahrhundert* (Augsburg, 1980).

Kreutz, Wilhelm, *Die Deutschen und Ulrich von Hutten. Rezeption von Autor und Werk seit dem 16. Jahrhundert* (Munich, 1984).

Kriedte, Peter, *Spätfeudalismus und Handelskapital. Grundlinien der europäischen Wirtschaftsgeschichte vom 16. bis zum Ausgang des 18. Jahrhunderts* (Göttingen, 1980).

Kroll, Jerome and Bachrach, Bernard, 'Sin and the Etiology of Disease in Pre-Crusade Europe', *Journal of the History of Medicine and Allied Sciences* 41 (1986), pp. 395–414.

Kümmel, Werner Friedrich, *Medizin und Musik* (Munich, 1977).

—, 'Der Puls und das Problem der Zeitmessung in der Geschichte der Medizin', *Medizinhistorisches Journal* 9 (1974), pp. 1–22.

Künast, Hans-Jörg, *"Gedruckt in Augsburg". Buchdruck und Buchhandel in Augsburg zwischen 1468 und 1555* (Tübingen, 1997).

Kunzel-Runtscheiner, Monica, *Töchter der Venus. Die Kurtisanen Roms im 16. Jahrhundert* (Munich, 1995).
Kuriyama, Shigehisa, 'Interpreting the History of Bloodletting', *Journal of the History of Medicine* 50 (1995), pp. 11–46.
—, *The Expressiveness of the Body and the Divergence of Greek and Chinese Medicine* (New York, 1999).
Kusukawa, Sachiko, 'Aspectio divinorum operum. Melanchthon and Astrology for Lutheran Medics', in Ole Peter Grell and Andrew Cunningham (eds), *Medicine and the Reformation* (London and New York, 1993), pp. 33–56.
—, *The Transformation of Natural Philosophy: The Case of Philipp Melanchton* (Cambridge, 1995).
Labisch, Alfons, *Homo Hygienicus. Gesundheit und Medizin in der Neuzeit* (Frankfurt, 1991).
—, 'The Social Construction of Health: From Early Modern Times to the Beginning of Industrialization', in Jens Lachmund and Gunnar Stollberg (eds), *The Social Construction of Illness: Illness and Medical Knowledge in Past and Present* (= *Medizin, Gesellschaft und Geschichte*, 1) (Stuttgart, 1992), pp. 85–104.
—, 'Zur Sozialgeschichte der Medizin. Methodologische Überlegungen und Forschungsbericht', *Archiv für Sozialgeschichte* 20 (1980), pp. 431–69.
—, and Spree, Reinhard, 'Neuere Entwicklungen und aktuelle Trends in der Sozialgeschichte der Medizin in Deutschland – Rückschau und Ausblick', *Vierteljahrschrift für Sozialund Wirtschaftsgeschichte* 84 (1997), pp. 171–210; S. 305–21.
—, 'Neuere Ergebnisse und Entwicklungen einer Sozialgeschichte der Medizin und des Gesundheitswesens in Deutschland im 19. und 20. Jahrhundert. Bericht über eine internationale Arbeitstagung im Zentrum für interdiziplinäre Forschung der Universität Bielefeld, 25. bis 28. 2. 1982', *Berichte zur Wissenschaftsgeschichte* 5 (1996), pp. 13–28.
Lambacher, Hannes, *Das Spital der Reichsstadt Memmingen* (Memmingen, 1991).
Lammel, Hans-Uwe, *Klio and Hippocrates: Eine Liason littéraire des 18. Jahrhunderts und die Folgen für die Wissenschaftskultur bis 1850 in Deutschland* (Stuttgart, 2006).
Lange, L., 'Woman is not a Rational Animal: On Aristotle's Biology of Reproduction', in S. Harding und M. Hintikka (eds), *Discovering Reality* (Dortrecht, 1983).
Laqueur, Thomas, *Making Sex: Body and Gender from the Greeks to Freud* (Cambridge, MA, 1992).
Latour, Bruno, 'Haben auch Objekte eine Geschichte? Ein Zusammentreffen von Pasteur und Whitehead in einem Milchsäurebad', in Michael Hagner (ed.), *Ansichten der Wissenschaftsgeschichte* (Frankfurt a. M., 2001), pp. 272–97.
—, 'On the Partical Existence of Existing and Non-Existing Objects', in Lorraine Daston (ed.), *Biographies of Scientific Objects* (Chicago, 2000), pp. 247–69.

Lederer, David, 'The Dishonorable Dead: Perception of Suicide in Early Modern Germany', in Sibylle Backmann et al. (eds), *Ehrkonzepte in der frühen Neuzeit. Identitäten und Ausgrenzungen* (Berlin, 1998), pp. 349–65.

—, *Madness, Religion and the State in Early Modern Europe* (Cambridge, 2006).

Lehnhardt, Friedrich, 'Blutschau. Untersuchungen zur Entwicklung der Hämatoskopie' (dissertation, Hannover, 1986).

Lengle, Peter, 'Heilig-Geist-Spital', in Wolfgang Baer et al. (eds), *Augsburger Stadtlexikon* (Augsburg, 1985), pp. 156.

—, 'Spitäler, Stiftungen und Bruderschaften', in Gunther Gottlieb et al. (eds), *Geschichte der Stadt Augsburg von der Römerzeit bis zur Gegenwart* (Stuttgart, 1984), pp. 202–8.

Lenk, Leonhard, *Augsburger Bürgertum im Späthumanismus und Frühbarock (1580–1700)* (Augsburg, 1968).

Lerner, Michel-Pierre and Verdet, Jean-Pierre, 'Copernicus', in Norriss Hetherington (ed.), *Cosmology: Historical, Literary, Philosophical, Religious, and Scientific Perspectives* (New York, 1993), pp. 147–73.

Lesky, Erna, 'Die Arbeiter und das Quecksilber', *Ciba-Zeitschrift* 8 (1959), pp. 3191–3200.

—, 'Quecksilber und Quecksilberverbindungen im Wandel der Zeit', *Ciba-Zeitschrift* 8 (1959), pp. 3202–8.

—, 'Von Schmier- und Räucherkuren zur modernen Syphilistherapie', *Ciba-Zeitschrift* 8 (1959), pp. 3174–89.

—, *Die Wiener medizinische Schule im 19. Jahrhundert* (Graz, 1965).

Leven, Karl-Heinz, *Die Geschichte der Infektionskrankheiten. Von der Antike bis ins 20. Jahrhundert* (Landsberg, 1997).

—, 'Krankheiten – historische Deutung versus retrospektive Diagnose', in Norbert Paul and Thomas Schlich (eds), *Medizingeschichte: Aufgaben, Probleme, Perspektiven* (Frankfurt and New York, 1998), pp. 153–85.

—, 'Zur Problematik moderner Deutungsversuche historischer Krankheitsfälle', in F. Hofmann (ed.), *Infektiologie, Diagnostik, Therapie, Prophylaxe. Handbuch und Atlas für Klinik und Praxis* (Landsberg, 1991).

—, 'Syfilis in de twintigste weersiegeld in de wassen beelden', *Geschiedenis der Geneskunde* 2 (1995) 5, pp. 260–65.

Lieb, Norbert, *Die Fugger und die Kunst im Zeitalter der hohen Renaissance* (Munich, 1958).

Lieburg, Maries J. van, 'De syfilitische patiënt in de geschiedenis van het Nederlandse ziekenhuiswezen vóór 1900', *Tjdschrift voor Soziale Geschiedenis* 8 (1982), pp. 156–79.

Liermann, Hans, 'Zur Rechtsgeschichte der Fuggerschen Stiftungen', *Zeitschrift für bayerische Landesgeschichte* 19 (1955), pp. 395–407.

Lindberg, Carter, 'The Lutheran Tradition', in Ronald L. Numbers, and Darrel W. Amundsen (eds), *Health and Medicine in Western Religious Traditions* (New York, 1986), pp. 173–203.

Lindberg, David C., *The Beginnings of Western Science: The European Scientific Tradition in Philosophical Religious, and Institutional Context, 600 B. C. to A. D. 1450* (Chicago, 1992).

—— and Numbers, Ronald L. (eds), *God and Nature: Historical Essays on the Encounter between Christianity and Science* (Berkeley, 1984).

Lindemann, Jean, 'Siegel, Schaudinn, Fleck and the Etiology of Syphilis', *Studies of History and Philosophy of Biological and Biomedical Sciences* 32 (2001), pp. 435–55.

Lindemann, Mary, *Health and Healing in Eighteenth-Century Germany* (Baltimore, 1996).

——, *Medicine and Society in Early Modern Europe* (Cambridge, 1999).

Lint, E. J. G., 'Eine der ersten Guajakschriften', *Janus* 36 (1932), pp. 384–91; p. 37; (1933), pp. 320–22.

Lömker-Schlögell, Annette, 'Prostituierte "umb vermeydung willen merers übels in der cristenhait"', in Bernd Ulrich Hergemöller (ed.), *Randgruppen der spätmittelalterlichen Gesellschaft. Ein Hand- und Studienbuch* (Warendorf, 1990), pp. 52–84.

Loetz, Francisca, *Vom Kranken zum Patienten. 'Medikalisierung' und medizinische Vergesellschaftung am Beispiel Badens 1750–1850* (Stuttgart, 1993).

Löwy, Ilana, 'Ludwik Fleck on the Social Construction of Medical Knowledge', *Sociology of Health and Illness* 19 (1988), pp. 133–55.

——, 'Testing for a Sexually Transmitted Disease 1907–1970: The History of the Wassermann Reaction', in Virginia Berridge and Philipp Strong (eds), *AIDS and Contemporary History* (Cambridge, 1993), pp. 74–92.

López Terrada, María Luz, 'El mal de siment en la Valencia del siglo XVI: Imágenes del morbo gallico en una ciudad mediterránea europea', *Dynamis* 11 (1991), pp. 119–46.

——, 'El Tratamiento de la sifilis en un hospital renacentista: La sala del mal de siment del hospital general de Valencia', *Asclepio* 41 (1989), pp. 19–50.

Lorenz, Maren, *Leibhaftige Vergangenheit. Einführung in die Körpergeschichte* (Tübingen, 2000).

MacDonald, Michael, *Mystical Bedlam: Madness, Anxiety, and Healing in Seventeenth-Century England* (Cambridge, 1981).

Maclean, Ian, *Logic, Signs and Nature in the Renaissance: The Case of Learned Medicine* (Cambridge, 2002).

——, *The Renaissance Notion of Women: A Study in the Fortunes of Scholasticism and Medical Science in European Intellectual Life* (Cambridge, 1980).

Malamani, Anita, 'Notizie sul mal franscese e gli ospedale degli incurabilie in età moderna', *Critica Storica* 15 (1978), pp. 193–216.

Mandrou, Robert, *Die Fugger als Grundbesitzer in Schwaben, 1560–1618* (Göttingen, 1997).

Martin, Alfred, *Deutsches Badewesen in vergangenen Tagen* (Jena, 1906).

——, 'The Patrons of Syphilis and the Pilgrimage of Syphilitics', *Urologic and Cutaneous Review* 27 (1923), pp. 69–75.

Martz, Elisabeth, 'Gesundheitswesen und Ärzte in Augsburg im 16. Jahrhundert' (dissertation, Munich, 1950).

Maschke, Erich, 'Die Unterschichten der mittelalterlichen Städte Deutschlands', in Erich Maschke, and J. Sydow (eds), *Gesellschaftliche Unterschichten in den südwestdeutschen Städten* (Stuttgart, 1967).

Mauer, Benedikt, *'Gemein Geschrey' und 'teglich Reden'. Georg Kölderer – ein Augsburger Chronist des konfessionellen Zeitalters* (Augsburg, 2001).

Meadow, Mark A., 'Merchants and Marvels: Hans Jacob Fugger and the Origins of the Wunderkammer', in Pamela Smith, and Paula Findelen (eds), *Merchants & Marvels: Commerce, Science, and Art in Early Modern Europe* (London, 2002), pp. 182–200.

McVaugh, Michael, *Medicine Before the Plague: Practitioners and Their Patients in the Crown of Aragon, 1285–1345* (Cambridge, 1993).

—, 'Quantified Medical Theory and Practice at Fourteenth-Century Montpellier', *Bulletin of the History of Medicine* 43 (1969), pp. 397–413.

—, 'Theriac at Montpellier, 1285–1325', *Sudhoffs Archiv* 56 (1972), pp. 113–43.

Mehl, Jürgen, *Aussatz in Rottweil. Das Leprosenhaus Allerheiligen der Siechen im Feld (1298–1810)* (Rottweil, 1993).

Mertens, Klaus, 'Die Landschlösser der Familie Fugger im 16. Jahrhundert', *Welt im Umbruch. Augsburg zwischen Renaissance und Barock.* Austellungskatalog (3 vols, Augsburg, 1981).

Merzenbacher, Friedrich, *Das Juliusspital in Würzburg vol. 2: Rechts- und Vermögensgeschichte* (Würzburg, 1976).

Meyer, Christian, *Chronik der Familie Fugger 1599* (Munich, 1902).

Meyer-Ahrens, *Geschichtliche Notizen über das erste Auftreten der Lustseuche in der Schweiz* (Zurich, 1841).

Midelfort, Erik H. C., 'Sin, Melancholy, Obsession: Insanity and Culture in Sixteenth-Century Germany', in Steven L. Kaplan (ed.), *Understanding Popular Culture: Europe from the Middle Ages to the Nineteenth Century* (Berlin, 1984), pp. 113–45.

—, *A History of Madness in Sixteenth-Century Germany* (Stanford, 1999).

Mikkeli, Heikki, *Hygiene in the Early Modern Medical Tradition* (Helsinki, 1999).

Mischlewski, Adalbert, 'Alltag im Spital zu Beginn des 16. Jahrhunderts', in Alfred Kohler and Heinrich Lutz (eds), *Alltag im 16. Jahrhundert. Studien zu Lebensformen in mitteleuropäischen Städten* (Wien, 1987), pp. 152–73.

Moeller, Bernd, 'Stadt und Buch. Bemerkungen zur Struktur der reformatorischen Bewegung in Deutschland', *Stadtbürgertum und Adel in der Reformation. Studien zur Sozialgeschichte der Reformation in England und Deutschland* (Stuttgart, 1979).

—, *Stadt und Kirche im 16. Jahrhundert* (Gütersloh, 1978).

Mörke, Olaf, 'Die Fugger im 16. Jahrhundert: Städtische Elite oder Sonderstruktur?', *Archiv für Refomationsgeschichte* 174 (1983), pp. 141–62.

Moll, Albert, *Doktor Alexander Seitz aus Marbach und seine Schrift über die Lustseuche vom Jahre 1509* (Stuttgart, 1825).

Moran, Bruce T., 'Paracelsus und seine internationale Rezeption in der frühen Neuzeit: Beitrage zur Geschichte des Paracelsismus', *Bulletin of the History of Medicine* 75 (2001), pp. 125–7.

Moreno Rodriguez, Rosa Maria and García-Ballester, Luis, 'El dolor en la teoria y la practica medicas de Galeno', *Dynamis* 2 (1982), pp. 3–24.

Morris, David B., *The Culture of Pain* (Berkeley, 1991).

Morton, R. S., 'Another Look at the Morbus Gallicus', *British Journal of Venereal Disease* 44 (1968), pp. 174–7.

—–, 'Some Aspects of the Early History of Syphilis in Scotland', *British Journal of Venereal Diseases* 38 (1962), pp. 175–80.

Moulin, Anne-Marie, 'L'ancien et le nouveaeu. La réponse médicale à l'épidemie de 1493', in Neithard Bulst and Robert Delort (eds), *Maladies et société (XIIe–XVIIIe siècle). Actes du colloque de Bielefeld, novembre 1986* (Paris, 1989), pp. 121–31.

Mummenhoff, Ernst, *Die öffentliche Gesundheits- und Krankenpflege im alten Nürnberg* [1889] (reprint Neustadt, 1986).

—–, *Zur Geschichte der Seuchenhäuser. Festschrift für die 65. Versammlung der Naturforscher und Ärzte 1892* (Nuremburg, 1892).

Müller, Ingo Wilhelm, *Humoralmedizin. Physiologische, pathologische und therapeutische Grundlagen der galenistischen Heilkunst* (Heidelberg, 1993).

Müller-Jahncke, Wolf-Dieter, *Astrologische-magische Theorie und Praxis in der Heilkunde der Frühen Neuzeit* (Stuttgart, 1985), pp. 193–207.

—–, 'Die Krankheit aus dem Gestirn. Syphilis und Astrologie', *Ulrich von Hutten (1488–1988). Akten des internationalen Ulrich-von-Hutten Symposions 15.–17. Juli in Schlüchtern* (Munich, 1989), pp. 117–27.

Munger, Robert S., 'Guaiacum, the Holy Wood from the New World', *Journal of the History of Medicine* 4 (1949), pp. 196–229.

Muschel, Heinz, *Das Spital der Reichen Siechen zu St. Katharina in Ulm. Eine rechtsgeschichtliche Untersuchung zur Interpretation von Wohlfahrtseinrichtungen durch die Reichsstadt im ausgehenden Mittelalter* (Ulm, 1965).

Nance, Brian, *Turquet de Mayerne as Baroque Physician: The Art of Medical Portraiture* (Amsterdam and New York, 2001).

Nauck, Ernst Theodor, 'Dr. Sigmund Grimm – Arzt und Buchdrucker zu Augsburg', *Zeitschrift des Historischen Vereins für Schwaben und Neuburg* 60 (1969), pp. 311–39.

Nelkin, Dorothy and Gilman, Sander, 'Placing Blame for Devastating Disease', *Social Research* 55 (1988) 3, pp. 361–7.

Neuburger, Max, 'An Historical Study of the Concept of Nature from a Medical Viewpoint', *Isis* 35 (1944), pp. 16–22.

Nicolson, Malcolm, 'The Metastatic Theory of Pathogenesis and the Professional Interests of the Eighteenth-Century Physician', *Medical History* 32 (1988), pp. 277–300.

Niebyl, Peter H., 'The Non-Naturals', *Bulletin for the History of Medicine* 45 (1971), pp. 486–92.

North, John D., 'Medieval Concepts of Celestial Influence: A Survey', in Patrick Curry (ed.), *Astrology, Science and Society: Historical Essays* (Woodbridge, 1987), pp. 5–17.

Nübel, Otto, 'Das Geschlecht Occo', *Lebensbilder aus dem Bayerischen Schwaben*, 10 (1973), pp. 77–113.

Numbers, Ronald L. and Amundsen, Darrel W. (eds), *Caring and Curing: Health and Medicine in the Western Religious Traditions* (New York and London, 1986).

—— (ed.), *Medicine in the New World: New Spain, New France, and New England* (Knoxville, 1987).

Nutton, Vivian, 'Beyond the Hippocratic Oath', in Andrew Wear, Johanna Geyer-Kordesch and Roger K. French (eds), *Doctors and Ethics: The Earlier Historical Setting of Professional Ethics* (Amsterdam, 1993), pp. 10–37.

——, 'Humoralism', in William F. Bynum and Roy Porter (eds), *Companion Encyclopedia of the History of Medicine*, vol. 1 (London, 1993), pp. 281–91.

——, 'Greek Science in the Sixteenth-Century Renaissance', in J. V. Field and A. J. L. James (eds), *Renaissance and Revolution: Humanists, Scholars, Craftsmen and Natural Philosphers in Early Modern Europe* (Cambridge, 1993), pp. 15–28.

——, 'Perception of Fracastoro's Theory of Contagion: The Seeds that Fell Among Thorns?', *Osiris* 6 (1990), pp. 196–234.

Öhlschlegel, Rudolf Christian Ludwig, 'Studien zu Lorenz Fries und seinem "Spiegel der Arznei"' (dissertation, Tübingen, 1985).

Oexle, Otto Gerhard, 'Armut, Armutsbegriff und Armenfürsorge im Mittelalter', in Christoph Sachße and Florian Tennstedt (eds), *Soziale Sicherheit und soziale Disziplinierung. Beiträge zu einer historischen Theorie der Sozialpolitik* (Frankfurt, 1986), pp. 73–100.

Oriel, J. David, *The Scars of Venus: A History of Venereology* (London and Berlin, 1994).

Osler, Margaret J., 'Mixing Metaphors: Science and Religion or Natural Philosophy and Theology in Early Modern Europe', *History of Science* 36 (1998), pp. 91–113.

Ottosson, Per-Gunnar, *Scholastic Medicine and Philosophy: A Study of Commentaries on Galen's Tegni (ca. 1300–1450)* (Naples, 1984).

O'Shea, J. G., '"Two Minutes with Venus, Two Years With Mercury" – Mercury as an Anti-Syphilitic Chemotherapeutic Agent', *Journal of the Royal Society of Medicine* 83 (1990), pp. 392–5.

Ozment, Steven, *The Age of Reform, 1250–1550: An Intellectual and Religious History of Late Medieval and Reformation Europe* (New Haven, 1980).

Pagel, Walter, *Paracelsus: An Introduction to Philosophical Medicine in the Era of the Renaissance*, 2nd edn (Basel and New York, 1982).

—, *Das medizinische Weltbild des Paracelsus. Seine Zusammenhänge mit Neuplatonismus und Gnosis* (Wiesbaden, 1962).

Palmer, Richard, 'The Church, Leprosy and Plague in Medieval and Early Modern Europe', in W. J. Sheils (ed.), *The Church and Healing* (Oxford, 1982), pp. 79–100.

Panhorst, Karl Heinz, *Deutschland und Amerika. Ein Rückblick auf das Zeitalter der Entdeckungen und die ersten deutsch-amerikanischen Verbindungen unter besonderer Beachtung der Fugger und Welser* (Munich, 1928).

Park, Katharine, *Doctors and Medicine in Early Renaissance Florence* (Princeton, 1985).

—, 'Healing the Poor: Hospitals and Medical Assistance in Renaissance Florence', in Jonathan Barry and Colin Jones (eds), *Medicine and Charity Before the Welfare State* (London and New York, 1991), pp. 26–37.

—, 'Medicine and Society in Medieval Europe, 500–1500', in Andrew Wear (ed.), *Medicine in Society* (Cambridge, 1992), pp. 59–90.

—, *Secrets of Women: Gender, Generation, and the Origin of Human Dissection* (Cambridge, MA, 2006).

Paschkis, Heinrich, 'Über Quecksilber-Räucherungen', *Vierteljahresschrift für Dermatologie und Syphilis* (1878), pp. 415–32.

Pawletz, Alois, 'Lepradiagnostik im Mittelalter und Anweisungen zur Lepraschau' (dissertation, Leipzig, 1915).

Pelling, Margret, 'Appearance and Reality: Barber-Surgeons, the Body and Disease', in A. L. Beier und R. Finlay (eds), *London 1500–1700: The Making of Metropolis*, (London, 1986) pp. 82–112.

—, 'Contagion/Germ Theory/Specificity', in William F. Bynum and Roy Porter (eds), *Companion Encyclopedia of the History of Medicine* (London, 1993), vol. 1, pp. 309–34.

—, 'Healing the Sick Poor: Social Policy and Disability in Norwich 1550–1640', *Medical History* 29 (1985), pp. 115–37.

—, 'Medical Practitioners', in Charles Webster (ed.), *Health, Medicine and Morality in the Sixteenth Century* (Cambridge, 1979), pp. 165–235.

—, 'Occupational Diversity: Barber-Surgeons and the Trades of Northwich 1550–1640', *Bulletin of the History of Medicine* 56 (1982), pp. 484–511.

— and Smith, Richard M. (eds), *Life, Death, and the Elderly: Historical Perspectives* (London and New York, 1992).

Peschke, Michael, *Ulrich von Hutten (1488–1523) als Kranker und als medizinischer Schriftsteller* (Cologne, 1985).

—, 'Ulrich von Hutten und die Syphilis', *Ulrich von Hutten. Ritter, Humanist, Publizist, 1488–1523. Katalog zur Ausstellung des Landes Hessen anläßlich des 500. Geburtstages* (Kassel, 1988), pp. 309–19.

Pfleger, Luzian, 'Das Auftreten der Syphilis in Straßburg, Geiler von Kaysersberg und der Kult des hl. Fiakrius', *Zeitschrift für Geschichte des Oberrheins* 72 (1918), pp. 153–73.

Pflummern, Joachim, 'Das Biberacher Spital vor der Reformation', *Heimatkundliche Blätter für den Kreis Biberach* 12 (1989) pp. 22–7.

Pölnitz, Götz von, *Anton Fugger* (4 vols, Tübingen, 1957/71).

—, *Die Fugger*, 2nd edn (Tübingen 1970).

—, 'Die Fuggerschen Stiftungen', in *Lebensbilder deutscher Stiftungen* vol. 2 (Tübingen, 1971), pp. 3–21.

—, *Jakob Fugger. Kaiser, Kirche und Kapital in der oberdeutschen Renaissance* (2 vols, Tübingen, 1949/1951).

— and Kellenbenz, Hermann, *Anton Fugger* (Tübingen, 1986).

Porter, Dorothy and Porter, Roy, *Patient's Progress: Doctors and Doctoring in Eighteenth-Century England* (Cambridge, 1989).

Porter, Roy, *The Greatest Benefit to Mankind: A Medical History of Humanity* (New York and London, 1997).

—, 'The Patient's View: Doing Medical History from Below', *Theory and Society* 14 (1985), pp. 175–98.

— (ed.), *Patients and Practitioners: Lay Perceptions of Medicine in Pre-Industrial Society* (Cambridge, 1985).

—, 'What is Disease?', in Roy Porter (ed.), *The Cambridge Illustrated History of Medicine* (Cambridge, 1996), pp. 82–117.

Pomata, Gianna, *Contracting a Cure: Patients, Healers, and the Law in Early Modern Bologna* (Baltimore and London, 1998).

Pomian, Krystof, 'Astrology as a Naturalistic Theology of History', in Paola Zambelli (ed.), *'Astrologi hallucinati': Stars and the End of the World in Luther's Time* (Berlin and New York, 1986), pp. 29–43.

Pouchelle, Marie-Christine, *The Body and Surgery in the Middle Ages* (New Brunswick, 1990).

Preysing, Maria von and Simnach, Georg (eds), *Die Fugger Testamente des 16. Jahrhunderts* (Weißenhorn, 1992), pp. 158–65.

Probst, Christian, 'Das Hospitalwesen im hohen und späten Mittelalter', *Sudhoffs Archiv* 50 (1966), pp. 246–58.

Proksch, Johann Karl, *Die Antimercurialisten des XV. und XVI. Jahrhunderts* (Wien, 1880).

—, 'Ein Beitrag zu den Sammelwerken der ältesten Schriften über Syphilis', *Medicinisch-chirurgisches Central-Blatt* 11 (1876), p. 7.

—, 'Einige Dichter der Neuzeit über die Syphilis. Ein Beitrag zur Geschichte und Literatur dieser Krankheit', *Medicinisch-Chirurgisches Central-Blatt* 16 (1881), pp. 349–51.

—, *Die Geschichte der venerischen Krankheiten* (2 vols, Bonn, 1895).

—, *Die Litteratur über die venerischen Krankheiten von den ersten Schriften über Syphilis aus dem Ende des fünfzehnten Jahrhunderts bis zum Jahre 1889* (5 vols, Bonn, 1989–1900).

——, *Die Quecksilbersublimatcuren gegen Syphilis. Eine literaturhistorische Studie* (Wien, 1876).

——, 'Das "Regiment wider die Frantzosen" von Magnus Hundt II. Ein Beitrag zu den Sammelwerken der ältesten Schriften über Syphilis', *Medicinisch-Chirurgisches Central-Blatt* 15 (1880), 37–50.

——, *Beiträge zur Geschichte der Syphilis* (Bonn, 1904).

Puff, Helmut, 'Das Hamburger Hiobshospital in der frühen Neuzeit', *Hamburger Zustände: Jahrbuch zur Geschichte der Region Hamburg* 1 (1988), pp. 183–207.

——, '"Von der Gutthätigkeit" und ihrem "stärcksten Bewegungs-Grund". Jobst von Overbeck (1663–1726) am Hamburger Hiobshospital', *Zeitschrift des Vereins für Hamburgerische Geschichte* 77 (1991).

Pusey, W. M. A., *The History and Epidemiology of Syphilis* (London, 1933).

Putman, Hilary, 'Sense, Nonsense and the Senses: An Inquiry Into the Powers of the Human Mind', *The Journal of Philosophy* 91 (1994), pp. 415–517.

Pschyrembel, *Klinisches Wörterbuch.* Bearbeitet von der Wörterbuch–Red. des Verlages unter der Leitung von Helmut Hildebrandt, 258, edn (Berlin, 1998).

Quétel, Claude, *History of Syphilis* (Baltimore, 1992).

Rabisch-Bey, J., 'Zur Geschichte der Quecksilbertherapie', *Wiener medizinische Wochenschau* 43 (1898), p. 487; 552; 599.

Rajkay, Barbara, 'Die Bevölkerung (Augsburgs) von 1500–1750', in Gunther Gottlieb et al. (eds), *Geschichte der Stadt Augsburg von der Römerzeit bis zur Gegenwart* (Augsburg, 1984), pp. 252–8.

Rath, Brigitte, 'Prostitution und spätmittelalterliche Gesellschaft im österreichisch-süddeutschen Raum', in *Frau und spätmittelalterlicher Alltag* (Wien, 1986), pp. 553–71.

Rather, L. J., 'The Six Things "Non-natural": A Note on the Origins and Fate of a Doctrine and Phrase', *Clio Medica* 3 (1968), pp. 337–47.

Rawcliffe, Carole, *Leprosy in Medieval England* (Woodbridge, 2006).

Reicke, Siegfried, *Das deutsche Spitalwesen und sein Recht im Mittelalter* [1932] (2 vols, reprint Amsterdam, 1970).

Reinhard, Wolfgang (ed.), *Augsburger Eliten des 16. Jahrhunderts. Prosographie wirtschaftlicher und politischer Führungsgruppen 1500–1620* (Berlin, 1996).

Rey, Roselyne, *The History of Pain*, 2nd edn (Cambridge, MA, 1998).

Richards, Peter, *The Medieval Leper and His Northern Heirs* (Cambridge, 1977).

Richter, Paul, 'Beiträge zur Geschichte des Aussatzes', *Archiv für Geschichte der Medizin* 4 (1911), pp. 323–52.

——, 'Noch ein altes Rezept "vor die Blatern male franzose"', *Archiv für Geschichte der Medizin* 5 (1912), pp. 412–13.

Riha, Ortrun, 'Medizin für Nichtmediziner. Die Popularisierung heilkundlichen Wissens im Mittelalter', *Medizin, Gesellschaft und Geschichte* 13 (1994), pp. 9–34.

Risse, Guenter B., 'Epidemics and History: Ecological Perspectives and Social Responses', in Elisabeth Fee and David M. Fox (eds), *AIDS: The Burden of History* (Berkeley, 1988), pp. 33–66.

—, 'History of Diagnostics', in Yosio Kawakita (ed.), *Proceedings of the 9th International Symposium on the Comparative History of Medicine – East and West, September 23–29, 1984* (Osaka, 1987), pp. 115–47.
—, 'The History of Therapeutics', in William F. Bynum and Vivian Nutton (eds), *Essays in the History of Therapeutics* (Amsterdam, 1991), pp. 3–11.
—, 'Medicine in New Spain', in Ronald L. Numbers (ed.), *Medicine in the New World: New Spain, New France, and New England* (Knoxville, 1987), pp. 12–63.
—, *Mending Bodies, Saving Souls: A History of Hospitals* (Oxford, 1999).
—, 'Transcending Cultural Barriers: The European Reception of Medical Plants from the Americas', in *Botanical Drugs of the Americas in the Old and New Worlds* (Stuttgart, 1983), pp. 31–42.
Rodekirchen, Dirk and Fleddermann, Heike, *Karl Sudhoff 1853–1938. Zwei Arbeiten zur Geschichte der Medizin und der Zahnheilkunde. Mit einem Essay 'Paracelsus und der gläserne Mensch'* (Cologne, 1991).
Rodenwaldt, Ernst, *Pest in Venedig 1575–1577. Eine Frage der Infektkette bei den Pestepidemien West-Europas* (Heidelberg, 1553).
Roeck, Bernd, '"Arme" in Augsburg zu Beginn des 30 jährigen Krieges', *Zeitschrift für bayerische Landesgeschichte* 46 (1983), pp. 515–58.
—, *Bäcker, Brot und Getreide in Augsburg. Studien zur Geschichte des Bäckerhandwerks und zur Versorgungspolitik der Reichsstadt im Zeitalter des Dreißigjährigen Krieges* (Sigmaringen, 1987).
—, 'Kollektiv und Individuum beim Entstehungsprozeß der Augsburger Architektur im ersten Drittel des 17. Jahrhunderts', *Elias Holl und das Augsburger Rathaus* (Ausstellungskatalog) (Regensburg, 1985), pp. 37–54.
—, *Eine Stadt in Krieg und Frieden. Studien zur Geschichte der Reichsstadt Augsburg zwischen Kalenderstreit und Parität* (2 vols, Göttingen, 1989).
Rödel, Walter G., 'Mensch und Gesundheit in der Geschichte der Neuzeit. Notizen zu einem Forschungsprojekt', *Medizinhistorisches Journal* 19 (1984), pp. 138–47.
Roller, Otto, 'Der Kampf gegen die Syphilis in Überlingen im Jahre 1581', *Sozialhygienische Mitteilungen* 12 (1928), pp. 10–18.
Roper, Lyndal, *The Holy Household: Women and Morals in Reformation Augsburg* (Oxford, 1989).
—, 'Luther: Sex, Marriage and Motherhoods', *History Today* 33 (1983), pp. 33–8.
Ropertz, Hans Peter, *Kleinbürgerlicher Wohnungsbau vom 14. bis 17. Jahrhundert in Deutschland und im benachbarten Ausland* (Frankfurt, 1976).
Rosen, George, *A History of Public Health* (New York, 1958).
Rossiaud, Jacques, *Dame Venus. Prostitution im Mittelalter* (Munich, 1989).
Rosenberg, Charles E., 'Disease in History: Frames and Framers', *The Milbank Quarterly* 67 (1989), pp. 1–15.

—, *Explaining Epidemics and Other Studies in the History of Medicine* (Cambridge, 1992).

—, and Golden, Janet (eds), *Framing Disease: Studies in Cultural History* (New Brunswig, 1991).

Roth, Friedrich, *Augsburgs Reformationsgeschichte*, 2nd edn (4 vols, Munich, 1901–1911).

Roth, F. W. E., 'Hieronymus Brunschwyg und Walter Ryff: zwei deutsche Botaniker des XVI. Jahrhunderts', *Zeitschrift für Naturwissenschaften* 75 (1903), pp. 102–23.

Rothschuh, Karl Eduard, *Konzepte der Medizin in der Vergangenheit und Gegenwart* (Stuttgart, 1978).

—, 'Der Krankheitsbegriff (was ist Krankheit?)', *Hippocrates* 43 (1972), pp. 3–17.

Rückert, M., 'Zur Geschichte der Syphilis in Franken', in Rückert (ed.), *Analecten zur Geschichte des fränkischen Medizinal-Wesens* (Würzburg, 1840), pp. 24–6.

Rudeck, Wilhelm, *Geschichte der öffentlichen Sittlichkeit in Deutschland* (Jena, 1897).

Rummel, Erika, 'Voices of Reform from Hus to Erasmus', in Thomas A. Brady, Heiko A. Oberman and James D. Tracy (eds), *Handbook of European History 1400–1600: Late Middle Ages, Renaissance and Reformation*, vol. II*: Visions, Programs and Outcomes* (Leiden, 1995), pp. 61–93.

Rummel, Peter, *Katholisches Leben in der Reichsstadt Augsburg (1605–1806). Sonderdruck aus dem 18. Jahresband des Vereins für Augsburger Bistumsgeschichte 1984* (Augsburg, 1984).

Russell, Paul A., 'Syphilis, God's Sourge or Nature's Vengeance? The German Printed Response to a Public Problem in the Early Sixteenth Century', *Archiv für Reformationsgeschichte* 80 (1989), pp. 286–307.

Rütten, Thomas, 'Karl Sudhoff and the "Fall" of German Medical History', in Frank Huisman and John Harley Warner (eds), *Locating Medical History: The Stories and Their Meaning* (Baltimore and London, 2004), pp. 95–114.

Ryan, Michael T., 'The Power of Tradition and the Shock of the New', *Comparative Studies in Society and History* 23 (1981), pp. 519–38.

Safley, Thomas Max, *Charity and Economy in the Orphanages of Early Modern Augsburg* (Atlantic Highlands, 1996).

Salzbrunn, Ingeborg, 'Das Ende des Augsburger Collegium Medicum', *Bayerisches Ärzteblatt* 28 (1973), pp. 156–62.

Sander, Sabine, *Handwerkschirurgen. Sozialgeschichte einer verdrängten Berufsgruppe* (Göttingen, 1989).

Santing, Catrien, *Geneeskunde en Humanisme. En intellectuele biografie van Theodericus Ulsenius (c. 1460–1508)* (Rotterdam, 1992).

—, 'Medizin und Humanismus: Die Einsichten des Nürnbergischen Stadtarztes Theodoricus Ulsenius über Morbus Gallicus', *Sudhoffs Archiv* 79 (1995), pp. 139–49.

—, 'Van Apollo, Aesculapius en Chiron: Theodericus Ulsenius (Dirk van Ulsen, c. 1460–1508). Medicus en humanist uit de noordelijke nederlanden', *Tijdschrift voor de geschiedenis der geneeskunde, naturwetenschappen, wiskunde en techniek* 13 (1990), pp. 129–40.

Sauerteig, Lutz, 'Die Eroberung des Gesundheitsmarktes: Pharmazeutische Industrie und Gesundheitswesen um die Jahrhundertwende', *Wirtschaft und Wissenschaft* 4 (1996).

—, *Krankheit, Sexualität, Gesellschaft. Geschlechtskrankheiten und Gesundheitspolitik in Deutschland im 19. und 20. Jahrhundert* (Stuttgart, 1999).

—, 'Medizin und Moral in der Syphilisbekämpfung', *Jahrbuch des Instituts für Geschichte der Medizin der Robert Bosch Stiftung* 19 (2000), pp. 55–70.

Sawday, Jonathan, *The Body Emblazoned: Dissection and the Human Body in Renaissance Culture* (London, 1995).

Scarry, Elaine, *The Body in Pain: The Making and the Unmaking of the World* (New York, 1985).

Schäfer, Lothar and Schnelle, Thomas, 'Ludwik Flecks Begründung der soziologischen Betrachtungsweise in der Wissenschaftstheorie', *Ludwik Fleck: Entstehung und Entwicklung einer wissenschaftlichen Tatsache. Einführung in die Lehre vom Denkstil und Denkkollektiv* (Frankfurt, 1993), pp. 7–49.

Schenda, Rudolf, 'Der "gemeine Mann" und sein medikales Verhalten im 16. und 17. Jahrhundert', in Joachim Telle (ed.), *Pharmazie und der gemeine Mann. Hausarznei und Apotheke in der Frühen Neuzeit*, 2nd edn (Weinheim, 1988), pp. 9–20.

Schilling, Heinz, *Aufbruch und Krise. Deutschland 1517–1648*, 4th edn (Berlin, 1998).

—, 'Gab es in Deutschland im späten Mittelalter und in der frühen Neuzeit einen Stadt-Republikanismus? – Zur politischen Kultur des europäischen Stadtbürgertums', in H. G. Koenisberger (ed.), *Republiken und Republikanismus, 15. bis frühes 17. Jahrhundert* (Munich, 1987), pp. 101–43.

Schipperges, Heinrich, 'Ernährung III: Diätetisch-medizinisch', *Lexikon des Mittelalters* (Munich, 1986), vol. 3, pp. 2169–71.

—, *Die Kranken im Mittelalter* (Munich, 1990).

Schleiner, Winfried, *Medical Ethics in the Renaissance* (Washington, 1995).

—, 'Moral Attitudes Towards Syphilis and Its Prevention in the Renaissance', *Bulletin of the History of Medicine* 68 (1994), pp. 389–410.

Schlich, Thomas, 'Die Herstellung wissenschaftlicher Fakten als Thema der Geschichtsforschung', in Norbert Paul and Thomas Schlich (eds), *Medizingeschichte: Aufgaben, Probleme, Perspektiven* (Frankfurt and New York, 1998), pp. 107–29.

Schmitt, Charles B., 'Aristoteles Among the Physicians', in Andrew Wear, Roger K. French and I.M. Loni, *The Medical Renaissance of the Sixteenth Century* (Cambridge, 1985), pp. 2–15.

—, *Aristotle in the Renaissance* (Cambridge, MA, 1983).

Schmölzer, Hilde, *Die Pest in Wien: "Des wütenden todts ein umbständig Beschreibung ..."* (Vienna, 1985).

Schmoller, Gustav, 'Entstehung, Wesen und Bedeutung der neueren Armenpflege', *Sitzungsberichte der Königlich preußischen Akademie der Wissenschaften* (Berlin, 1902), pp. 916–25.

Schneider, Anton, 'Otto, Truchseß v. Waldburg', in Wolfgang Baer et al. (eds), *Augsburger Stadtlexikon* (Augsburg, 1985), p. 275.

Schnelle, Thomas, *Ludwik Fleck – Leben und Denken. Zur Entstehung und Entwicklung des soziologischen Denkstils in der Wissenschaftsphilosophie* (Freiburg, 1982).

Schöner, Erich, *Das Viererschema in der antiken Humoralpathologie* (Wiesbaden, 1964).

Schönfeld, J., 'Zum Ursprung der Krankheitsbezeichnung "Syphilis"', *Offenburger Gesundheitswesen* 46 (1984), pp. 104–5.

——, 'Wandlungen in der Einstellung der Moral zu den Geschlechtskrankheiten (STD)', *Zentralblatt Haut* (1986), pp. 203–8.

Schönfeld, Walther, *Kurze Geschichte der Dermatologie und Venerologie und ihrer kulturgeschichtlichen Spiegelung* (Hannover, 1954).

Schottenloher, Karl, *Doktor Alexander Seitz und seine Schriften. Ein Kleinbild aus dem Münchner Ärzteleben des XVI. Jahrhunderts* (Munich, 1925).

Schrank, Josef, *Die Geschichte der Prostitution in Wien, in historischer, administrativer und hygienischer Beziehung* (Wien, 1886).

Schreiner, Klaus, 'Si homo non pecasset... Der Sündenfall Adams und Evas in seiner Bedeutung für die soziale, seelische und körperliche Verfaßtheit des Menschen', in Klaus Schreiner and Norbert Schnitzler (eds), *Gepeinigt, begehrt, vergessen. Symbolik und Sozialbezug des Körpers im späten Mittelalter und in der frühen Neuzeit* (Munich, 1992), pp. 41–84.

Schuster, Beate, *Die freien Frauen. Dirnen und Frauenhäuser im 15. und 16. Jahrhundert* (Frankfurt and New York, 1995).

Schuster, Peter, *Das Frauenhaus. Städtische Bordelle in Deutschland 1350–1600* (Paderborn, 1992).

Schwarz, Maureen Trudelle, 'The Explanatory and Predicitive Power of History: Coping with the "Mystery Illness"', *Ethnohistory* 42 (1995), pp. 375–401.

Scribner, Robert W., *The German Reformation* (Houndmills, 1986), pp. 3–4.

——, 'How Many Could Read? Comment on Moeller's "Stadt und Buch"', in *Stadtbürgertum und Adel in der Reformation. Studien zur Reformation in England und Deutschland* (Stuttgart, 1979), pp. 44–54.

Sebeok, Thomas A., 'Symptome, systematisch und historisch', *Zeitschrift für Semiotik* 6 (1984), pp. 37–50.

Seida und Landensberg, *Franz Eugen von, Historisch-statistische Beschreibung aller Kirchen-, Schul-, Erziehungs- und Wohlthätigkeitsanstalten in Augsburg. Von ihrem Ursprunge an bis auf die neuesten Zeiten* (2 vols, Augsburg, 1812).

Seidler, Eduard, 'An Historical Survey of Children's Hospitals', in Lindsay Granshaw and Roy Porter (eds), *The Hospital in History* (London and New York, 1989), pp. 181–97.

Seiz, Anneliese, 'Das Ulmer Blatter-Haus im Seelhaus im Gries. Ein Beitrag zur Geschichte des öffentlichen Gesundheitswesens in Ulm', *Ulm und Oberschwaben. Zeitschrift für Geschichte und Kunst* 44 (1982), pp. 366–71.

Settipane, Guy (ed.), *Columbus and the New World: Medical Implications* (Providence, 1995).

Shapin, Steven, *Social History of Truth: Civility and Science in Seventeenth-Century England* (Chicago, 1994).

Shyrock, Richard H., 'The History of Quantification in Medical Science', in *Isis* 52, 2 (1961), pp. 215–37.

Siebenthal, W. V., *Krankheiten als Folge der Sünde. Eine medizinhistorische Untersuchung* (Hannover, 1950).

Siegel, Rudolph S., *Galen's System of Physiology and Medicine: An Analysis of His Doctrines and Observations on Bloodflow, Respiration, Tumors and Internal Diseases* (Basel, 1968).

—, *Galen on Sense of Perception: His Doctrines, Observations and Experimentations in Vision, Hearing, Smell, Taste, Touch and Pain, and Their Historical Sources* (Basel, 1970).

Sieh-Burens, Katharina, *Oligarchie, Konfession und Politik im 16. Jahrhundert. Zur sozialen Verpflechtung der Augsburger Bürgermeister und Stadtpfleger 1518–1618* (Munich, 1986).

Siena, Kevin (ed.), *Sin of the Flesh: Responding to Sexual Disease in Early Modern Europe* (Toronto, 2005).

—, *Venereal Disease, Hospitals, and the Urban Poor: London's "Foul Wards", 1600–1800* (Rochester, 2004).

Siraisi, Nancy G., *Avicenna in Renaissance Italy: The Canon and Medical Teaching in Italian Universities after 1500* (Princeton, 1987).

—, *The Clock and the Mirror: Girolamo Cardano and Renaissance Medicine* (Princeton, 1997).

—, 'Disease and Symptom as Problematic Concepts in Renaissance Medicine', in Eckhard Kessler and Ian Maclean (eds), *Res et Verba in der Renaissance* (Wiesbaden), pp. 217–40.

—, 'Medieval and Early Renaissance Medicine', *Introduction to Knowledge and Practice* (Chicago, 1990).

—, 'Medieval and Renaissance Medicine: Continuity and Diversity', *Journal of the History of Medicine and Allied Sciences* 41 (1986), pp. 391–4.

Slack, Paul, 'Introduction', in ibid. and Terence Ranger (eds), *Epidemics and Ideas: Essays on the Historical Perception of Pestilence* (Cambridge, 1992), pp. 1–20.

—, 'Mirrors of Health and Treasures of Poor Men: The Uses of the Vernacular Medical Literature of Tudor England', in Charles Webster (ed.), *Health, Medicine and Morality in the Sixteenth Century* (Cambridge, 1979), pp. 237–73.

—, 'Mortality Crisis and Epidemic Disease in England 1485–1610', in Charles Webster (ed.), *Health, Medicine and Morality in the Sixteenth Century* (Cambridge, 1979), pp. 9–59.

—, 'Responses to Plague in Early Modern Europe: The Implications of Public Health', *Social Research* 55 (1988), pp. 433–53.

Smith, Pamela and Findlen, Paula (eds) *Merchants & Marvels: Commerce, Science and Art in Early Modern Europe* (London, 2002).

Sorge, W., *Geschichte der Prostitution* (Berlin, 1920).

Staiano, Kathryn Vance, *Interpreting Signs of Illness: A Case Study in Medical Semiotics* (Berlin and New York, 1986).

—, 'The Semiotic Perspective', in Jens Lachmund and Gunnar Stollberg (eds), *Social Construction of Illness: Illness and Medical Knowledge in Past and Present* (Stuttgart, 1992), pp. 173–80.

Stein, Claudia, *Die Behandlung der Franzosenkrankheit in der Frühen Neuzeit am Beispiel Augsburgs* (Stuttgart, 2003).

—, 'The Function of the Quack as a Means of Group Distinction in the Medical Community of Sixteenth-Century Augsburg – Preliminary Thoughts', *Ludica, annli di storia del gioco* 5–6 (2000), pp. 192–200.

—, 'Der Leipziger Streit (1497–1501) über die Ursachen der Franzosenkrankheit und ihre Behandlung im Augsburger Blatterhaus' in Stefan Oehmig (ed.), *Medizin und Sozialwesen in Mitteldeutschland in der Reformationzeit* (Leipzig, 2007), pp. 156–178.

—, 'The Meaning of Signs: Diagnosing the French Pox in Early Modern Augsburg', *Bulletin of the History of Medicine* 80 (2006), pp. 617–48.

—, 'Sozialhistorische Aspekte der städitischen Prostitution in der Frühen Neuzeit am Beispiel Kölns', *Rheinisches Jahrbuch für Volkskunde* 31 (1995/96), pp. 7–80.

Steinhilber, Wilhelm, *Das Gesundheitswesen im alten Heilbron 1281–1871* (Heibronn, 1956).

Stettler, Antoinette, 'Zeichen lesen und Zeichen deuten', *Gesnerus* 44 (1987), pp. 33–45.

Sticker, Georg, 'Ulrich von Huttens Buch über die Franzosenseuche als heimlicher Canon für die Syphilistherapie im 16. Jahrhundert', *Archiv für Geschichte der Medizin* 3 (1910), pp. 197–222.

Stollberg-Rilinger, Barbara, 'Gut vor Ehre oder Ehre vor Gut? Zur sozialen Distinktion zwischen Adels- und Kaufmannsstand in der Ständeliteratur der Frühen Neuzeit', in Johannes Burkhardt (ed.), *Augsburger Handelshäuser im Wandel des historischen Urteils* (Berlin, 1996), pp. 31–45.

Strauss, Gerald, 'Ideas of REFORMATIO and RENOVATIO from the Middle Ages to the Reformation', in *Handbook of European History 1400–1600*, vol. II*: Visions, Programs and Outcomes* (Leiden, 1995), pp. 1–28.

Strauß, David Friedrich, *Ulrich von Hutten* (Bonn, 1895).

Strieder, Jakob, 'Die Fugger und die Guajakholzkur', *Dermatologische Wochenschrift* 99 (1934), pp. 888–90.

Stuart, Kathy, *Defiled Trades and Social Outcasts: Honor and Ritual Pollution in Early Modern Germany* (Cambridge, 1999).
Stuckenbrock, Karin, *'Der zerstückte Cörper.' Zur Sozialgeschichte der anatomischen Sektionen in der frühen Neuzeit (1650–1800)* (Stuttgart, 2001).
Sudhoff, Karl, 'Amerikanischer Ursprung und "mal franzoso" um die Mitte des 15. Jahrhunderts in Italien', *Dermatologische Zeitschrift* 20 (1913), pp. 325–30.
—, 'Anfänge der Syphilisbeobachtung und Syphilisprophylaxe zu Frankfurt a. M., 1496–1591', *Dermatologische Zeitschrift* 20 (1913), pp. 95–116.
—, *Aus der Frühgeschichte der Syphilis. Handschriften- und Inkunabelstudien. Epidemiologischer Untersuchung und kritische Gänge* (Leipzig, 1912).
—, 'Aus meiner Arbeit', *Sudhoffs Archiv* 21 (1929), pp. 333–87.
—, 'Aussatzproben', *Archiv für Geschichte der Medizin* 3 (1910), p. 80.
—, 'Art. Prostitution I (Geschichte)', in M. Marcuse (ed.), *Handwörterbuch der Sexualwissenschaften* (Bonn, 1923), pp. 365–71.
—, 'Behördliches Einschreiten gegen Kurpfuscher am Ende des 15. Jahrhunderts', *Münchner medizinische Wochenschrift* 59 (1912), p. 2424.
—, 'Eine Blutprobe zur Erkennung der Lepra', *Archiv für Geschichte der Medizin* 6 (1913), p. 159.
—, 'Dokumente zur Ausübung der Lepraschau in Frankfurt am Main im 15. Jahrhundert', *Lepra Bibl. int.* 13 (1913), pp. 141–70.
—, 'Drei historische Fixpunkte im Bekanntwerden der Syphilis', *Dermatologische Wochenschrift* 80 (1925), pp. 361–5.
—, 'The Earliest Printed Literature on Syphilis: Being Ten Tractates from the Years 1495–1498', *Complete Facsimile With an Introduction and Other Accessory Material by K. S., adapted by Charles Singer* (Florence, 1925).
—, 'Die ersten Maßnahmen der Stadt Nürnberg gegen die Syphilis in den Jahren 1496 u. 1497. Aktenstudien', *Archiv für Dermatologie und Syphilis* 116 (1911), pp. 1–30.
—, *Graphische und typographische Erstlinge der Syphilisliteratur aus den Jahren 1495 und 1496* (Munich, 1912).
—, 'Geschichte der Geschlechtskrankheiten', in Max Marcuse (ed.), *Handwörterbuch der Sexualwissenschaft*, 2nd edn (Bonn, 1926), pp. 594–601.
—, 'Geschichte der Prostitution', in Max Marcuse (ed.), *Handwörterbuch der Sexualwissenschaft*, 2nd edn (Bonn, 1926), pp. 365–71.
—, 'Die geschichtliche Entwicklung der Beziehungen zwischen ärztlichem Beruf und dem Krankenhaus. Ein Einführung', *Nosokomeion* 2 (1931), pp. 1–8.
—, 'Das Gotteslästerermandat, Berthold von Henneberg und die Syphilis', *Mitteilungen zur Geschichte der Medizin und der Naturwissenschaften* 12 (1913), pp. 1–9.
—, 'Grundfragen der historischen Epidemiologie', *Münchner medizinische Wochenschrift* 59 (1912), p. 2480.
—, 'Historia und curatio morborum', *Mitteilungen der Geschichte der Medizin und der Naturwissenschaften* 19 (1920), p. 2109.

—, 'Lepraschaubriefe aus dem 15. Jahrhundert', *Sudhoffs Archiv* 4 (1910), pp. 370–378; 5 (1911), pp. 154–156, 434f; 6 (1912), p. 392f.

—, 'Maßnahmen zu Leipzig, nachdem die Syphilis dort Beachtung gefunden hatte', *Dermatologische Wochenschrift* 95 (1932), pp. 1397–9.

—, 'Neue Probleme in der Geschichte der Syphilis', *Münchner medizinische Wochenschau* 59 (1912), pp. 560; 616.

—, 'Eine neue Krankheit, "nuwe krenckte" im Juni 1494 zu Düsseldorf', *Archiv für Geschichte der Medizin* 7 (1913–1914), pp. 43–5.

—, 'Was geschah mit den (nach erneuter Schau) als leprafrei erklärten und aus den Leprosorien wieder Freigelassenen von behördlicher Seite?', *Archiv für Geschichte der Medizin* 6 (1912), pp. 149–54.

—, 'Rat und Ärzte der Stadt Nürnberg und ihr Vorgehen gegen die Syphilis. Maßnahmen einiger westdeutscher Städte', *Studien zur Geschichte der Medizin* 9 (1912), pp. 20–41.

—, 'Seuchenschutzmaßregeln in der Vergangenheit', *Zeitschrift für ärtzliche Fortbildung* 17 (1920), pp. 53–6.

—, 'Sorge für die Syphiliskranken und Luesprophylaxe zu Nürnberg. Weitere Aktenstudien', *Archiv für Dermatologie und Syphilis* 118 (1913), pp. 285–318.

—, 'Ein spätmittelalterliches Epileptikerheim (Isolier- und Pflegespital für Fallsüchtige) zu Rufach im Oberelsaß', *Archiv für Geschichte der Medizin* 13 (1912), pp. 449–55.

—, 'Syphilis in den Jahren 1494 und 1495. Der Brief des Scillacio und der Reisebericht des Monetarius', *Dermatologische Wochenschrift* 57 (1913), p. 79.

—, 'Syphilis und Pest in München am Ende des 15. und zu Anfang des 16. Jahrhunderts. Eine Urkundenstudie', *Münchner Medizinische Wochenschrift* 60 (1913), pp. 1439–43.

—, 'Syphiliserfahrung zweier Augsburger beamteter Ärzte, Johannes und Ambrosius Jung in den Jahren 1497 und 1498', *Pharmazeutische Monatshefte* 4 (1923), pp. 142–3.

—, 'Über Hohenheims Syphilisschriften', *Münchner medizinische Wochenschrift* 59 (1902), p. 1899.

—, 'Vorsorge für die Syphiliskranken in Würzburg und Augsburg zu Ende des 15. und bis ins zweite Viertel des 16. Jahrhunderts', *Dermatologische Wochenschrift* 97 (1933), pp. 1431–45.

—, 'Wendepunkt im Krankenhauswesen des Abendlandes', *Archiv für Geschichte der Medizin* 21 (1929), pp. 246–7.

—, *Zehn Syphilisdrucke aus den Jahren 1495–1498* (Milan, 1924).

—, and Sticker, Georg (eds), *Zur historischen Biologie der Krankheitserreger. Materialien, Studien und Abhandlungen, Heft 1: Karl Sudhoff: Historik und Seuchenforschung; Heft 2: Georg Sticker: Parasitologie und Loimologie* (Gießen, 1910).

Tanner, Jakob, 'Körpererfahrung, Schmerz und die Konstruktion des Kulturellen', *Historische Anthropologie* 2 (1994), pp. 489–502.

Telle, Joachim, 'Arzeikunst und der "gemeine Mann" Zum deutschen-lateinischen Sprachenstreit in der frühneuzeitlichen Medizin', in Telle (ed.), *Pharmazie und der gemeine Mann. Hausarznei und Apotheke in der Frühen Neuzeit*, 2nd edn (Weinheim, 1988), pp. 43–50.

—, 'Latein und Deutsch im Spiegel der Arzneiliteratur des 16. und 17. Jahrhunderts', *Beiträge zur Geschichte der Pharmazie* 30 (1978), pp. 1–2.

—, 'Wissenschaft und Öffentlichkeit im Spiegel der deutschen Arzneibuchliteratur. Zum deutsch-lateinischen Sprachenstreit in der Medizin des 16. und 17. Jahrhunderts', *Medizinhistorisches Journal* 14 (1979), pp. 32–52.

—, 'Wolfgang Thalhauser. Zu Leben und Werk eines Augsburger Stadtarztes und seinen Beziehungen zu Paracelsus und Schwenkfeld', *Medizinhistorisches Journal* 7 (1972), pp. 1–30.

Temkin, Owsei, 'On the History of "Morality and Syphilis"', in Owsei Temkin, *The Double Face of Janus* (London, 1977), pp. 472–84.

—, 'The Role of Surgery in the Rise of Modern Medical Thought', *Bulletin of the History of Medicine* 25 (1951), pp. 248–59.

—, 'The Scientific Approach to Disease: Specific Entity and Individual Sickness', *Scientific Change* (London, 1963), pp. 629–47.

—, 'Therapeutic Trends and the Treatment of Syphilis before 1900', in Owsei Temkin, *The Double Face of Janus* (London, 1977), pp. 518–24.

Terrien, S., 'Job', in M. Eliade (ed.), *The Encyclopedia of Religion* (New York, 1987) vol. 8, pp. 97–100.

Thivel, Antoine, 'Diagnostic and Procnostic à l'époque d'Hippocrate à la notre', *Gesnerus* 42 (1985), pp. 479–97.

Thomas, Keith, *Religion and the Decline of Magic: Studies in Popular Beliefs in the Sixteenth and Seventeenth Centuries* (London, 1973).

Tietz-Strödel, Marion, *Die Fuggerei in Augsburg. Studien zur Entwicklung des sozialen Stiftungsbaus im 15. und 16. Jahrhundert* (Tübingen, 1982).

Toellner, Richard, 'Mattäus Kardinal Lang von Wellenburg und Paracelsus. Zur Polemik des Paracelsus gegen Kardinal Lang und die Fugger', in R. Blaser and H. Buens (eds), *Aktuelle Probleme der Geschichte der Medizin. Verhandlungen des XIC. Internationalen Kongresses zur Geschichte der Medizin* Basel (Basel, 1964), pp. 489–97.

Trometer, Johann, 'Das Augsburger Pilgerhaus' (MA dissertation, Augsburg, 1997).

Trueb, Paul C., 'Die geschichtliche Entwicklung des ärztlichen Standeswesens in Deutschland', *Medizinische Monatsschrift* 15 (1961), pp. 478–88.

Tsouyopoulos, Nelly, 'Auf der Suche nach einer adäquaten Methode für die Geschichte und Theorie der Medizin. Auseinandersetzunge mit Ludwik Flecks "Entstehung einer wissenschaftlichen Tatsache"', *Medizinhistorisches Journal* 17 (1982), pp. 20–36.

Tuana, Nancy, 'Der schwächere Samen. Androzentrismus in der Aristotelischen Zeugungstheorie und der Galenischen Anatomie', in Barbara Orland and Elvira Scheich (eds), *Das Geschlecht der Natur. Feministische Beiträge zur Geschichte und Theorie der Naturwissenschaften* (Frankfurt a. M., 1995), pp. 203–23.

Uexküll, Thure von, 'Historische Überlegungen zu dem Problem einer Medizin-Semiotik', *Zeitschrift für Semiotik* 6 (1984), pp. 53–8.

——, 'Semiotics and Medicine', *Semiotica* 38 (1982), pp. 205–15.

Uhlig, Walter, 'Ein Beitrag zur Geschichte der Holzkur in der zweiten Hälfte des 16. Jahrhunderts' (dissertation, 1913).

Ulbricht, Otto, 'Pesterfahrung. Das "Sterben" und der Schmerz in der Frühen Neuzeit', *Medizin, Geschichte, Gesellschaft* 15 (1997), pp. 9–36.

Ulrich, Hans-Peter, *Das Heilig-Geist-Hospital zu Biberach an der Riß* (Biberach, 1965).

Vasold, Manfred, 'Nürnberger Blatterhäuser und Cholerahäuser im 19. Jahrhundert', *Würzburger medizinische Mitteilungen* 12 (1994), pp. 225–43.

——, *Pest, Not und schwere Plagen. Seuchen und Epidemien vom Mittalter bis heute* (Munich, 1999).

Vetter, Johannes, '"Bedenkhen Württembergischer Physicorum"" betreffend die Holzkur für Herzog Christoph. Ein Betrag zur Syphilistherapie um die Mitte des 16. Jahrhunderts' (dissertation, Leipzig, 1914).

Virchow, Rudolf, 'Beitrag zur Geschichte der Lues', *Dermatologische Zeitschrift* 3 (1896), pp. 1–9.

Vöttiner-Pletz, Patricia, *Lignum sanctum. Zur therapeutischen Verwendung des Guajak vom 16. bis zum 20. Jahrhundert* (Frankfurt, 1990).

Vorberg, Gaston, *Über den Ursprung der Syphilis* (Stuttgart, 1924).

Vries, Jan de, *European Urbanization* (London, 1984).

Wackes, G.L., *Constructivist Medicine* (Maastricht, 1994).

Waddington, Ivan, 'General Practitioners and Consultants in Early Nineteenth-Century England: The Sociology of an Intra-Professional Conflict', in J. Woodward and D. Richards (eds), *Health Care and Popular Medicine in Nineteenth-Century England* (London, 1977), pp. 164–88.

Wagner, Hans-Joachim, 'Zur Geschichte des Biberacher Spital. Seine Leistungen in der Kranken- und Armenpflege', *Sudhoffs Archiv* 37 (1957), pp. 422–7.

Walsham, Alexandra, 'Miracles and the Counter Reformation Mission to England', *Historical Journal* 46 (2003), pp. 779–815.

——, 'Miracles in Post-Reformation England', in Kate Cooper and Jeremy Gregory (eds), *Signs, Wonders, Miracles: Representations of Divine Power in the Life of the Church* (London, 2005).

Walter, Tilmann, *Unkeuschheit und Werk der Liebe. Diskurse über Sexualität am Beginn der Neuzeit in Deutschland* (Berlin, 1998).

Warmbrunn, Paul, *Zwei Konfessionen in einer Stadt. Das Zusammenleben von Katholiken und Protestanten in den paritätischen Reichsstädten Augsburg, Biberach, Ravensburg und Dinkelsbühl von 1548–1648* (Wiesbaden, 1983).

Watson, Gilbert, *Theriac and Mithridatium: A Study in Therapeutics* (London, 1966).

Watts, Sheldon, *Epidemics and History: Disease, Power and Imperialism* (New Haven, 1997).

Waugh, M.A., 'Venereal Disease in Sixteeth-Century England', *Medical History*, 17 (1973), pp. 192–9.

Wear, Andrew, 'Galen in the Renaissance', in Vivian Nutton (ed.), *Galen: Problems and Prospects* (London, 1981), pp. 229–67.

——, *Knowledge and Practice in English Medicine, 1550–1680* (Cambridge, 2000).

——, 'Puritan Perceptions of Illness in Seventeenth Century England', in Roy Porter (ed.), *Patients and Practitioners: Lay Perceptions of Medicine in Pre-Industrial Society* (Cambridge, 1985), pp. 55–99.

——, 'Religious Beliefs and Medicine in Early Modern England', in Hilary Marland and Margaret Pelling (eds), *The Task of Healing: Medicine, Religion and Gender in England and the Netherlands, 1450–1800* (Rotterdam, 1996), pp. 145–69.

——, Roger K. French and I. M. Lonie (eds), *The Medical Renaissance of the Sixteenth Century* (Cambridge, 1985).

Webster, Charles, 'Alchemical and Paracelsian Medicine', in ibid. (ed.), *Health, Medicine and Morality in the Sixteenth-Century* (Cambridge, 1979), pp. 300–333.

——, 'Paracelsus: Medicine as Popular Protest', in Ole Peter Grell and Andrew Cunningham (eds), *Medicine and the Reformation* (London, 1993), pp. 57–77.

Weeks, Andrew, *Paracelsus: Speculative Theory and the Crisis of Early Modern Reformation* (Albany, 1997).

Wehrli, Gustav A., 'Die Krankenanstalten und die öffentlich angestellten Ärzte und Wundärzte im alten Zürich', *Mitteilungen der Antiquarischen Gesellschaft in Zürich* 31 (1934), pp. 5–94.

Weidenbacher, Josef, *Die Fuggerei in Augsburg. Die erste deutsche Kleinhausstiftung. Ein Beitrag zur Geschichte des deutschen Kleinhauses* (Augsburg, 1926).

Weimann, Karl-Heinz, 'Paracelsus und Kardinal Mattäus Lang als Gegner im Guajak-Streit', *Sudhoffs Archiv für Geschichte der Medizin und der Naturwissenschaften* 45 (1961), pp. 193–200.

Weindling, Paul, 'From Infections to Chronic Diseases: Changing Patterns of Sickness in the Nineteenth and Twentieth Centuries', in Andrew Wear (ed.), *Medicine in Society: Historical Essays* (Cambridge, 1992), pp. 303–16.

——, 'The Politics of International Co-Ordination to Combat Sexually Transmitted Diseases, 1900–1980s', in Virginia Berridge and Philipp Strong (eds), *AIDS and Contemporary History* (Cambridge, 1993), pp. 93–117.

Weiss, M., *Diagnose und Prognose aus dem Harn* (Wien, 1936).

Wendelhorst, Alfred, *Das Juliusspital in Würzburg, Bd. 1: Kulturgeschichte* (Würzburg, 1976).

Wenninger, Marcus (ed.), *'du guoter tot'. Sterben im Mittelalter – Ideal und Realität* (Klagenfurt, 1998).

Werner, Anton, 'Der ungarische Ochsenhandel und das Augsburger Metzgergewerbe', *Der Sammler* 74 (1911), pp. 3–5.

—, *Die örtlichen Stiftungen für die Zwecke des Unterrichts und der Wohltätigkeit in der Stadt Augsburg: Historisch und systematisch dargestellt* (Augsburg, 1899).

Westman, Robert S., 'The Copernicans and the Churches', in David C. Lindberg and Ronald L. Numbers (eds), *God and Nature. Historical Essays on the Encounter Between Christianity and Science* (Berkeley, 1986).

Wickersheimer, Ernest, 'Les débuts à Strasbourg de l'hospitalisation des syphilitiques', *Scalpel* 10 (1960), pp. 185–95.

—, 'Le Gaiac à Strasbourg au XVIe siècle', *Analecta Medico-Historica* 1 (1965), pp. 55–66.

Wiesflecker, Hermann, *Kaiser Maximilian I. Das Reich, Österreich und Europa an der Wende der Neuzeit* (4 vols, Munich, 1971–1975)

Wilson, Adrian, 'On the History of Disease-Concepts: The Case of Pleurisy', *History of Science* 38 (2000), pp. 271–319.

Windemuth, Luise, *Das Hospital als Träger der Armenfürsorge im Mittelalter* (Stuttgart, 1995).

Winau, Rolf, 'Bakteriologie und Immunologie im Berlin des 19. Jahrhunderts', *Naturwissenschaftliche Rundschau* 43 (1990), pp. 369–77.

—, 'Körperkonzepte und Krankheitskonzepte in der neuzeitlichen Medizin', *Jahrbuch des Deutschen Medizinhistorischen Museums* 5 (1983–1985), pp. 67–71.

Winkelmann, Otto, *Das Fürsorgewesen der Stadt Straßburg vor und nach der Reformation bis zum Ausgang des 16. Jahrhunderts. Ein Beitrag zur deutschen Kultur- und Wirtschaftsgeschichte* (Leipzig, 1922).

—, 'Über die ältesten Armenordnungen der Reformationszeit (1522–25)', *Historische Vierteljahrszeitschrift* 17 (1914/1915), pp. 187–228; 361–400.

Winkle, Stefan, *Geißeln der Menschheit. Kulturgeschichte der Seuchen* (Düsseldorf and Zurich, 1997).

Witt, Ronald G., 'The Humanist Movement', in Thomas A. Brady, Heiko A. Oberman and James D. Tracy (eds), *Handbook of European History 1400–1600. Late Middle Ages, Renaissance and Reformation, vol. 2: Visions, Programs and Outcomes* (Leiden, 1995), pp. 93–126.

Wolf, J.H. (ed.), *Lepra, Hansen-Krankheit. Ein Menschheitsproblem im Wandel.* 1. Teil: Katalog (Munich, 1982); 2. Teil: Aufsätze (Würzburg, 1986).

Wood, Corinne Shear, 'Syphilis in Anthropological Perspective', *Social Sciences and Medicine* 12 (1978), pp. 47–55.

Wright, Peter and Treacher, Andrew (eds), *The Problem of Medical Knowledge: Examining the Social Construction of Medicine* (Edinburgh, 1982).

Zacharias, S., 'Die Pest und das Böse. Oder: Was Seuchen bedeuten können', *Frankfurter Allgemeine Zeitung* vom 23.07.1988.

Zaundik, Rudolph, 'Bibliographie Karl Sudhoffs. Nachtrag für die Jahre 1933–1938', *Sudhoffs Archiv* 31 (1938), pp. 343–4a.

Zimmermann, Ernest L., 'The French Pox of That Great Clerke of Almayne, Ulrich von Hutten, Knyght', *Janus* 36 (1932), pp. 235–50.

Zoepfl, Friedrich, *Das Bistum Augsburg und seine Bischöfe im Reformationsjahrhundert* (Augsburg and Munich, 1969).

Zorn, Wolfgang, *Augsburg. Geschichte einer deutschen Stadt* (Augsburg, 1972).

Index